To our husbands, Chris and Jeff,
for their encouragement and belief in our abilities,
and to colleagues who mentored and supported us
in our clinical research journeys.
—*Bradi B. Granger*
Marianne Chulay

And to my parents and heros,
Ed and Larrie Bartrug.

—*Bradi*

Contents

Preface

Having learned a great deal about research methods and statistics in school, we returned to positions in the clinical setting thinking we possessed the tools to conduct research that would have a direct impact on patient care. We were not prepared, though, for the obstacles that seemed to pop up every step of the way. Roadblocks to conducting and using research included finding time to review the literature and write a protocol, getting support for the project from administration, finding money to conduct the study, collecting and analyzing data, and finding the best ways to disseminate the results. Our formal research education did not give us practical information on how to do research while employed in a full-time clinical position.

Now, after years of doing nursing research while employed in clinical positions, we have found a number of different approaches to overcoming the roadblocks to doing nursing research in clinical practice. *Research Strategies for Clinicians* fills the gap between research theory and making research "do-able" in real-life, clinical practice situations. You will find new ways to:

- Select important clinical research questions with significant clinical importance and high organizational priority.
- Develop a research team where every member truly "owns" the research project and maintains momentum throughout the research process.
- Simplify the protocol development process to fit into the busy clinician's day.
- Successfully get protocols approved in a clinical facility.
- Conduct research studies without ever filling out a grant request.
- Find resources (money, people, and equipment) to complete your study.
- Deal with data analysis needs.
- Communicate research findings both within your facility and throughout the nursing profession.

Sample protocols, data collection forms, consent documents, and approval forms, included in the helpful appendix section, provide "templates" to use in developing a study of your own. Guidelines for investigational review boards (IRB) are also included, detailing required elements of an informed consent, circumstances under which written informed consent can be eliminated, and research activities which may be reviewed through an expedited process.

We hope the information in *Research Strategies for Clinicians* will help you, as it has helped us, overcome common roadblocks to research completion in clinical practice.

Bradi B. Granger
Marianne Chulay

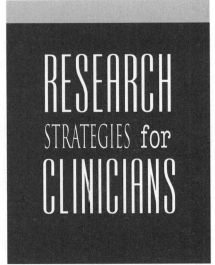

RESEARCH
STRATEGIES for
CLINICIANS

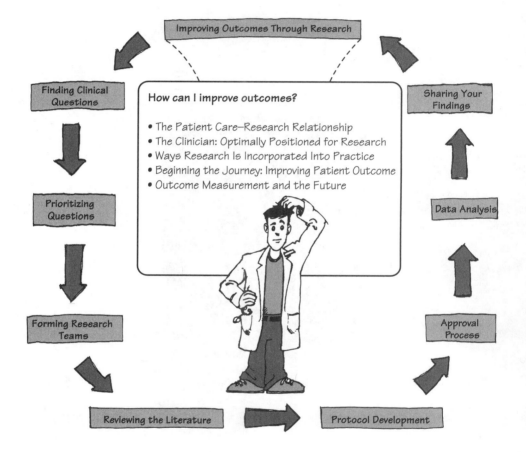

Improving Outcomes Through Research

▶ THE PATIENT CARE–RESEARCH RELATIONSHIP

What is excellence in patient care? It is any number of things we do as nurses every day to meet the needs of our patients. It is assessing, advising, and educating. It is careful monitoring and management of critical events such as stroke, childbirth, or myocardial infarction. It is skillful coordination of technologically advanced interventions, such as care of the patient dependent on extracorporeal membrane oxygenation (ECMO) or continuous arterial-venous hemodialysis (CAVHD). It is continuous communication, understanding and caring, hand-holding and therapeutic touch. Excellence in patient care is broad, personal, and individual. It is seemingly unrelated to research, yet it is the axis on which clinical nursing research spins.

The purpose of clinical nursing research is to inquire, investigate, and inform about patient care. We inquire each time we ask, "Why do we do it this way?"; each time a new product surfaces, and we ask is it really better, or is it only "glitzier"? Each time nurses come into a new environment with a fresh perspective and question the rationale for routines and practice standards, we are inquiring. We inquire based on what we know, what we read, and what we have experienced. When we use research to inquire, we inquire better.

Another purpose of research is to investigate solutions. By doing research to answer clinical questions, nurses generate solid, science-based answers. Investigating clinical questions through the research process also requires using existing research. A study that answers one question generally leads to another question, which generates further research. This circular process for investigation results in a stronger foundation for practice because a body of science is built around the topic or clinical question. *Do* research, learn from it, and then ask again. Investigation is a piece of the research cycle, whereby we truly gain and achieve by asking the question, learning from the answer, using the new information, then asking again. And again, and again.

A third purpose of clinical nursing research is to inform practice. To "inform" is to use research for providing information that improves the care we deliver to patients every day. Research informs our practice by helping clinicians understand how, when, and why nursing interventions benefit the patient, and what interventions might be more beneficial than others. Informing practice using research creates opportunities for improving patient outcomes by improving the interventions intended to achieve those outcomes.

Research enables us to improve outcomes by enlightening our understanding of outcomes. Without it, Florence Nightingale would not have discovered that hand-washing would lead to decreased mortality in the Crimean War. Without it, we would not understand the benefits of music therapy during stress, the needs of families in critical care situations, or the best way to oxygenate a premature infant during suctioning. Without research, we would not understand how to move from identifying a clinical problem, to testing an intervention, to changing practice, to improving clinical outcome for our patients (Fig. 1–1).

Improving patient outcomes is dependent on the process of improving our understanding of the problem and testing various solutions. This process is research.

▶ THE CLINICIAN: OPTIMALLY POSITIONED FOR RESEARCH

Research begins with the patient. As a principal and consistent caregiver in myriad settings, the nurse has a keen grasp on the needs of patients, the limita-

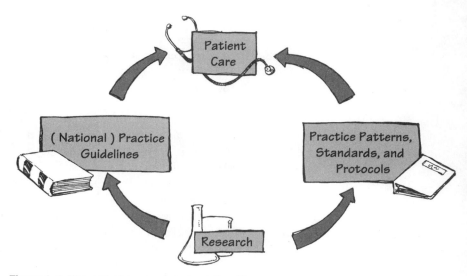

Figure 1–1. The patient care–research relationship.

tions of the health care delivery system, and the opportunities for improvement in providing the best care to patients. The clinician is in an excellent position to process problems and generate possible solutions. You do it every day.

"Problem Processors"

The clinician identifies and processes problems for patients every day. For example, think about the patient you cared for yesterday, or last week. Beyond the patient's diagnosis, what were some of the issues you addressed in his or her care? Did the patient require a bedpan and have trouble, either logistically or psychologically, with using the bedpan? Did the patient have family members who were concerned and who seemed to be asking the same questions over and over and over? Was the patient difficult to wean from ventilatory support, or unable to eat? Almost everything you did to care for that patient involved processing a problem. How many of the solutions were based on research?

Each problem mentioned above has been the basis for research by nurses. How frequently is what we do based on research? Not frequently enough! Nurses process problems every day, yet much of what we do is still based on tradition or consensus rather than science.

"Solution Generators"

The clinician generates solutions to patient problems every day. Examples include small solutions, such as creatively affixing fecal incontinence bags or using ingenuity to tape a Foley bag for easier ambulation. Other examples are big solutions that may be broadly applied, such as revising practice standards, implementing quality improvement projects, and conducting research. The spectrum of issues that challenge nurses in the clinical setting is vast. Research is used to resolve questions along this entire spectrum. Clinicians are optimally positioned for research because clinicians are creative "solution generators."

Consumers of Research

As principal caregivers and key players on clinical practice committees, policy and procedure committees, standards development committees, and ethics committees, clinicians are continual consumers of research. For example, each time a clinical question is discussed in a clinical practice council or committee meeting, research should be used to answer the question or solve the problem. Each time new standards are written or revised, or new critical pathways are generated, clinicians should be using research to determine best practices. When you read recent articles or books or consult experts to solve a practice problem, you are probably using research. Is current literature on the topic generally reviewed as a part of these discussions at *your* facility?

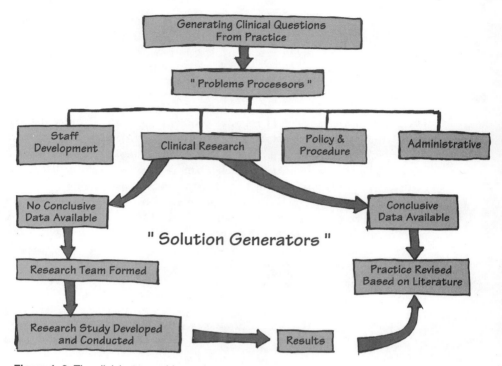

Figure 1–2. The clinician as problem solver.

As noted in Fig. 1–2, nurses encounter and process problems, making decisions that then drive practice. Those decisions are informed by research. When decisions are made without a scientific basis, we are less confident in the solution and frequently must reconvene to generate solutions again. As consumers of research, we review the literature and implement research-based solutions to improve patient care. Nursing practice, at its very best, is research in motion.

▶ WAYS RESEARCH IS INCORPORATED INTO PRACTICE

As the patient's care coordinator, the nurse frequently uses and develops tools for guiding and/or measuring the effectiveness of health care delivery and the resulting patient outcome. Some of the tools we use along these lines are forums, such as clinical practice committees or councils that set standards that guide practice. Some of the tools are more concrete instruments, such as critical pathways, variance tracking tools, quality or process improvement tools, nursing and medical practice guidelines, patient care standards, and policies and procedures. Current research should be incorporated into each of these tools to ensure the best patient outcomes. When research is used as a foundational building block, each of these forums or tools is an example of research in practice (Table 1–1).

Table 1–1	Examples of Using Research in Practice

Practice Forum or Tool	Definition	How Research Is Used
Clinical Practice Committee or Practice Council	Representative group of nurses that evaluates and makes decisions regarding acceptable standards for clinical practice.	a. Research is reviewed and evaluated to determine state of the science and evidence for practice. b. Benchmarking surveys are conducted to compare practice patterns across geographic regions and determine best practice.
Quality Improvement Committee	Usually a unit- or division-based multi-disciplinary group that evaluates care delivery processes and identifies opportunities for improvement.	a. Research is reviewed and evaluated to determine state of the science and evidence for practice. b. Benchmarking surveys are conducted to compare practice patterns across geographic regions and determine best practice.
Process Improvement Protocol	A formalized tool to measure and evaluate processes of health care delivery.	Tool should be developed using evidence-based indicators to measure identified outcomes. Evidence-based indicators are variables in the process that affect the end result.
Policy	Written statement regarding the acceptable processes and limits surrounding an issue, usually for legal substantiation or standardization.	a. Should be based on review of current literature and research. b. Benchmarking surveys may be conducted to identify policies being used in similar facilities.
Procedure	Step-by-step instructions on how to perform a psychomotor skill for a specific task.	Should be based on review of current literature and research.
Standard	Written statement defining an acceptable level of practice. The acceptable level of practice may be "standard" across or within regions or institutions.	Should be based on review of current literature and research.
Critical Pathway	Plans of care for a patient population, generally including time frames, identified outcomes, and indicators for achieving those outcomes or goals.	a. Should be based on review of current literature and research. b. Review focuses on what expected outcomes and quality indicators should be for various phases and levels of care.
Protocol	Defines the care and management of a broad patient care problem or issue in five categories: non-invasive and invasive equipment; diagnostic, prophylactic, and therapeutic measures; physiologic and psychological states; and nursing diagnosis.	Should be based on review of current literature and research. Research Based Practice Protocols are published by the American Association of Critical Care Nurses (AACN) with supporting levels of evidence for each recommendation, similar to the AHCPR guidelines.

(continued)

Table 1–1	Examples of Using Research in Practice (continued)	
Practice Forum or Tool	**Definition**	**How Research Is Used**
Guideline (ie, National Guidelines)	Defines recommendations for care and management of a broad patient population problem or issue. Lists level of evidence or research basis for each recommendation.	Is based on review of current literature and research. Currently national guidelines are published by the Agency for Health Care Policy and Research (AHCPR), and specialty organizations such as the American College of Cardiology (ACC), American College of Surgeons, and a growing number of others. These guidelines are typically adapted and individualized to a specific unit or institution.
Journal Club	A forum for review of research and current literature in identified topical areas.	Usually a single article or study is reviewed, but all contributing background literature/research is typically discussed as well.
Product Review Committees	A facility-wide multidisciplinary group responsible for reviewing new products and devices for possible purchase.	Research supporting advantages or disadvantages of new products is reviewed and evaluated to determine the state of the science and evidence for product selection.

Tools like those in Table 1–1 use or generate information that guides practice, that results in, or has an impact on, a given patient outcome. You *are* *using* research because you are *practicing* nursing! Could you be using research better? Should you be generating better research? Perhaps so!

▶ BEGINNING THE JOURNEY: IMPROVING PATIENT OUTCOMES USING RESEARCH

Patients deserve the best that we can offer in terms of state-of-the-science nursing care. So where do we begin? The journey to improving patient outcome begins with the clinical question. Questions come in all shapes and sizes. Thankfully, so do solutions. Clinical questions range from very simple, such as, "Is refrigerator temperature consistently within an acceptable range?", to very complex, such as, "What factors influence mortality in premature infants?" The entire spectrum of clinical questions is depicted in Fig. 1–3. Solutions, or infor-

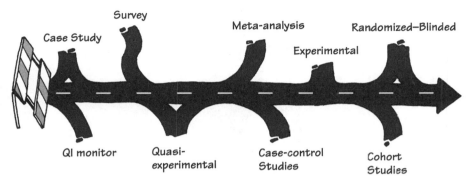

Figure 1–3. The spectrum of clinical problems and research approaches.

mation to guide solutions, can be generated using research at any point along this spectrum.

Because the research process is useful for problem solving, it is useful for improving patient outcomes. Research provides the framework and instruments to describe problems, implement interventions, and measure the change, or "outcome" resulting from those interventions.

What Is An Outcome?

Outcome can be defined as the end result of a process. It is usually quantifiable, reproducible, and objective. When outcomes are discussed in relation to patient care, the "process" is the plan of care for that patient, and the outcome is the end result of the plan of care. If the patient achieved the desired result of care within the appropriate time frame, with appropriate use of resources, and he/she was satisfied with the health care experience, then the desired "outcomes" were met. When something causes the patient to deviate from the expected plan of care, then the desired outcomes may not be achieved. These detours from the expected plan of care are called *variances*.

Outcomes can be measured at a number of different times or points in the process of delivering patient care. For example, patient education is a process. It is, in fact, an important piece of the overall process or plan for patient care. Education can be thought of as an intervention that we hope will increase patient knowledge and understanding. Increased knowledge, we hope, will give the patient more confidence to care for him- or herself and will change the patient's self-care behavior in a positive way. The changed behavior, frequently referred to as *compliance* or *adherence*, we hope will result in better health and/or improved functional status. We started with an intervention, patient education, and want to measure the outcome of education, but there are many intervals along the way at which "outcome" might logically be measured (Fig. 1–4). Does education result in increased knowledge? Does increased knowledge result in changed behavior? Does changed behavior in fact

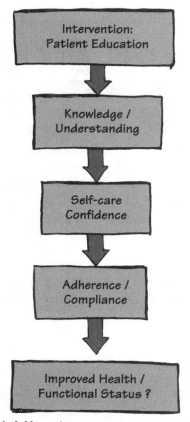

Figure 1–4. Measuring outcomes at various intervals.

result in improved health status? Some of these outcomes can be measured soon after the intervention, whereas others require many years before measurement is meaningful.

The result or outcome of patient education is an example of a clinical outcome that is of interest to nurses. Other clinical outcomes include mortality, morbidity, complications, psychosocial adjustment, activity progression, and measures of ability to provide self-care. In addition to clinical outcomes, financial and service outcomes are also of interest to nurses, because these outcomes are a reflection of the efficiency and effectiveness of the systems put in place to provide care. Many of the outcomes of interest to nurses are also of importance to payers and patients.

Table 1–2 lists common categories of outcomes and some examples of these in clinical practice. Changing or improving outcomes in each of the categories can be accomplished through the research process, even when, as with quality improvement projects, the simplest levels of research are used.

Tools to Measure Outcomes

As discussed in the previous section, many tools that are used to guide clinical practice are also useful for tracking and measuring outcomes. Examples include

Table 1–2	Categories of Outcome Measurement

Clinical Outcomes	Examples in Practice
Mortality	Intraoperative, surgical death rates, death at any specific point such as in hospital, 6 months, etc
Complications	Nosocomial infections, decubitus ulcer, patient falls, medication reactions
Functional status	Ability to navigate home requirements (ie, staircase) at discharge, return to pre-hospitalization exercise capacity
Psychosocial adjustment	Healthy perception of self following a limiting illness such as amputation or mastectomy
Quality of life	Patient reports "quality" of lifestyle, ability to participate in life activities, now as compared to before illness
Self-care	A new diabetic can give own insulin, a heart failure patient can limit sodium intake effectively and perform daily weights
Adherence	A new diabetic can give own insulin and DOES IT over an extended time period

Financial Outcomes	Examples in Practice
Length of stay (LOS)	Affects cost: Nursing care hours/day; supply usage, etc
Cost of care	Direct, indirect, variable, and fixed costs that are generated in delivering care
Charge for care	Patient billing, actual charge to patient for service provided (in some cases is less than cost)
Readmission rates	Affects cost (same issues as LOS)

Patient Service Outcomes	Examples in Practice
System process issues	Lab work "run and report" time Scheduling time for elective procedures
System access issues	Clinic waiting room time Phone response time
Patient satisfaction	Postdischarge satisfaction surveys

Table 1–3	Tools to Track or Measure Outcome

Clinical pathways

Variance tracking tools

Clinical complication worksheets/reports

Process improvement monitors (QI)

Administrative databases (cost-accounting systems)

Scorecards

Data collection forms from research protocols

Psychological scales: quality of life; coping; anxiety; etc.

Satisfaction surveys

Functional status scales

critical pathways, variance tracking tools, and process improvement measures. Table 1–3 lists a number of tools commonly used for measuring outcome in a practice setting.

Many issues ultimately affect patient outcome. As key players on the health care team, we have the job of questioning every aspect of patient care from the "patient outcome" perspective (Fig. 1–5). As we do so, many opportunities

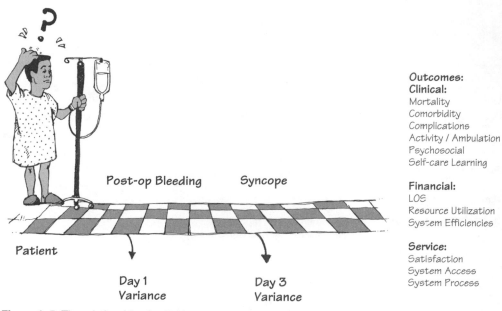

Figure 1–5. The relationship of patient care processes to outcomes.

will arise for tracking and measuring outcomes along the patient care trajectory. Often a tool for measuring a particular outcome will already be developed and in place. Sometimes you may be called upon to develop or implement a new tool. Either way, accurate statements about patient outcome are dependent upon sensitive, specific, valid, and reliable tools.

The Future of Outcomes

The practice of using outcome measures to evaluate health care and health care delivery is escalating. Accreditation bodies, such as the Joint Commission for Accreditation of Healthcare Organizations (JCAHO), are redesigning organizational reviews to focus more on *outcomes* and less on the *processes* used to achieve outcomes. Professional groups are coming together to standardize language around outcome measurement and improve consistency in reporting outcomes. Consumers are increasingly interested in outcomes, not only clinical outcomes related to personal illness, but also more global outcomes of the practitioners, payers, and health care plans they choose. As we move into the next century, outcome measurement will look more sophisticated in a number of ways. A few improvements and changes to expect include:

- Increased automation of data collection and analysis.
- Increased validation of outcome measurement by accreditation bodies.
- Increased investment in long-term clinical outcomes by payers.
- Increased value of outcomes data to consumers.
- Increased standardization of language surrounding outcome measures.
- Increased transdisciplinary collaboration to improve outcomes across all categories: clinical, financial, and service.

Our role as nurses in the evolution of outcomes measurement is not only to participate, but to lead. Clinicians are in key positions to assess and understand the needs of patients, the limitations of the health care delivery system, and the opportunities for improvement in providing the best care to patients. Our responsibility is to inquire, investigate, and inform practice for the benefit of patients. This responsibility requires diligent application of the research process in clinical practice.

A number of roadblocks will become evident as you move, and lead others to move, in the direction of more evidence-based practice (Fig. 1–6). These roadblocks are usually avoidable, or at least navigable, if approached from the right direction and with sufficient background information.

This book presents a practical approach for applying the research process in a clinical setting, to evaluate, measure, change, and improve patient outcome. An overview of the process is depicted in Fig. 1–7. Could YOU be using research better? Should YOU be generating better research? Perhaps so! Here's how.

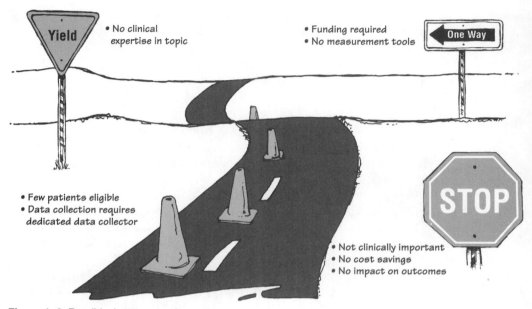

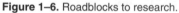

Figure 1–6. Roadblocks to research.

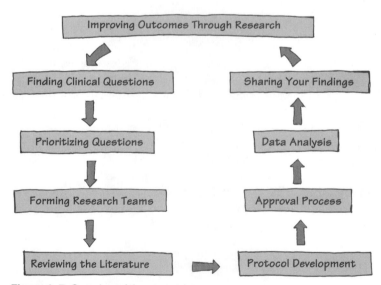

Figure 1–7. Overview of the research process.

▶ REFERENCES

RESEARCH TEXTBOOK SUGGESTED READINGS

Polit D, Hungler B. Chapter 1: Introduction to nursing research. Essentials of Nursing Research: Methods, Appraisal, and Utilization, 4th ed. Philadelphia: Lippincott–Raven Publishers, 1997, pages 4–28.

OTHER SUGGESTED READINGS

Bueno M, Hwang R. Understanding variances in hospital stay. Nursing Management 1993;24(11):41–57.

Mark B, Burleson D. Measurement of patient outcomes: Data availability and consistency across hospitals. Journal of Nursing Administration 1995;25:52–59.

Nelson E, Splaine M, Batalden P, Plume S. Building measurement and data collection into medical practice. Annals of Internal Medicine 1998;128:460–466.

Sackett, D. Evidence-based medicine: How to practice and teach evidence-based medicine. Pearson Professional Limited, London, 1997.

Sherer A. Designing Critical Pathways. American Association of Critical Care Nurses, Aliso Viejo, CA, 1997.

Spath P. Clinical Paths: Tools for Outcomes Management. American Hospital Publishing, Inc., Chicago, IL, 1994.

Smith-Marker C. Setting Standards for Professional Nursing: The Marker Model. St. Louis: Mosby, 1988.

Williams M. Benchmarking to improve financial performance. Health Management Technology 1995;Feb:10–12.

Wojner A. Outcomes management: From theory to practice. Critical Care Nursing Quarterly 1997;19(4):1–15.

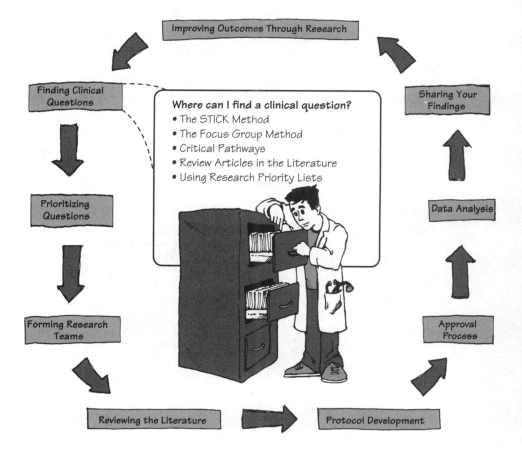

Improving Outcomes Through Research

Finding Clinical Questions

Where can I find a clinical question?
- The STICK Method
- The Focus Group Method
- Critical Pathways
- Review Articles in the Literature
- Using Research Priority Lists

Sharing Your Findings

Prioritizing Questions

Data Analysis

Forming Research Teams

Approval Process

Reviewing the Literature

Protocol Development

CHAPTER 2

Clinical Questions: Where Do You Find Them?

▶ INTRODUCTION

Where do you as a staff nurse identify the answers to questions that arise on a regular basis in the clinical setting? What sorts of questions? you may ask. Questions that are important to your patients. Questions that may affect your ability to deliver quality care to your patient. Questions that may arise in the course of pathway development.

Do any of the following situations sound familiar?

- Of the many types of telemetry electrodes on the market, which one can monitor patients for the longest period of time with optimal conductivity and without causing skin irritation or poor adherence in patients with oily skin or after bathing or diaphoresis?
- The new tympanic thermometers are wonderful, they are so fast! But are they as accurate as our current product? Do they really cut down on nosocomial infections transmitted via thermometers? Can we justify the added expense of this new technology?
- How can we optimize the CABG patient's length of stay in the ICU? Some hospitals are using "fast tracking" for early extubation. Should we try that? Would this change our CABG outcomes?

You have probably encountered similar questions in your own practice. Consider for a moment your own patient care setting. What examples have you encountered just this week that might give rise to questions like: What do we do, why do we do it that way, and is there a better way to do it?

If you are having trouble recalling a specific example, you are not alone. For the most part, the fast pace of patient care makes it difficult for us to recall ideas, problems, or creative thoughts from one minute to the next. Often the questions get "lost" in the course of the day, so that when nurses are asked, "What kinds of clinical questions can you think of that directly affect patients in your practice?" even expert staff are at a loss to think of one.

▶ THE STICK METHOD

One solution to this "thought-capture crisis" is the STICK method. STICK, Strategies to Investigate Clinical-Cost Kinetics, refers to the practice of investigating the "kinetics" or the interactive, dynamic relationship that exists between clinical practice and outcomes, and the costs associated with those outcomes. The STICK method is a simple approach to capturing clinical questions as they occur, in the midst of the dynamic patient care setting. Because this setting is where we are most interactive with patients, devices, technology, and new ideas, the bedside is an excellent forum for the generation of patient-centered research questions.

Often, however, the most creative, interesting thoughts come while we are in challenging situations and unable to leave the patient. The questions revolving around and affecting patients usually arise during actual delivery of patient care, on rounds, or in conversation with family members or other members of the health care team such as physicians, respiratory therapists, or pharmacists. The STICK method provides an easy avenue for capturing these questions at the bedside, without distracting the care nurse from his or her immediate situation. The following steps will help you get started with the STICK method:

1. Adhere a pad of Post-It Notes™ at the bedside or workstation at each bedside (Fig. 2–1). Anything that one calls into questions in the course of the shift can be written on these "stickies." For example, the question may be related to a procedure, diagnosis, teaching tool, nursing responsibility, or patient issue. Examples of typical questions generated by a coronary care unit are listed in Table 2–1.

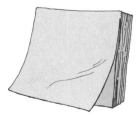

" Stickies " allow the clinician to jot down ideas or questions as they occur in the course of patient care, thereby preventing loss of clinical questions.

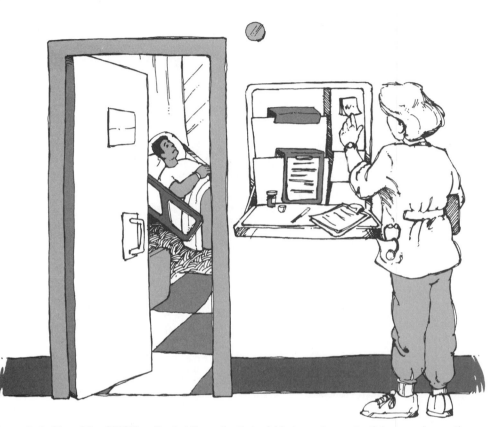

Figure 2–1. Use of the STICK method at the patient's bedside to capture potential research questions.

2. The second step is to post the stickies in a central location. The purpose of locating STICK questions in a central area is to stimulate interest of other staff members and to promote a forum for multidisciplinary discussion. General review and a systematic evaluation of each STICK question will be done at a later time. There are a number of ways to "centralize" the STICK questions:

   ▼ Identify a common gathering area on your unit, such as the coffee pot, a lounge, or a nursing station, and create a designated bulletin board for STICK!

   ▼ Identify a member of the staff, the charge nurse, the clinical specialist, or a member of the research committee, to collect the stickies and place them on the central board each day.

3. The third step is to determine which questions are best addressed with research methods. Some of the questions raised may actually be adminis-

trative, educational, or nonclinical issues. And some of the clinical questions may be beyond the scope of the staff's expertise at this time. It is imperative that some process be in place to narrow down the list of "clinical questions" into those that are most amenable to research interventions and have significant clinical priority. A systematic approach can assist you in this step of the process (Fig. 2–2).

The STICK method algorithm is used to assist clinicians to first categorize questions into various groups that have different functions, some of which will be amenable to research. Questions generally cross a myriad of disciplines, issues, and aspects of patient care. The most common categories for grouping are policy issues, staff development issues, administrative issues, and actual clinical practice questions. Depending on the issues listed with the STICK method, other categories may emerge and should be included in this sorting phase. The categorizing of the STICK questions can be done by members of the unit research committee, if one exists, or by a group of different staff members. Questions that can help guide this categorization process include:

- Is this issue/question easily resolved by creating a policy or does it indicate a need for policy change? If either is so, categorize as a policy issue and refer the issue/question to the appropriate unit or hospitalwide policy committee.
- Could this issue/question be easily resolved by an administrative decision or person? If yes, categorize as an administrative issue and consult the individual(s) with the power/authority to change the identified problem or concern.
- Could this issue/question be easily resolved by a simple explanation or in-service or educational session? If yes, categorize as a staff development issue and refer the issue/question to the clinical educator or appropriate committee/department.
- Remaining questions can be placed in the research category for further investigation (see Fig. 2–3).

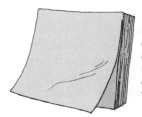

If you have limited resources or a very small working group of staff you may want to collect stickies from more than one unit, for example the coronary unit and the telemetry unit. By pooling STICK questions from a division or group of like units, you may generate enough interest in a single topic to have a larger working group.

Table 2–1	Clinical Questions Identified with the STICK Method in a Coronary Care Unit (CCU)

STICK! Questions of the Month for CCU

1. Do TEDS go under pneumatic stockings? Does this retard skin breakdown or not?

2. Do we really need Avo$_2$ differences done every 4 hours? Should we change our policy?

3. Is saline lavage useful for ETS or not? Recent article in *American Journal of Critical Care* indicates it is not helpful and may harm patients. Should we be using Mucomyst for thinning thick secretions instead?

4. Can bolus infusions be given via the PA port?

5. Can RBCs run on a pump?

6. Can more than one unit of blood be given through each filter?

7. For repeated K$^+$ checks, would it be cheaper to check K$^+$ with ABG analysis or K$^+$ pocket?

8. What should the level of care be for a patient on a continuous infusion of quinidine, for which there is no policy?

9. What is the rationale for crossing a patient's arms when giving morgue care? This is inconsistently done; what is the rationale?

10. Do we induce a prerenal state in AMI patients by maintaining a hypotensive BP for several days (ie, systolic BP of 100 mm Hg in a patient with a normal creatinine and usual systolic BP of 150–180 mm Hg)?

11. Do we adequately sedate and/or give proper "taper" therapy to patients as DTs are resolving?

12. What is the need for nutritional maintenance in long-term ventilator patients following extubation?

13. We always discontinue nasogastric tubes when endotracheal tubes are removed. Is this necessary? Should we change our policy on this?

14. Can nurses remove PA catheters?

Issues/questions in the research category should be evaluated to determine which ones are of clinical importance. This step is accomplished primarily by informal discussion with staff members and any easily accessible clinical expert. Any issues/questions that are not considered to be of high clinical importance are eliminated from the research category. Any eliminated items are discussed with the original contributor to validate this decision. An example of STICK categorization from the coronary care unit is presented in Table 2–2.

Questions remaining in the research category will be further evaluated and prioritized by the group at its next session. Information on how to accomplish this step will be covered in the next chapter.

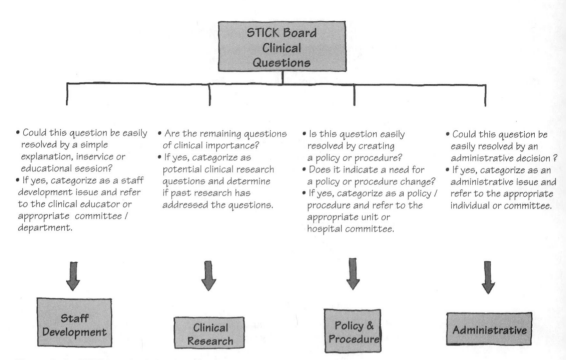

Figure 2–2. STICK method algorithm for categorizing clinical questions.

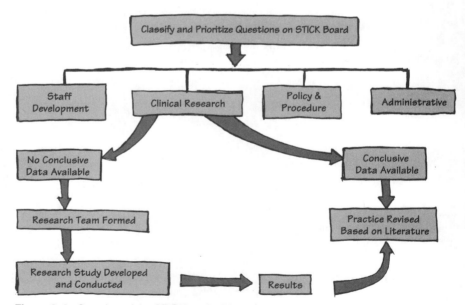

Figure 2–3. Overview of the STICK method for resolving clinical practice questions.

Table 2–2	Categorizing Clinical Issues/Questions Identified with the STICK Method in a Coronary Care Unit (CCU)

Policy Issues/Questions:

1. Do we really need Avo$_2$ differences done every 4 hours? Should we change our policy?

2. We always discontinue nasogastric tubes when endotracheal tubes are removed. Is this necessary? Should we change our policy on this?

3. Can RBCs run on a pump?

4. Can more than one unit of blood be given through each filter?

Administrative Issues/Questions:

1. What should the level of care be for a patient on a continuous infusion of quinidine, for which there is no policy?

2. Can nurses remove PA catheters?

Educational Issues/Questions:

1. Can bolus infusions be given via the PA port?

2. What is the need for nutritional maintenance in long-term ventilator patients following extubation?

3. What is the rationale for crossing a patient's arms when giving morgue care? This is inconsistently done; what is the rationale?

4. For repeated K$^+$ checks, would it be cheaper to check K$^+$ with ABG analysis or K$^+$ pocket?

Research Issues/Questions:

1. Do we adequately sedate and/or give proper "taper" therapy to patients as DTs are resolving?

2. Do TEDS go under pneumatic stockings? Does this retard skin breakdown or not?

3. Is saline lavage useful for ETS or not? Recent article in *American Journal of Critical Care* indicates it is not helpful and may harm patients. Should we be using Mucomyst for thinning thick secretions instead?

4. Do we induce a prerenal state in AMI patients by maintaining a hypotensive BP for several days (ie, systolic BP of 100 mm Hg in a patient with a normal creatinine and usual systolic BP of 150–180 mm Hg)?

In summary, the STICK method may help you to capture clinical questions more effectively by:

- Providing access to scrap paper during rounds.

- Designating a fixed place to write questions on, so they don't go home with the nurse on a patient worksheet or other "washable" item.

- Facilitating the collection and assimilation of the questions in an organized way, for group discussion, preventing the problem of eternally unanswered questions.

- Encouraging the nurse at the bedside to WRITE IT DOWN! Whatever you're thinking may be valuable or of interest to others.

- Providing a forum for entertaining ANY questions, thereby encouraging less-accomplished staff to get involved and emphasizing the philosophy that no question is a silly question.

▶ THE FOCUS GROUP METHOD

Another method to identify clinically important research questions is to gather clinicians from the unit and engage in a focus group to identify clinical research questions. Using this approach, it is possible for clinicians to easily identify 10 to 20 potential research questions after two or three 1-hour sessions.

The first phase of this process involves the identification of high-volume patient populations that are cared for on the unit and their needs/problems that require nursing intervention during hospitalization. The second phase involves brainstorming potential research questions that clinicians feel are important. The third and final phase involves prioritizing the research questions, which will be discussed in Chap. 3. Good research projects for busy clinicians, who often have limited research experience, are identified in this final phase using a set of criteria.

Phase I: Brainstorming High-volume Patient Care

The steps involved in the first phase include the following:

1. Gather some of the unit clinicians for a 1-hour meeting. Identify the purpose of the first meeting as brainstorming about common patient care problems/needs and nursing interventions that are often employed to address these needs/problems. Clarify the role of the facilitator.
2. Using a flip chart, have group members identify the following:

    ▼ High-volume patient populations and common needs/problems. List the major characteristics of the patients cared for on your unit:
    - age ranges of patients
    - medical diagnoses
    - nursing diagnoses
    - symptoms
    - problems/needs
    - other

    ▼ Frequent nursing interventions. List the most common nursing interventions prescribed for your patient population. For example,

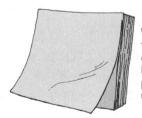

While the facilitator's role is to guide the group through the steps, it is helpful for this individual to have a strong clinical expertise with the patient population. This background will allow the facilitator to more easily identify patient care needs and realistic research questions if members of the group get hung up along the way.

- catheter management
- education (discharge teaching, preparation for procedures, symptom management, technology care)
- symptom management (interventions targeted to specific symptoms, such as pain or dyspnea)
- drug administration
- psychosocial support
- family support

▼ Common technologies:
- infusion pumps
- monitoring devices (blood pressure, temperature, EKG, oxygenation)
- bedside laboratory testing (blood glucose, coags, K^-, ABGs)

Examples of a completed session with clinicians from an oncology and critical care unit are provided in Tables 2–3 and 2–4.

3. Typically, in a 1-hour session, groups can easily identify most of the information required in all these categories. At the next session, prior to beginning Phase II, have the group revisit the listings and add or delete from the list as needed.

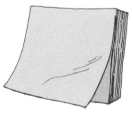

After the session, type up the information on the flip charts so it can be given out at the next session. This gives the group a sense of accomplishment, having a " product " of their efforts. It also serves as a visual reminder of high volume patient care situations as the group moves into the next phase where research questions or topics will be identified.

Phase II: Identification of Potential Research Topics or Questions

Using these high-volume patient care situations as a foundation, have the group members begin questioning their practice. Some questions that can be asked to stimulate this phase would be:

- Do we know that X nursing intervention is effective to treat Y? How often should we be performing this intervention to achieve maximal benefit? For example, does mouth care every 4 hours decrease the incidence of mucositis and oral discomfort in chemotherapy patients? Would every-2-hour use of mouth care improve patient outcomes? Another example is related to chest PT. If chest PT is one of the frequently performed nursing interventions, one might question if it has ever been shown to be effective in postoperative patients. If it has been effective, do we know what frequency of treatment is best?

Table 2–3	Example of the First Phase of the Focus Group Method from an Oncology Unit

Phase I: Brainstorming

High-Volume Patient Populations & Patient Needs/Problems
Cancer (ovarian, breast, prostate, lymphoma)
Bone marrow transplants (lymphoma, breast CA)
Neutropenia
Fever
Alterations in skin integrity (sloughing, pruritus, etc), particularly associated with IL-1 administration
Self-care common
Deep vein thrombosis
Depression
Nausea/vomiting
Chronic pain

Common/Frequent Nursing Interventions
CVC care (Hickman's, Broviac, etc)
   flushing
   dressings
   assessment for infection
Blood withdrawal for therapeutic and research specimens
Symptom management
   mucositis (mouth pain, infection)
   diarrhea
   nausea & vomiting
   pain (fentanyl common for analgesia)
   constipation
   skin problems R/T IL-1
   alopecia
   neuropathies
Patient education
   research protocol related
   symptom management
   lifestyle changes
   disease information
   side effects of chemotherapy
   subcutaneous injections
   catheter care
Shivering/rigors R/T amphotericin administration
   different types of treatment for symptom management
   premedication and postmedication
   mechanical treatments (heat lamps, wrapping)
Blood product administration
Chemo administration
Various electrolyte administrations (potassium, magnesium chloride)
Skin care (sitz baths, medicated lotions/creams)
Psychosocial support
Caring for immobilized patients (use of Hoyer lift, single/two nurses and transfers, high-energy expenditure of staff)
Antibiotic administration

Table 2–3	Example of the First Phase of the Focus Group Method from an Oncology Unit (continued)

Heparin administration—subcutaneous
Premedication for various therapies (benadryl, Zofran, compazine)

Technologies Commonly Used
Automated noninvasive blood pressure devices
Portable infusion pumps
Catheters of all sizes and shapes
Pulse oximetry
Hypothermia
Apheresis catheter (new, increased use expected)

- Have previous studies on X nursing intervention been done in a variety of patient populations, specifically your high-volume patients? For example, if mouth care with Peridex™ has been shown to be effective with total body irradiation for bone marrow transplant patients, is it effective for mucositis caused by Cisplatin in ovarian cancer treatment? Another example is regarding brief hyperoxygenation periods before and after endotracheal suctioning. Does this practice prevent hypoxemia in cardiac surgical patients, and if so, has it also been shown to be effective in patients with severe respiratory failure on high levels of Fio_2?

- How do different nurses intervene with Y symptom? Here you want to elicit discussion about different approaches that clinicians use and begin to question if we know which approach is best. For example, what approaches do staff use to control shivering associated with chemotherapy? Another example may be, what approaches do staff think are best to reduce fever in postoperative patients? Is antipyretic therapy used more than cooling methods (sponge baths, hypothermia blankets, ice packs, fans)? Which methods do staff think work the best?

- Have the previous studies on X used techniques (methods) that are similar to the way interventions are done in real practice? If not, a great research question might be the use of clinically relevant methods. For examples, if the past studies on hyperoxygenation in endotracheal suctioning used a second ventilator to deliver the hyperoxygenation, is that similar to how it is typically done in real practice? If the answer is no, then would similar results be found if we repeated the study using a manual resuscitation bag for the hyperoxygenation?

Examples of research questions identified with this approach are listed in Tables 2–5 and 2–6.

| Table 2–4 | Example of Phase I of the Focus Group Method from a Medical Intensive Care Unit |

Phase I: Brainstorming

High-Volume Patient Populations & Patient Needs/Problems
Sepsis—with/without shock
Respiratory failure
Renal failure
Cardiac failure R/T chemotherapy
Cardiac arrhythmias R/T chemotherapy, Taxol, suramin
Pediatric HIV—admissions to unit as well as for procedures
Pancreatitis
GCD patients with respiratory failure or sepsis
Fever
Tumor lysis syndrome

Common/Frequent Nursing Interventions
Assisting/monitoring patients during short-term procedures (bone marrows, bronchoscopy, CVC line insertions, lumbar punctures, bone biopsy)
Specimen collections for therapeutic or research purposes (urine, blood, stool, sputum, etc)
Endotracheal suctioning—with/without normal saline instillation, open method only, manual resuscitation bag for hyperoxygenation
Pain management—mainly IV drug administration (prn or continuous infusion); some new approaches being seen (TENS)
Transports
Medication administration (antibiotics, vasopressors, neuromuscular blockers, chemo)
IV tubing and dressing changes
Patient/family teaching (ICU routines, admission information, procedures, transfer planning, visiting)
Computer interventions (putting in orders, etc)
Temperature control measures
Dressing changes
Chest tubes

Technologies Commonly Used
Special beds—different types
Ventilators—common modes these days are pressure control with fairly normal PEEP levels
Physiologic monitoring—invasive and noninvasive (BP, Sao_2, $Paco_2$)
Sequential compression devices
CVVH (and his uncles)
Blood glucose monitoring
Hypothermia units
Smart needles
Sonogram for catheter insertion
Pacemakers
Capnography
12 lead EKG
Fluoroscopy
Cardiac monitoring
Portable suction
Syringe pumps

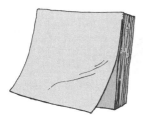

The facilitator will need to go into the session with some ideas of practice areas where the current techniques are not based on scientific information, are out of date, or where some controversy exists on the best approach.

▶ USING CARE PATHS OR CRITICAL PATHWAYS FOR GENERATING RESEARCH

Increasingly, nursing is leading the health care team in developing, implementing, and refining collaborative patient care guidelines or pathways for various patient populations. Whether your institution refers to these guidelines as care maps, care pathways, critical paths, or some other term, the purpose is the same. These care paths are used to provide consistency of care for specific patient populations. This allows complications and variances to be tracked and facilitates the measurement of clinical and financial outcomes.

As paths become increasingly sophisticated, refined, and computerized, using care paths to identify research ideas will facilitate the research process . This approach ensures that the research you choose to engage in is pertinent to your clinical area and consistent with the goals and objectives of the institution. In addition, the framework of most care paths lends itself easily to construction of a research proposal, data collection forms, and elementary levels of data analysis.

How can clinical questions be identified from care paths? Three of the most common ways are by:

- Examining variances or common complications identified for a specific pathway.
- Comparing observed institutional outcomes to national/regional benchmarked outcomes, identifying areas of practice where change is indicated.
- Questioning if more efficient/effective approaches to patient management are available using new technology or processes.

Examining Clinical Pathway Variances or Complications

Optimally, care paths are designed to reflect "best practice" in that they represent guidelines for patient management that are based on the results of carefully reviewed research. In any given patient population, however, variances from the expected or desired outcome occur. Because a clinical path is designed to meet the needs of about 70–80% of the patients in a diagnostic group, 20% (or more) can be expected to experience complications that cause

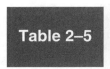

| Table 2–5 | List of Potential Research Topics or Questions Generated during Phase II of the Focus Group Method from an Oncology Unit |

1. Does the use of PCA pumps for the administration of morphine sulfate improve pain/discomfort in patient with mucositis?
   Dependent variables: level of pain/discomfort
   total amount of morphine required/24 h
   compliance with oral hygiene routine
   cost
   condition of oral mucosa

2. Is double-dose Zofran more effective than the traditional dose of Zofran in controlling nausea and vomiting?
   Dependent variables: level of nausea
   frequency of retching
   caloric intake

3. Does the administration of Zofran decrease nausea and vomiting?
   Dependent variables: as above

4. Can blood withdrawn for discard prior to obtaining laboratory specimens be safely returned to the patient?
   Dependent variables: clot formation in discarded blood
   catheter dysfunction (ease of withdrawal, injection)
   amount of blood/24 h removed

5. Is heparin necessary in the flush solution of Hickman catheters?
   Dependent variable: catheter function (ease of withdrawal, injection)

6. What educational strategies are effective in decreasing Hickman complications (infection, clotting)?
   Dependent variables: catheter function
   infection

7. Does the wearing of masks by the patient and care provider alter infection incidence?
   Dependent variables: infection rates
   blood/skin cultures

8. Which oral hygiene method is the best for mucositis: current regime vs saline only vs topical analgesic vs placebo?
   Dependent variables: cost (drugs & nursing time)
   pain/discomfort
   oral cavity condition

9. Is the use of a hypothermia blanket better than other methods for fever reduction (antipyretics only vs antipyretics & ice packs)?
   Dependent variables: shivering
   temperature
   discomfort

10. What is the most effective treatment for perineal skin excoriation (sitz bath vs whirlpool vs nothing vs topical medication vs combination)?
    Dependent variables: pain/discomfort
    cost
    skin integrity assessment

Table 2–6	List of Potential Research Topics or Questions Generated during Phase II of the Focus Group Method from a Medical Intensive Care Unit

1. What are the risks and benefits associated with the use of normal saline with endotracheal suctioning?

   Dependent variables: amount of mucous
                                consistency of mucous
                                O_2 Sat, Pao_2
                                cost
                                patient comfort

2. Are portable glucose meters as accurate as plasma glucose levels for managing critically ill patients?

   Dependent variables: serum glucose level
                                  cost

3. Which method (manual or mechanical) is better for the delivery of hyperoxygenation breaths during endotracheal suctioning? Which patients benefit from closed-system suctioning (high PEEP, Fio^2, etc)?

   Dependent variables: ABGs
                                  MAP
                                HR
                                peak airway pressure during delivery
                                patient comfort

4. Which methods of temperature control work best with fever (prn vs scheduled antipyretic medications vs hypothermia unit vs ice packs vs tepid baths)?

   Dependent variables: core temperature
                                  shivering
                                  patient comfort

the patient to deviate from normal expectations. This deviation is commonly referred to as a "variance." A fruitful area for investigation into changes in practice may emerge when variances exceed the 20% expectation. For example, on a Same-day Angioplasty Pathway the number of patients meeting expectations for LOS (36 hours) might only be 50%. This leads one to ask, "What factors are causing prolonged LOS?" A number of variables may be identified, such as patients' inability to perform groin incision care, and based on these variables research questions may be derived to more carefully examine and evaluate the issues.

Another example of research ideas that can be generated from clinical path variances emerges when most or all patients are achieving expected outcomes. If 100% of the patients on a given clinical path are achieving an identified objective or outcome, such as length of stay or discharge time, the goal may be too graciously set. For example, consider ambulation following sheath removal in catheterization patients. The traditional time to ambulation following sheath removal post-cardiac catheterization is 6 hours. If 100% of patients meet this expected outcome, the 6-hour standard may be inappropriate and more aggressive ambulation routines may be safe. This leads one to ask a research question such as, "Can early ambulation (3 hours) after sheath removal be done safely without an increase in bleeding complications?"

Variances trigger clinical questions in that the care nurse is continually driven to ask the question, "Why did this complication or deviation from the expected outcome occur?" Examination of variances provides an opportunity to reevaluate practice and to identify potential areas in which changing practice may be appropriate. Examples of how clinical questions can be identified from examination of variances on clinical pathways is presented in Table 2–7. Exercise 2–1 is an example of how to identify clinical questions using variance analysis. Complete Exercise 2–2 to tailor this concept to a pathway example at your institution.

Using National and Regional Benchmark Data

"Benchmark data" refers to data that are generally accepted by experts in a particular field as being the standard by which others can and should be measured. "Benchmarks" can be institutions, studies, or specific outcomes such as length of stay or mortality rate in a given patient population. Clinicians often use various benchmarks or benchmarked data to design, develop, and evaluate clinical paths.

Table 2–7	Examining Variances and Locating Fruitful Areas for Research
Variance Situations	**Questions to Ask**
Exceeding expected outcomes	Could the outcome be safely changed to occur at an earlier time? Are system processes creating unnecessary delays?
Not achieving expected outcomes	Is the expected outcome based on scientific and/or national standards? Are there any aspects of patient management that could interfere with achieving the outcomes (eg, drugs, confounding variables, technical problems with equipment, breaks in technique or routines)? Would increasing the frequency or timing of key interventions be likely to improve outcomes?
Challenging acceptable outcomes	Would a different approach or method be likely to improve patient outcomes (eg, comfort, satisfaction, physiologic stability, mobility, communication, complications)? Would a different approach or method be a more efficient or effective use of resources (eg, personnel, supplies, time, services)?

▶ **Exercise 2-1**

**Using Variance Analysis to Identify Clinical Questions
from a Cardiovascular Pathway**

Joe, a patient on an MI path, is now on day 4 post cath and has a groin bleed. Joe
has moved smoothly thus far from one day or "phase" to the next on his MI care
path. Today he has a groin complication, which prevents him from progressing to
day 5 (discharge day) on schedule. Consider the following questions:

1. What is the reason(s) for groin complications in patients like Joe?
   a. Coagulopathy?
   b. Compression pressure inadequate?
   c. Compression time inadequate?
   d. Patient noncompliant or inadequately educated regarding bedrest instruc-
      tions?
2. Identify the percentage of patients falling into each of the above categories of reasons in your facility.
3. What is the most common reason? Is one reason more prevalent than all the
   others?

If the patients experiencing groin complications are relatively equally distributed
among a number of different "reasons," the variance is less likely to be useful or con-
ducive to a study, because the incidence of complication for any given reason is
small. On the other hand, if the majority of patients fall into one or two "reasons" categories, further evaluation of that particular reason or practice parameter is warranted. This is a good starting point for a clinical study.

Where do benchmark data come from? A number of groups and organizations, private as well as public, at the federal, state, and local level, provide
health care data for the purposes of benchmarking. Examples of such groups
include Medicare's Cooperative Cardiovascular Project (CCP), which provides
regional and national data to its subscribers on a number of cardiovascular issues; the Agency for Health Care Policy and Research (AHCPR), which provides clinical practice guidelines for specific disease states and patient populations; and various specialty organizations, such as the American Association of
Critical Care Nurses (AACN), which provides research based practice protocols
useful for benchmarking practice patterns. Insurance agencies, such as Blue
Cross Blue Shield, have developed standards for "optimal" length of stay and
costs, and private enterprises such as Milliman and Rogers have established
guidelines that are marketed and sold to insurers and hospitals for use in establishing a "bench." Industry has joined the data-driven frenzy as well, and companies such as Genentech have set up national databases to be used by clients

▶ **Exercise 2–2**

Using Variance Analysis to Identify Clinical Questions

1. Identify a variance on one of your pathways that reflects one of the following:
   a. Exceeds expected outcome:

   b. Outcomes not met:

2. What are some potential reasons for the variance abnormality?

3. Ask yourself the following questions to identify approaches to manage the abnormality:
   a. Exceeds expected outcomes:
      (i) Could the outcome be safely changed to occur at an earlier time?
      (ii) Are system processes creating unnecessary delays? Is the expected outcome realistic?
   b. Not meeting expected outcomes:
      (i)   Is the expected outcome realistic?
      (ii) Is the expected outcome based on scientific and/or national standards?
      (iii) Are there any aspects of patient management that could interfere with achieving the outcomes (eg, drugs, confounding variables, technical problems with equipment, breaks in technique or routines)?
      (iv) Would increasing the frequency or timing of key interventions be likely to improve outcomes?

and nonclients in the health care community for purposes of benchmarking acute MI patient care outcomes. Other sources of benchmark data can be classic articles that have been accepted as the "gold standard" in a given field, and numerous private consultant groups that provide data on regional and national issues such as length of stay (LOS) and cost of care, which can be helpful for evaluating one's own costs and actual hospital days.

The process of obtaining and using benchmark data may be simplified by following these first steps:

1. Identify data sources currently being used by your institution. The first place to look is your nurse manager, department head, and/or divisional or administrative director. These individuals are most likely to be aware of the sources and types of data currently being used at your institution.
2. Identify the type of benchmarks you would like to use (ie, practice stan-

dards or patterns versus numerical data such as LOS or costs, or a combination of these types of benchmarks).

3. Identify how frequently these sources submit updated reports to your hospital, and how frequently you will be able to obtain updates on your own patient population that you are using for comparison (ie, monthly, quarterly). The purpose of this step is to ensure an "apples to apples" comparison, using fiscal years and patient populations that are similar.

Time to extubation following coronary artery bypass grafting is one example of a clinical question which may arise from a care path and for which ample benchmark data exist. Following the steps outlined above, identify sources of data used at your institution, as well as any specialty organizations or journals that may be able to offer data on this topic (ie, anesthesia, cardiovascular groups, or critical care groups). Collect data from a number of sources if possible and compare your institution with the national benchmark. Several sources cite 4–6 hours as being optimal for extubation. What is the time to extubation at your institution? Is it within the optimal range as identified by the experts? Do you see a discrepancy? Might this be an area for research at your institution?

Length of stay following acute myocardial infarction is one example of an area for research in which using benchmark data would be helpful to derive research questions. What is the LOS at your institution following MI? Does it compare favorably with the benchmark data in your region? In the country? A number of sources can be used to obtain bench data for this particular question. Following the steps above, identify which sources of information your hospital uses or has access to for acute MI patients. The AHCPR guidelines, NRMI database, and American Heart Association data are available to anyone; however, your particular institution may or may not participate in the NRMI program. Because of the large number of sources available to address this particular question, data regarding your particular institution may not be as important. The consensus of large numbers of experts is 4–5 days. How is your population tracked? Is your LOS within the range of optimal as defined by these national and regional databases (see Fig. 1–5 on page 10)?

Considering New Technologies or Approaches to Care

Another way to use care paths for identifying research questions is to compare traditional methods or techniques for patient care with new technologies. New technologies are generally created and marketed because they fulfill, or claim to fulfill, one of the following objectives: save time for clinicians, are easier for clinicians to use, provide an advanced approach to a problem (such as special beds for pressure ulcer management), and/or provide increased comfort or ease of use for patients.

Consider the example presented in Exercise 2–1 relating to groin bleeding. Is the mechanism for applying pressure after sheath removal optimal, not only for hemostasis but also for patient comfort? This groin-bleeding variance can be managed in a number of ways:

- RN holds manual pressure to the groin site until bleeding stops.
- Technician or UAP holds manual pressure to the groin site until bleeding stops.
- A special device is used to apply pressure to the groin site until bleeding stops:
  - C clamp
  - Femostop

Which of the above methods is best for patient comfort, as well as decreasing groin-bleeding complications? Ask yourself the following questions:

- What are the options for achieving hemostasis?
- What is the comfort range with the traditional method?
- What is the comfort range with a new device?
- Is the cost of the new device worth the difference in comfort provided to the patient?

Obviously a number of things must be considered before you have enough data to make an informed decision. What are some of the appropriate questions to ask and how should you go about asking them? Using a decision tree can help to sort out available information related to new products (Fig. 2–4). It will also help to point out areas where information is unavailable and should be investigated.

▶ GETTING RESEARCH IDEAS FROM THE LITERATURE

A wonderful way to get ideas for research projects is to read review articles on topics that are common in your unit. The authors, who are usually experts in that area of research, often suggest areas for future research. These suggestions may be based on problems with how the past studies were carried out, "holes" in the research, or new areas for research that are based on existing work.

Another place in the literature that you can find ideas for research projects is at the end of research studies. Typically, the authors list a few areas for future research based on the findings of their study.

▶ USING RESEARCH PRIORITIES IDENTIFIED BY PROFESSIONAL ASSOCIATIONS

Many professional nursing organizations have published lists of research priorities for clinical practice. Typically, the specialty nursing organizations have research priorities that are more clinically focused, narrow in scope, and specific

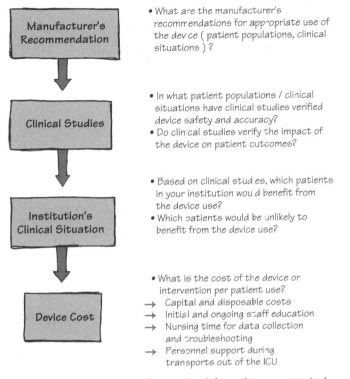

Manufacturer's Recommendation

- What are the manufacturer's recommendations for appropriate use of the device (patient populations, clinical situations) ?

Clinical Studies

- In what patient populations / clinical situations have clinical studies verified device safety and accuracy?
- Do clinical studies verify the impact of the device on patient outcomes?

Institution's Clinical Situation

- Based on clinical studies, which patients in your institution would benefit from the device use?
- Which patients would be unlikely to benefit from the device use?

Device Cost

- What is the cost of the device or intervention per patient use?
  → Capital and disposable costs
  → Initial and ongoing staff education
  → Nursing time for data collection and troubleshooting
  → Personnel support during transports out of the ICU

Figure 2–4. Decision tree for sorting information on new technology.

to patient populations. These research priorities can be an excellent source of ideas for your unit projects. Again, it's important to stay away from ideas/ questions that do not commonly occur in the patients you care for on your unit. Some examples of research priorities published by the American Association of Critical-Care Nursing (AACN) and the Oncology Nursing Society (ONS) are listed in Tables 2–8 and 2–9.

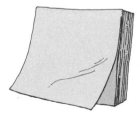

When considering research suggestions from experts in the field, avoid selecting topics that do not occur on a routine basis in your patient population. Data collection could take 20 years in your facility if a topic is not something that many of your patients experience!

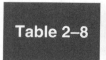

Table 2–8	Research Priorities for Critical Care Nursing from the American Association of Critical-Care Nurses

Priorities for clinical practice research in critical care nursing:

1. Techniques to optimize pulmonary functioning and prevent pulmonary complications

2. Weaning of mechanically ventilated patients

3. Effect of nursing activities/interventions on hemodynamic parameters

4. Techniques for real-time monitoring of tissue perfusion and oxygenation

5. Nutritional support modalities and patient outcomes

6. Interventions to prevent infection

7. Pain assessment and pain-management techniques

8. Accuracy and precision of invasive and noninvasive monitoring devices

9. Effect of nursing activities, environmental stimuli, and human interactions on intracranial and cerebral perfusion pressure

Priorities for research on the context within which critical care nursing takes place:

1. Incorporation of research findings into critical care nursing practice

2. Levels of nursing competence (eg, certification) and the effect on patient outcomes

3. Occupational hazards (eg, HIV, noise, substance abuse, premature delivery)

4. Ethical issues related to initiation, maintenance, and withdrawal of life support technology (eg, living wills)

5. Patient care delivery models for critical care

6. Collaboration and communication among health care professionals

7. Role of critical care nurses in decisions regarding resuscitation status of critically ill patients

Reference: Lindquist R, Banasik J, Barnsteiner J, et al. Determining AACN's research priorities for the 90's. American Journal of Critical Care 1993;2(2):110–117.

▶ REFERENCES

RESEARCH TEXTBOOK SUGGESTED READINGS

Wilson HS. Discovering research problems in clinical practice. In: Research in Nursing, Addison-Wesley Publishing Co: Menlo Park, CA, 1985, pages 110–126.

Polit D, Hungler B. Chapter 3: Research problems, research questions and hypotheses. In: Essentials of Nursing Research: Methods, Appraisal, and Utilization, 4th ed. Philadelphia: Lippincott–Raven, 1997, pages 65–88.

OTHER SUGGESTED READINGS

Beck C. Replication strategies for nursing research. Image: Journal of Nursing Scholarship 1994;26(3):191–194.

Brink H. Basic issues in clinical nursing research. Part 2: Identifying and demarcating the study area and framing research questions. Nursing 1994;9(6):31, 33–34.

Table 2–9	Research Priorities for Oncology Nursing from the Oncology Nursing Society

Top Ten Research Issues

1. Pain
2. Prevention
3. Quality of life
4. Risk reduction/screening
5. Ethical issues
6. Neutropenia/immunosuppression
7. Patient education issues
8. Stress, coping, and adaptation
9. Detection
10. Cost containment

Reference: Stetz KM, Haberman MR, Holcombe J, Jones LS. 1994 Oncology Nursing Society Research Priorities Survey. Oncology Nursing Forum 1995;22(5):785–789.

Chulay M, White T. Nursing research: Instituting chages in clinical practice. Critical Care Nurse 1989;9(5):106, 108, 110–113.

Connelly C. Replicating research in nursing. International Journal of Nursing Studies 1986;23:71–77.

Fitch M. Creating a research agenda with relevance to cancer nursing practice. Cancer Nursing 1996;19(5):335–342.

Kacuba A. Turning tradition upside down: Staff nurses and clinical research. American Journal of Nursing 1993;(suppl):5–10.

Johnson B. How to ask research questions in clinical practice. American Journal of Nursing 1991;91(3):64–65.

Lindquist R, Banasik J, Barnsteiner J, et al. Determining AACN's research priorities. American Journal of Critical Care 1993;2(2):110–117.

Munro B. Looking for a research question? Clinical Nurse Specialist 1996;10(3):130.

Stetz KM., Haberman MR, Holcombe J, and Jones LS. 1994 Oncology Nursing Society Research Priorities Survey. Oncology Nursing Forum 1995;22(5):785–789.

White S, Bartrug B, Bride W. Supporting nursing innovations in a cost-conscious environment. Critical Care Nursing Clinics of North America 1995;7(2):399–406.

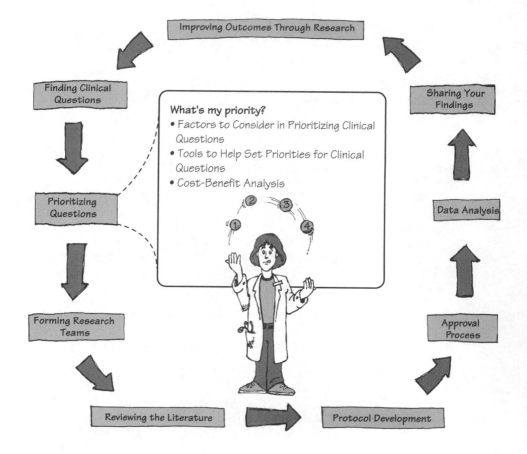

Improving Outcomes Through Research

Finding Clinical Questions

Sharing Your Findings

What's my priority?
- Factors to Consider in Prioritizing Clinical Questions
- Tools to Help Set Priorities for Clinical Questions
- Cost-Benefit Analysis

Data Analysis

Prioritizing Questions

Forming Research Teams

Approval Process

Reviewing the Literature

Protocol Development

Prioritizing Clinical Questions

▶ **THE IMPORTANCE OF SETTING PRIORITIES: WHY PRIORITIZE?**

Using the focus group or STICK method, it's easy to come up with many potential research questions. Which one should we choose for our project, you might ask? Does it really matter whether the question on symptom management or the question about accuracy of a new temperature device is chosen? The answer to the question is yes! It does matter which question you select for your research study, for a number of reasons.

Doing research is hard work. There will be many roadblocks along the way that you will want to avoid, if possible (Fig. 3–1). By keeping potential roadblocks in mind while you are selecting your research topic, you can cut down on the number of problems you will encounter along the way. This is especially important when there are limited resources available in your institution to support research. Prioritizing research questions based on the number of potential roadblocks each has will help you to select the best research question. Prioritizing in this way may also maximize your potential for success by differentiating clinically important and feasible research questions from those that may be more difficult to accomplish given current expertise and resources.

▶ **FACTORS TO CONSIDER WHEN PRIORITIZING**

Key factors to consider when attempting to prioritize your research question include staff expertise, patient population and setting, other projects currently in process in your unit or work area, institutional priorities, cost, availability of tools, and funding requirements (Table 3–1). Another factor that may be use-

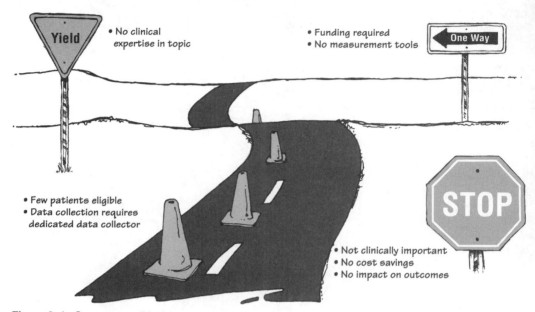

Figure 3–1. Common roadblocks to research completion.

ful in prioritizing is to consider research priorities that have been identified by professional groups or associations.

Staff Expertise

First, the ideal project would take advantage of the staff's area of clinical expertise. This allows the working group to concentrate on learning the research process instead of having to learn new practice skills, as well as the research process. Since most clinicians who carry out research have minimal research experience, this type of criterion is especially important. Building on staff's clinical expertise will also help them to recognize themselves as clinical experts, empowering them to have control over their own practice. Close alignment of the research topic with clinical practice expertise will ensure staff's ability to maintain interest through project completion.

Patient Population and Setting

Another criterion of ideal research studies is that large numbers of patients should be eligible for the study. This will assist in keeping the time required for data collection to a minimum and ensures that skills required for study enrollment and data collection are maintained at a high level, increasing reliability of the data collected. Enthusiasm and commitment will also be easier to maintain throughout data collection if there is a steady flow of patients into the study.

Table 3–1	Criteria for Ideal Research Topics

Criteria for Ideal Research Topics

1 Takes advantage of clinical expertise of the staff.

2. Maintains the interest of the staff through a potentially lengthy period to project completion.

3. Is important to clinical practice and patient outcomes.

4. Has potential cost-saving impact for the institution.

5. Includes large numbers of patients eligible for the study.

6. Has established tools for variable measurement.

7. Requires no additional funds for study completion.

8. Recognizes political priorities of the organization.

9. Allows data-collection procedures to be easily incorporated into daily nursing practice routines.

Another criterion for ideal research projects is having few barriers to enrollment of subjects. Barriers to enrollment that may occur owing to the setting of the study include:

- Logistical barriers. These are barriers such as limited access to specific patient populations or patient care facilities. For example, if your research question is related to a cardiac rehabilitation program, but the research team works in the acute care center, the team may have a difficult time carrying out data collection in the other site.

- Clinical/physiologic barriers. For example, patients require consent postoperatively, but the study is taking place in the Post Anesthesia Care Unit where patients are sedated and unable to give consent.

- Administrative barriers. For example, the research question requires monitoring infection from children visiting in an adult ICU, but children under 13 are not permitted in the unit. Another example would be a research question that would require the expenditure of fiscal resources that are not included in the unit budget.

Other Concurrent Projects

Another consideration when prioritizing research questions is how well the question would complement or conflict with other ongoing unit projects, such as quality improvement (QI) or staff development projects. Research that complements or builds on other, ongoing projects is desirable in that it contributes to an established or evolving body of science.

A body of science is valuable, especially long term, for what it can say about a given topic. For example, if your case managers have noted persistently high variance rates in respiratory complications in your CABG population, and the unit QI committee is monitoring compliance with pulmonary toilet protocols, then a significant contribution to the body of information might be a study pertaining to ventilation or respiratory issues. Rather than choosing to do work on a number of different and unrelated topical areas over time, see if several interest areas in your unit might complement or build on one another, and pursue this focus across working groups such as QI, staff development, and research.

Institutional Priorities

To maximize the chances that research will be viewed as valuable by the institution, it is important that projects deal with relevant clinical problems or issues. For projects to survive the political and economic realities of hospital organizations in the next century, close alignment to patient outcomes and institutional priorities is essential. Because administrators make difficult choices on the use of scarce resources, it is much easier to justify a project with potential cost savings to the institution or improved patient outcomes than one with no apparent benefit.

Cost Issues

Closely linked to institutional priorities are cost issues. The ability of a study to demonstrate a cost savings or an increase in quality for the same cost is invariably more valuable to both the patient and the institution than one that does not address these issues. Determining the impact of cost issues prior to selecting a topic or doing a study can be tricky! Specific variables that should be taken into consideration at this point in the process are discussed in more detail in the next section, "Tools to Help Set Research Priorities."

Availability of Measurement Tools

Another criterion for prioritizing research questions is the availability of tools to measure the dependent variables. If no established instruments to measure the variables exist, such as the variable "self-efficacy," the topic is *not* ideal for clinicians with minimal research expertise. Tool development is a research project in and of itself and is usually outside the scope of the average researcher.

Funding Requirements

The need to obtain funds for equipment or other resources for a study will almost certainly create a roadblock to study completion. Neophyte researchers do not compete well for funding because of a lack of experience managing research funds. Details on study funding are discussed in Chapter 10, but for the purposes of prioritizing research questions, the first-time researcher should select a project that requires little or no outside funding to complete the study.

What is funding for and how do you know at this stage what funding you may need? Funding is generally used for preparation of materials, such as printing data-collection forms and inservicing materials, purchase of equipment necessary to conduct the study, personnel for data collection (time reimbursement or designated personnel), and statistical consultation and analysis. The ideal research topic is one that has minimal requirements in each of these areas, especially in terms of free-standing data collectors and the purchase of equipment.

Preparation of Materials

Materials necessary for a study range from very elaborate, in the case of glossy patient-education materials or interactive video production for example, to very simple, involving only a data-collection tool or case report form. The ideal research topic would involve minimal material preparation, for example by using an existing bedside computer screen for documentation and collection of data points rather than printing data-collection forms, using existing or donated educational materials, or using an available copy machine for making study forms.

Data Collection

The ideal research topic would not require a group member to be released from patient care responsibilities to be a data collector but would incorporate data collection into the usual nursing practice routines of the unit. For example, when examining the accuracy of a new temperature device, the procedure for data collection can be set up so it coincides with the usual times that temperatures are measured. Creating research studies that require free-standing data collectors is outside the fiscal realities of most institutions.

Statistical Analysis

Statistical consultation fees range from $70 to $150 dollars per hour. As with free-standing data collectors, an expense of this magnitude is typically outside of the budget for first-time researchers, most of whom have no budget! Options for avoiding statistical consultation and analysis charges are discussed in more detail in Chapters 8 and 10; however, when prioritizing research questions the ideal study is one that requires minimal professional consultation in its design.

For most unit-based research projects, the majority of these funding roadblocks can be circumvented by using creativity and careful project selection. At this stage, the most important point is to be aware of the possible funding roadblocks that exist—and don't bite off more than you can fiscally chew!

Research Priorities of Professional Groups

Professional groups and associations generally publish listings of research areas or topics that are of importance to the association or professional group (see

Table 2–8 and 2–9). While these priorities may be useful for generating ideas for research and reinforcing the importance of a particular topic or question, they should not take precedence over other ideas that pertain more directly to the patients and staff interests in your particular unit or institution.

Other Criteria

In addition to these criteria, there may be others that are specific to your institution that should also be included in the evaluation process. For example, if staff have had little prior experience as principal and associate investigators themselves, it may be prudent to avoid topics having potential political ramifications associated with them. Spending a little time at the beginning of the topic review process determining evaluation criteria that will maximize the selection of good projects will definitely pay off later.

▶ TOOLS TO HELP SET RESEARCH PRIORITIES

Although each of the criteria listed above is an important consideration, some will pertain more than others to your particular situation; therefore, each of the criteria should be considered individually when attempting to prioritize research topics. Using a tool to score or rank the topics you have identified can be invaluable. This section will review one such tool, a rating worksheet, which is a comprehensive tool used to rank or prioritize research topics. Cost and care paths, two additional criteria listed on the rating worksheet, are discussed in more detail later as these particular criteria have a number of underlying factors to consider and require a slightly more detailed explanation.

Rating Worksheet for Research Priorities

An easy way to prioritize clinical research questions is to develop an evaluation tool that group members can use as they objectively evaluate each question or topic. The tool discussed here is a simple rating worksheet that can be adapted to fit your particular setting or situation (Table 3–2). The criteria discussed above are used in the rating worksheet to evaluate each potential study question. Use of such a tool will help maximize success in the research process by differentiating clinically important and feasible research questions from those that may be more difficult to accomplish given current staff or researcher expertise and resources.

The ideal research topic would meet a variety of the criteria discussed above. As shown in Table 3–2, criteria used for evaluation of the idea or topic are listed down the left side and the topics or questions being evaluated are listed across the top of the chart. Each topic is evaluated and scored on how well it fulfills or meets each of the criteria. By using such a tool, the advantages and disadvantages of each research question are clarified. One might think of the

Table 3–2	Rating Worksheet for Prioritizing Research Questions

Scoring System: 0 = not present   + = present/yes   ++ = highly present/strong yes

Criteria	Topic	Topic	Topic	Topic
Area of staff interest				
Staff have clinical expertise				
Important to clinical practice, patient outcomes				
Large number of pts eligible				
No political landmines				
Potential financial impact				
No additional $ required				
Measurement tools available				
Data collection fits with unit routines				
Data collection could be finished quickly				
Miscellaneous				

rating worksheet as an organized version of a pros and cons list. To use the worksheet follow these steps:

- List each research question or topic in the left-hand column of the evaluation sheet.
- Add any criteria that may be individual to your institution to the list across the top of the sheet.
- Taking one topic at a time, begin the evaluation process by briefly summarizing for the group what the proposed research topic would address.
- Have group members vote on each of the criteria. It might be helpful for the criteria dealing with staff interest to record the exact number of staff interested, rather than coming up with an overall score for that item.
- If the group is unsure about cost issues, complete the worksheets in the next section and then come back to complete the rating worksheet.
- Once the topics have been scored individually, delete from the list those that scored poorly.
- Once you have narrowed the list down to four or fewer, proceed to the next step.
- To complete the ranking process, it may be necessary to gather more in-

formation on the topics by performing a limited literature review in each topic area. Identify one or two articles for the group to read related to each of the remaining topics and discuss each of these at the next meeting. The main objective during this step is to assess for feasibility and availability of tools necessary to do the study. Go for simple!

- A final selection of topic is done by having the group vote on a topic. This voting can be accomplished through a variety of techniques, such as nominal group process, consensus-building strategies, or merely asking each member to cast a vote and allow majority rule to decide the project.

An example of the rating worksheet used in an oncology unit is given in Table 3–3. Try plugging your research question or idea into the blank worksheet in Table 3–2. Before you begin, consider whether there are other criteria specific to your site that need to be added to the table.

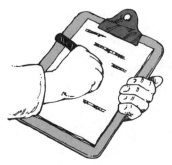

- If your list of topics includes some overlapping or similar topics, combine those ideas or topics.
- If other criteria specific to your topic or site are identified add these to the left hand column of table.
- To save meeting time, consider having group members fill in their own table and bring it in for a " group consensus " meeting.

Cost Evaluation Worksheet

Cost and cost implications are important criteria to consider when selecting a project for research. Accurate assessment of cost issues can have implications for your research project on a number of fronts, including assessing how your project lines up with institutional priorities, lobbying for administrative buy-in, identifying short- and long-term clinical impact, and plotting the generalizibility of the findings. Perhaps most important, cost issues and your ability to articulate them clearly and accurately may affect the degree to which your project is able to influence both the state of the science and other members of the health care team regarding implications for practice.

Cost issues can be complex and difficult to sort out, especially given the large number of often hidden variables related to costs and charges. At this stage in project selection only a broad, general idea of cost implications should be identified and discussed. Later, during the analysis of results, final cost implications of the project should be investigated and delineated in much greater detail to appropriately define and emphasize the impact of the study results.

Table 3–3	Example of a Rating Worksheet from an Oncology Unit

Scoring System:	0 = not present	+ = present/yes	++ = highly present/strong yes	
Criteria	**Use of PCA vs Nurse-controlled Analgesia**	**Single vs Double Dose Zofran**	**Zofran vs Traditional Antiemetic**	**Blood Discard**
Area of staff interest	++	++	++	+
Staff have clinical expertise	++	++	++	++
Important to clinical practice, patient outcomes	++	++	++	++
Large number of pts eligible	3–4/month	8/month (ovarian) 3/month (other)	Same as previous	Tons
No political landmines	0	?	?	?
Potential financial impact	?	+	+	0
No additional $ required	Possibly (pumps)	0	0	0
Measurement tools available	++	++	++	+/++
Data collection fits with unit routines		++	++	++
Data collection could be finished quickly	+	+/++	+/++	++
Miscellaneous		Anticipatory N/V	Addresses pt concern	

Two steps are important in evaluating the impact of cost as it relates to your research question. The first is to understand and use correct descriptive terms when referring to cost. The second is to understand the interaction of cost with clinical benefit or effectiveness. This step allows the researcher to assign weight to either side of the cost–benefit ratio "scale" to ascertain the overall impact of cost as it relates to patient outcome.

Step One: Key Terms

A number of key terms are commonly used when discussing cost issues. Understanding these terms will help you correctly articulate which types of cost issues you are addressing and why. It will also give you a broader understanding of many cost issues you may not be able to address at this time without help from a nurse administrator or an economic consultant (Table 3–4). After reading through the list of terms, complete Exercise 3–1 to test your skill with cost terminology.

Table 3–4	Cost Terms and Definitions	
Cost Terms	**Definition**	**Example**
Direct	Costs for a specific product or service	Medications, procedural devices such as catheters
Indirect	Costs that cannot be traced directly to a specific product or service	Cost of the salary for the administration of a unit or hospital
Fixed	Costs that do not change with changes in patient volume	Overhead such as building electricity and water
Semifixed	Costs that change with changes in patient volume, not in a continuous or gradual fashion but in intervals or steps over time	Incremental changes in staffing patterns and ratios
Variable	Costs that change with changes in patient volume	Sterile gloves
Semivariable	Costs that start as fixed, but that increase on acontinuous basis with increases in volume	Electricity when the lab is open more than regular hours (nights or weekends for example)
Marginal	The incremental cost of producing (or saving) one extra unit of service	Preventing (saving) a patient visit to radiology for enteral feeding tube placement
Incremental	Cost of producing (or saving) a unit of service for an entire population	Preventing (saving) an entire patient population from needing feeding tube placed (due to some new intervention)
Induced	Costs associated with subsequent use of resources in the future	Cost of readmissions for 1 year in class IV heart failure patients
Bottom-up	A method of measuring costs that enumerates cost for each individual resource necessary to provide a service or product	Listing each individual item, from gloves to room charges, for figuring cost related to suctioning
Top-down	A method of measuring costs that uses hospital billing or care summary descriptors, such as DRG assignment, to retrospectively assess cost	Using DRG reimbursement for pneumonia and hospital bill itemization to figure cost related to suctioning (for pneumonia population)

Once you have a basic understanding of terms used to discuss and define costs, the next hurdle is being able to use the terms accurately and effectively. For example, a clinical question related to a more rapid method for nitroglycerin titration may save costs by cutting nursing hours per patient day. To measure these cost issues accurately you must first know (1) how nursing hours per patient day are calculated at your institution and (2) how the time saved from tapering the IV nitroglycerin will be used by the nurses. While time saved for any given task or procedure does theoretically save money, the time savings will probably not result in a net decrease in nursing hours per patient day since alternative activities will be carried out in lieu of tapering the medication. Be-

► Exercise 3–1

Cost terms: Matching

Match the letter of the example with the correct term.

Cost Terms	Match All Examples That Fit
1. Direct	
2. Indirect	
3. Fixed	
4. Semifixed	
5. Variable	
6. Semivariable	
7. Marginal	
8. Incremental	
9. Induced	

Examples
a. One full-time RN
b. A ventilator
c. One hospital day in ICU (room rate)
d. Salary of nurse manager or administrator
e. One pair sterile gloves
f. Per diem or prn nursing staff
g. Dose of aspirin
h. Normal saline flushes (for saline locks)
i. Housekeeping services
j. An angioplasty catheter
k. A bedpan
l. Meal tray
m. Fluoroscopy machine
n. The catheterization lab (building/space)
o. An appendectomy procedure
p. Patient readmissions (or lack thereof)
Add examples from your own question:

cause other activities will consume the time saved, an actual full-time employee (FTE) will probably not be cut. Therefore actual costs for the unit will remain the same regarding nursing hours per patient day because this is a direct, fixed cost, rather than a direct, variable cost.

Understanding the specific terms of direct, indirect, fixed, and variable costs will enable you to correctly articulate the cost variables you hope to address with your particular question. Using your clinical question, complete Exercise 3–2. Use this exercise to begin to list and investigate cost issues that you may want to consider for your study. Remember the following key points when completing Exercise 3–2:

- Usually only direct, variable costs will be able to be influenced by your study.

- Indirect costs should be kept in mind as influential, but don't sweat over identifying specific numbers for these costs.

- Often patient care items and services are costed and charge differently based on geographic region and vendor contract negotiation. Keep this in mind when generalizing your findings.

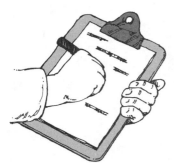

How can indirect costs be identified?
- Indirect costs, both fixed ones and variable ones, can be identified by checking with an administrator or your hospital accounting department.
- Sometimes it is impractical to track down the specific indirect costs, especially during the project prioritization / identification phase. Don't waste time doing this now! Keep in mind that indirect costs exist and will probably not change based on your study, unless your intervention would close an entire building or wing, or negate the need for housekeeping, heat, electricity, water, et cetera!

Step Two: Determining Cost and Clinical Benefit

Most nurses (or any health care researcher for that matter) would like to do a study and be able to report findings related to cost that sound like these:

- The (X intervention) was found to be safer and more cost effective than (Y standard therapy); or

- The (X intervention) was equally effective for (purpose of intervention) and significantly more cost effective than (Y standard or comparison intervention).

Statements such as these are repeatedly found in the literature; however, they are frequently in error. The reason is that "cost-effectiveness" is a form of analysis known as economic efficiency analysis. This type of analysis is a theory-

► **Exercise 3–2**

Cost Evaluation Worksheet

Direct Costs (All fixed and variable)	Costs For My Clinical Question (Or charges if unable to identify cost)
Health Professional Time	
Nursing time—patient care activities	
Nursing time—research team activities	
Physician time	
Pharmacist time	
Respiratory therapist time	
Physical/Occupational therapy time	
Other professional/technical time:	
1.	
Equipment and Materials Costs	
Equipment cost (large equipment may be financed over time and be indirect)	
Equipment maintenance cost	
Disposable materials consumed:	
1.	
2.	
3.	
Cost of funded or donated materials:	
1.	
Educational Costs	
Instructor/personnel time	
Educational materials:	
1. Printing	
2. Audiovisuals	
3. Computer equip/disks	
4.	
Other Direct Costs Expected in Your Study	
Labs	
Patient room rate	
Medications	
Indirect Costs (All fixed and variable)	
Building/equipment capital investment	
Building/equipment depreciation	
Overhead	

based analysis, done predominantly by economists for the purpose of making decisions regarding allocation of resources across major sectors of the population, including defense and education spending as well as health care. Economic efficiency attempts to identify what intervention or therapy has the most benefit to society for the least cost. There are three types of economic efficiency analysis: cost-effectiveness, cost-utility, and cost–benefit. Each type uses the same general formula $[Cost_{(new)} - Cost_{(standard)}]$ divided by $[Effectiveness_{(new)} - Effectiveness_{(standard)}]$ and the same general calculation for determining cost differences (cost of new intervention – cost of usual or standard intervention). The three types differ in the way that "effectiveness" is determined.

Determining effectiveness of an intervention requires more than simply observing and measuring whether or not the intervention "works." Determining effectiveness accurately requires an evaluation and measurement of health benefit in terms of quality of life and/or "life-years." For example, suctioning without using normal saline may be less costly in terms of resources used, and it may also "work" in terms of clearing the airway. It may work "better" than suctioning with saline in that it results in less deoxygenation and desaturation in the perisuctioning period. However, to claim that the intervention (suctioning without saline) is more cost-effective or has a better cost–benefit ratio you would have to translate the benefit (less deoxygenation and desaturation) into life-years.

Measurement of cost-effectiveness, utility, or benefit is usually beyond the scope of novice or even seasoned researchers owing to the difficulty of accurately measuring or projecting life-years and quality of life in terms of life-years saved.

Though "cost-effectiveness" is often what small, individual researchers would like to claim, we are usually inaccurate in making such a claim because we are limited in our ability to measure, project, and generalize the construct of life-years.

How then should you most accurately report cost issues related to your study? As a legitimate second best to true cost-effectiveness or cost–benefit analysis, simply report your findings related to effectiveness, or exactly how the intervention worked, and then report your findings related to cost. Cost can be accurately reported by reporting all resources required to provide the intervention compared to all resources required to provide the standard intervention $[Cost_{(new)} - Cost_{(standard)}]$.

Using the suctioning example, report that the intervention successfully cleared the airway while producing lower levels of deoxygenation and desaturation in the perisuctioning period. Then report the cost of suctioning without saline minus the cost of suctioning with saline $[Cost_{(new)} - Cost_{(standard)}]$. You have now accurately reported your results without extrapolating that suctioning without normal saline was or is more cost-effective.

One other important cost point to consider when choosing your research project or topic is the factors that might affect or "drive" cost, either up or down, in your particular patient scenario. These factors are called cost drivers. Because cost drivers are important variables to monitor or measure in the

Table 3–5	Factors That Drive Cost

Categories of Medical Cost Drivers

Patient-related factors
Age
Sex
Disease severity
Comorbidities

Treatment-related factors
Aggressive versus conservative management
Complications

Provider-related factors
Quality of care
Efficiency of care
Preferred management styles

Geographic and economic factors
Labor costs
Supply costs

Reprinted with permission from Mark, D. Medical economics in cardiovascular medicine. In: Topol, E.J. ed. Textbook of Cardiovascular Medicine. Philadelphia: Lippincott–Raven, 1998, page 1039.

study, they should be given serious thought in the project selection and development phase. Table 3–5 lists common cost drivers for medical studies. Consider the role these variables may play in your patient population or clinical question. Are there others that you feel should be added to the list for your question? Using Exercise 3–3, practice accurately stating the cost concepts measured or evaluated in various clinical situations and what factors may be cost drivers for those clinical questions.

At this stage you are simply trying to select a project; therefore, a gross cost assessment may be helpful for visualizing the outcomes you hope to demonstrate with any given project. One way to "eyeball" a gross assessment of cost as it relates to the clinical benefit of your project is by using a 2 × 2 grid and plotting gross cost (more expensive or less expensive) on the *y* axis and projected clinical effectiveness (more effective or less effective) on the *x* axis. Inexpensive and effective interventions would be most desirable; expensive and ineffective interventions would be least desirable (Fig. 3–2). Using this grid allows you to quickly evaluate a project in terms of overall cost, taking into account the variable of effectiveness. In Fig. 3–3 (page 56) a number of common interventions are listed in each quadrant of the tool. The examples in the upper left-hand box are interventions that are very effective and cost very little. The examples in the lower right corner are interventions that have not been shown to be particularly effective and at the same time are very expensive.

Because you don't know the "answer" to your clinical question at this point, you won't know exactly how expensive or effective your variables are. Try to

▶ **Exercise 3–3**

Cost Application to Clinical Situations

Identify the measurable costs and cost drivers associated with each of the following clinical questions.

Clinical Question	Measurable Costs	Associated Cost Drivers
1. Is continuous cardiac output useful information and less costly than standard intermittent cardiac output measurement?		
2. Is in-line continuous blood sampling accurate and less costly than standard blood sampling techniques?		
3. Can in-line suctioning catheters be safely used for greater than 24 hours before changing the circuit?		
4. Chest P.T. versus triflow versus cough and deep breath: is there a difference in atelectasis?		
5. Is bolus feeding or continuous feeding better for nutritional absorption and gastric tolerance?		
6. Should antiemetic medications be given prophylactically or episodically in oncology patients receiving chemotherapy?		
7. *Your questions:*		
8.		
9.		

predict or project what you *think* the cost and effectiveness will be. For example if you wanted to test or compare two types of telemetry patches, you would be able to find out the cost differences, but you would have to project their effectiveness. Another example might be use of pneumatic stockings for prevention of thromboembolism. *Not* using the stockings will obviously cost less; however, you could project that this strategy would be less effective because of

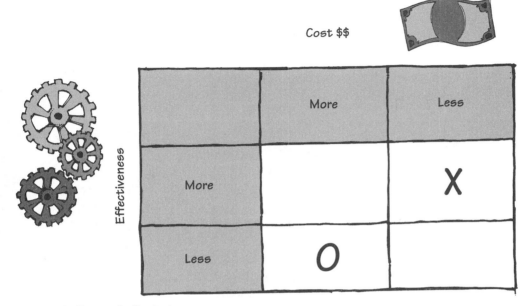

Figure 3–2. Cost-evaluation tool.

an increase in complications incurred. By plotting this example on the grid you might decide that the cost of the stockings is much cheaper than the "cost" of the sequelae from thromboembolism. Using your research question, plot your projected cost and clinical effectiveness in the grid in Fig. 3–2.

If you haven't already done so, complete Exercise 3–3 to begin an assessment of the variables affecting cost as they relate to your research question. Some blanks in the exercise may have to be completed later when the results of your study are available. Striking a balance that optimizes quality and cost often poses a challenge for team members when identifying research priorities. Investigation into and clarification of cost issues can help the team to identify research priorities on the unit.

Care Paths

As discussed in Chapter 1, care paths serve to establish a standard or guideline for a particular patient population or procedure. Care paths should describe efficient and effective management practices, with periodic measurements for determining progress toward desired outcomes. Most patients for whom a path has been developed are considered high volume or high cost/risk. As such, if a particular variance is observed to occur repeatedly in patients on a given path, then that issue or topic will rank as high priority for all of the following reasons:

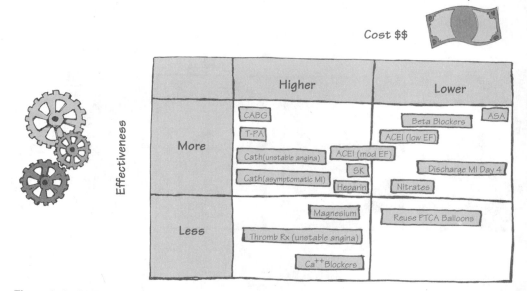

Figure 3–3. Assessment of several cost-evaluation interventions.

- High institutional priority
- Opportunity to improve efficiency of care
- Patients readily available (high-volume groups)
- Staff experienced in the care of these patients
- Necessary data collection (or tools) already a part of daily documentation

As you can see, the criteria don't change from those identified in Table 3–1. A different tool, the care path, is simply used for help in prioritizing. Because the variance has been observed to occur repeatedly, this is probably a good topic to study, and the study would probably have a very valuable effect on patient care.

If your unit or institution is measuring a variable for a given patient population on a care path and *no* variance has ever been noted, then you may want to consider changing the threshold (if you are not happy with the current threshold) or discontinuing measurement of that particular variable (if you are happy with the current threshold). For example, if the length of stay threshold for CABG patients is 5 days, and all patients always meet this target, then consider shortening the threshold to 4 days, or if you are happy with 5 days as the optimal length of stay for patients, then discontinue measurement of the variable because it has been consistently achieved over an acceptable period of time. If your research question involves patients on a care path, complete Exercise 3–4 to help assess priority. (See Chapter 2 for more examples using care paths.)

▶ **Exercise 3–4**

Considering the Priority of a Study Involving Patients on a Care Path

1. My clinical question is _____
   _____

2. The care path patient population involved is _____

3. The path variable being tested is _____

4. The defined path standard for this variable is _____
   (At least 80% of patients should be meeting this defined goal.)

5. The current variance for this variable or issue is :

   a. ___% of patients **meet** the defined threshold each quarter.

   OR b. ___% of patients are **above** the defined threshold each quarter.

   OR c. ___% of patients are **below** the defined threshold each quarter.

Example: Can patients undergoing diagnostic cardiac catheterization ambulate earlier than 6 hours following sheath removal and be discharged the same day?

2. Care path involved is Cardiac Catheterization.

3. Variable being tested is time to ambulation following sheath removal.

4. Defined path standard is 80% of patients should be ambulating at 6 hours.

5. Current variance at our institution for this variable is 98% of patients ambulate at 6 hours without complication.

Researchable question: All patients are meeting the standard. Can the standard be tightened without increasing rates of complication (bleeding)?

▶ **REFERENCES**

Campbell G, Chulay M. Establishing a clinical nursing research program. In: Spicer J, Robinson MA, eds. Environmental Management in Critical Care Nursing. Baltimore: Williams & Wilkins, 1990, pages 52–60.

Cronin S, Owsley V. Identifying nursing research priorities in an acute care hospital. Journal of Nursing Administration 1993;23(11):58–62.

Estabrook C, Hodkins M. Clinical significance: Play it again, Sam . . . Clinical Nursing Research 1996;5(4):371–375.

Fitch M. Creating a research agenda with relevance to cancer nursing practice. Cancer Nursing 1996;19(5):335–342.

Mark D. Medical economics in cardiovascular medicine. In: Topol E, ed. Textbook of Cardiovascular Medicine. Philadelphia: Lippincott–Raven, 1998, pages 1033–1061.

Sheree A. P. Designing Critical Pathways. American Association of Critical Care Nurses, 1997.

White S, Bartrug B, Bride W. Supporting nursing interventions in a cost-conscious environment. Critical Care Nursing Clinics of North America 1995;7(2):399–406.

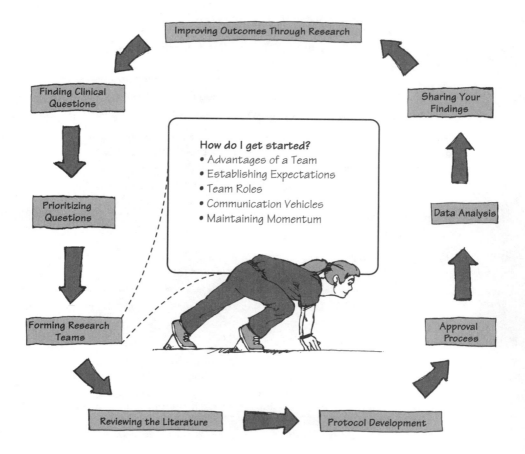

Improving Outcomes Through Research

Finding Clinical
Questions

Prioritizing
Questions

Forming Research
Teams

Reviewing the Literature

Protocol Development

Approval
Process

Data Analysis

Sharing Your
Findings

How do I get started?
- Advantages of a Team
- Establishing Expectations
- Team Roles
- Communication Vehicles
- Maintaining Momentum

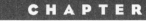
Research Teams: Getting Started and Keeping Momentum

Often, research and the "how to's" of conducting research are taught from the perspective of one individual as the primary researcher. Even if others are involved in the project, the primary researcher really "owns" the project, usually because it was this individual's idea. The study, in this situation, is designed and carried out by the primary researcher or individuals hired by the primary researcher. Though this model works well in academic situations, the "lone ranger" approach is very difficult for a clinician in a service setting. The benefits of an interdependent team approach are as important in clinical research as they are to patient care in general. This chapter discusses why, and then highlights ways to develop and make the most of a team.

▶ THE ADVANTAGE OF A TEAM APPROACH

Beginning the research process is an exciting and busy time! It is also the point at which a well-laid plan and a cohesive working team will be invaluable. So what does a "cohesive working team" look like? In the course of this chapter we outline the necessary steps for building a research team and give some insight into common misconceptions of working with a team or workgroup.

The purpose of a team approach to clinical research is to allow for a variety of conceptual and creative contributions to enhance the overall product, your research project. The value of contributions from many people is inestimable and will become increasingly clear as you move toward completion of the project. The advantages of a team, in addition to providing more brain power, include more people to spread the word about the project, improved morale during the slow phases of the project, and more people among whom to divide the work. While a team can also be more work when it comes to keeping communication open and minimizing conflict, the advantages far outweigh the extra work sometimes required.

▶ WHO SHOULD BE ON A TEAM?

Once a research question has been identified, it's time to define the working group of nurses and other team members who will carry the project through to completion. Who will be involved with the project and to what extent will those individuals be involved? To begin your project, assemble the group of people who are interested and willing (for whatever reason!) to work on the project. For our purposes we will call this group the Research Team; however, you may call them anything you like, as long as everyone has a common understanding of the group and its purpose. When gathering team members, keep the following points in mind:

1. Identify individuals interested in the project. Both volunteers and solicited participants are valuable to the project.
2. Don't allow the team to be so large that it becomes unproductive (usually more than eight to ten people), or so small that the work can't get done (about one to three people). These numbers are only a guide and may differ in your group. If you have too few people, try to recruit more. If you have a large group, ask people to share roles. Roles that commonly require lots of time, commitment, and manpower are data collectors, data monitors, and people to enter data.
3. Multidisciplinary teams can be helpful. Again, remember that different backgrounds and perspectives are complementary and advantageous to the team, as long as everyone is on the same wavelength regarding the overall plan and research objectives.
4. Some people are good at some things; other people are good at other things. Proper positioning of team players optimizes efficient progress and outcomes. We will address this point more in the next section.

Anyone interested and willing to contribute some extra time to a project should be a viable candidate for inclusion in the research team. Examples include:

- Staff nurses. Any staff nurse who works with the patient population being studied should feel comfortable participating on the research team. As the care provider, the nurse has a significant contribution to make to the effort regardless of academic credentials or level of expertise.
- Consultants. Consultants may be advanced practice nurses, physicians, statisticians, administrators or managers, or other members of the health care

team (see below). Regardless of title, consultants can be invaluable as reviewers for your protocol, as clinical experts to contribute expertise to an area, as ad hoc group members to provide supporting data for the development of your argument, and/or to guide or mentor the team in the research process.

- Other health care team members. Other members of the health care team should also be included on the research team when their expertise is well matched to the topic under study. Participation of these individuals will vary based on the topic you choose for your protocol. For example, a tube feeding study should include a dietician, or a study on ambulation after hip replacement should include a physical therapist if possible. Other disciplines with expertise relevant to nursing research topics include pharmacists, physicians, and respiratory therapists.

▶ ESTABLISHING EXPECTATIONS OF THE TEAM

Before getting started it is helpful to establish a few expectations and discuss any sensitive issues, especially publication and authorship, up front. Even if the thought of making presentations or submitting a final manuscript seems far, far away, discussing these issues in the beginning will prevent one source of conflict down the road and prevent every member of the working group from considering him- or herself to be first author. Any number of expectations can be discussed up front, depending on the individual setting. The three "Ps," participation, publication, and presentation, are generally the most sensitive and are usually a good place to start.

- Participation. Participation of all members throughout the process is key to getting the job done! Establishing this ground rule up front gives everyone in the group an opportunity to hear the expectation and hold one another accountable for role responsibilities throughout the research process.

- Publication. The entire team can be listed on a publication. In general, there are two approaches to listing authors for the publication: listing each person as an author or giving the research study group a name that becomes the "author." When listing individual names for authorship, typically the team leader or the individual with the original idea is first author and primary writer on the manuscript. Following first author, those contributing most to the body of work and content of the manuscript should be listed in descending order. The "anchor" or last author is typically the faculty sponsor or mentor, assuming this individual has made significant contributions throughout the process of the project. When using the group name approach as the author of the publication, such as the Endotracheal Suctioning Research Group, an asterisk is placed at the end of the group name and a footnote appears that lists each member of the group in alphabetical order. This approach is especially useful when there is no one person who "owns" the research idea or when the workload has been equally shared by all group members.

- Presentation. Presentations are a good opportunity to "spread the wealth," giving a number of team members a chance at center stage. Usually the project can be presented in more than one forum or professional meeting and, optimally, the team can rotate the speaking role to various members in the group so that a number of people have a chance to be recognized.

Roles and responsibilities of each team member should also be discussed in the early stages of the group formation. Some suggestions for defining roles and optimizing the contribution of individuals in those roles are discussed below.

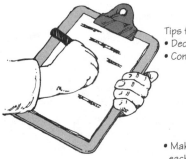

Tips for Discussing the " Three P's "
- Decide prior to the meeting who will raise the the issue
- Consider one of the following non-threatening approaches
  - have a flip chart with the " three P's " outlined
  - pass the hat (members randomly read and discuss each " P ")
  - initiate a group discussion of things to consider with each " P "
  - have a third party come to discuss the " P's "
- Make sure the group can come to agreement regarding each " P "

▶ TEAM ROLES: MATCHING PEOPLE AND ROLES FOR OPTIMAL PRODUCTIVITY

Delineate role responsibilities from the start!! This will eliminate confusion along the way and will allow the team members to hold one another accountable for getting things done in a timely and appropriate manner. Another advantage of delineating role responsibilities up front is that it will become clear whether or not you have enough people-resources to get the job done. If your team of three people are all primarily interested in one role, then you know you have work to do to recruit new members with different strengths.

Roles and Responsibilities

Roles and responsibilities of a research team will vary slightly depending on the nature of the study and the size of your group. In general however, the following roles are necessary for the group to get the job done and function smoothly:

- Team leader or project director
- Data collector(s)
- Mentor or facilitator

A number of other "roles" are important and required; however, on small teams these roles and responsibilities can be assumed by all members of the group. These roles include the "forms supervisor," the public relations role, and several additional roles that require input from everybody on the team.

Team Leader or Project Director

The team leader is generally the principal investigator and/or the one who "started the engine" so to speak in getting the idea and the project off the ground. Responsibilities of the team leader typically include:

- Establishing the meeting schedule and timeline, in conjunction with the group
- Running the meetings
- Delegation of work assignments
- Oversight of the research process

Data Collector(s)

The data collector role typically involves *everyone* on the team! Other staff who are not necessarily a part of your research team may also be data collectors. Training and requirements for data collectors should be discussed and developed by the entire team. Responsibilities include:

- Patient consent, screening, and enrollment
- Data collection
- Monitoring of collected data to ensure completeness and reliability

Mentor or Facilitator

Since many research teams lack research expertise, having an individual who can mentor the team throughout the process can be invaluable. The mentor is generally someone who has participated in the research process before. If no such person is available, a nurse manager, advance practice nurse, administrator, or physician colleague can be helpful. Responsibilities include:

- Providing research expertise as needed
- Oversight of the protocol development process, especially data collection, analysis, and presentation
- Assisting investigators to avoid or anticipate potential roadblocks related to the conduct of research
- "Cheerleading" or helping maintain momentum throughout the process

"Forms Supervisor"

A number of activities are required related to forms. Development of the data collection form or case report form is one major activity that generally requires input from the entire team and possibly a statistical consultant. A point person for forms-related issues is a great asset to the team. Responsibilities include:

- Creation of forms for consent and data collection
- Assembly of enrollment packets
- Oversight of supply/data form availability throughout the study

The individual responsible for forms can make his or her job much easier by recruiting staff from each shift to pitch in with the last two of these responsibilities.

Public Relations Role

Another role that the team may benefit from, if you have a large enough group, is the public relations role. If you have a relatively small working group, the whole group will have to pitch in to get this done. This PR person is responsible for the following:

- Publicizing the project from start to finish
- Ensuring that key formal and informal unit leaders are kept informed about the project
- Facilitating the various mechanisms for communication, as discussed later

Roles That Need Everybody

The following are key roles that require the participation of the entire team:

- Writing and editing the protocol
- Training data collectors
- Participation in presentation of study results

Matching People Types and Role Responsibilities

The best thing about a team is that everyone is different. In most groups, even small groups of three or four, individual strengths vary considerably. Typically this is evident from the beginning, especially in groups of adults who tend to be more aware of their various work habits, preferences, and idiosyncracies. "Personalities" with regard to work tend to fit into the following general categories

- Creative/conceptual
- Objective/analytical
- Detail oriented

- Goal oriented
- "Starters"
- "Finishers"

Differences in work habits can be a source of conflict; however, they can also be used to the advantage of the team and the overall project if individuals' strengths are recognized from the start. *MATCH THE PERSON WITH THE NEED!* Personality trait or strength should complement the research role or responsibility chosen by that individual.

As will become evident, certain personality types tend to be more effective at accomplishing certain responsibilities. Often "people types" match with "responsibility types" as in Fig. 4–1.

Things to remember:

- *EVERYBODY* is important to the process!
- This is a guideline only, certainly not a rule.
- Generally people are more effective when doing things they are enthusiastic about.

Complete Exercise 4–1 using members of your own team. What are your strengths and weaknesses in terms of available talent?

▶ ADDING PEOPLE TO THE TEAM

In the course of most research projects, team members will need to leave and new members may become available and interested in joining. Regardless of the circumstances for either of these events, it is important to remember that significant contributions of members should not go unrecognized, even if a team member has moved on or moved away when the project is complete. These contributors should still be recognized in presentations or publications according to their commitment and contribution to the overall project. Likewise, new members, be they new staff members or additional consultants invited "midstream," should be updated on the overall project, its progress, and their specific responsibilities, and then readily incorporated into the team.

▶ DEALING WITH CONFLICT

Sometimes even the most synchronous working groups encounter conflict. Conflict in small groups can, of course, be devastating because each member is vital to the progress of the project. Typically when group members don't see eye to eye on one issue or another, there has been a breakdown in either the understanding of the common goal or the communication necessary to accomplish that goal. Conflict in a group, regardless of the source and scope, should

" People Type "	Characteristics	Examples in the Workplace	Possibilities for Responsibilities
Creative / Conceptual	Risk-taker Outgoing Open Imaginative / inventive Self-reliant Independent thinker	Chaos at the bedside doesn't influence this individual's ability to work effectively.	Topics generator Team leader role Public relations role
Objective / Analytical	Realistic Perceptive Mentally active " thinker " Discriminating Concrete	Works best in a neat, orderly environment. Distracted by clutter.	Study design role Form development Data collector
Detail Oriented	Accurate Particular Exacting Scrupulous Concrete Factual	Documentation is always impeccable, even if this requires staying late.	Excellent data collectors Form development Editor Data monitor
Goal Oriented	Active / busy Pragmatic Assertive Strong willed	Patient care is always priority, documenting the specifics of that care, such as frequent vitals or hourly output, takes a back seat.	Team leader Facilitator
" Starter "	Tenacious Self-starter Independent thinker Leader Courageous	Always ready to start a new project, not always tuned in for the " long haul ".	Study developer / design Public relations role
" Finisher "	Detail oriented (see above) Precise Systematic Concrete Orderly	Committed to achieving closure or completion of a project. Does whatever it takes to complete tasks for the shift.	Data collector Writing / publications Director Editor Data monitor

Figure 4–1. Matching people types with responsibility types.

always be managed as quickly and directly as possible, minimizing the escalation time for frustrations and tempers. Should you experience conflict within your team, consider the following as sources of that conflict and problem solve from there:

- Primary goal is unclear. This is evident when group members are not "singing off the same page" so to speak. Group members may have "hidden agendas" or may frequently suggest dramatic changes in direction for

▶ **Exercise 4-1**

Matching People Types with Roles and Responsibilities

" People Type "	Our Representative Team Member(s) Is:	This Team Member's Role on Our Team Is:
Creative / Conceptual		
Objective / Analytical		
Detail Oriented		
Goal Oriented		
" Starter "		
" Finisher "		
Other:		

the group, such as changing the research question, not doing a research project, or pursuing an administrative decision rather than an investigation into the problem. In a team meeting, clarify the goal and establish buy-in from every member of your team before going any further. It is OK for some group members to opt out if they cannot agree with the primary goal.

- Ongoing communication ineffective. This is evident when "the right hand doesn't know what the left hand is doing." Sometimes everyone is moving toward the goal, but not in concert. Things get overlooked or done twice. If this is the case, general systems of communication for the group need to be strengthened. Strategies for strong group communication will be discussed in the next section.

- An individual is problematic. A number of authors have addressed constructive ways to deal with problematic individuals (see reference list). In general, commitment of every team member to the goal is critical, and personal imperfections beyond this primary requisite should not detract from the progress of the group. However, if conflict is generated because of an individual, consider some of the strategies suggested by Brinkman and Kirschner for dealing with this source of conflict.

▶ COMMUNICATION VEHICLES

Communication is key to a successful research team and a successful project. When staff and others are aware of the project, who's involved, study progress, and accomplishments, they feel a part of the study even if they have not participated directly. A research project that is well communicated all along can be a source of pride for the entire unit.

Obviously, direct communication in person is an ideal approach to keeping everyone involved and updated. Other methods of communication should be considered for situations in which group members may not be able to attend meetings. The following suggestions may help:

- Circulate brief "minutes" from the meeting highlighting key points and actions taken. This vehicle is also helpful for the group to ensure a historical recording of decisions.
- Tape record the meeting for others to listen to later.
- Assign specific team members to summarize the meeting for absent members.
- E-mail a summary of meeting to members.
- Update a project/study notebook after each meeting with key points and actions taken.

Communication Within the Team

The most important communication that occurs within the team is related to planning and discharge of responsibilities among team members. For the most part, this refers to setting schedules and meetings and holding members accountable for being there. The following section will help you address the most important considerations in advance.

How Often and Where Does the Team Meet?

In general it is nice to meet at regular intervals and in the same location, so that all members of the group have the opportunity to plan ahead. The location of meetings should optimally take place on the unit, so that staff on duty can participate as patient care allows. The exception to this general rule of thumb is discussed at the end of this chapter—the times when celebration is in order! For these occasions a different location or special time, such as an evening out, may supersede the regular meeting.

What Does the Team Discuss When They Meet?

The following key points should be on the meeting agenda each time: The timeline for the project and where you stand on that timeline; patient enrollment update; overview of what needs to be done next and the responsible team member (Table 4–1). Any new issues or concerns should be added as they come up. The goals and objectives, as well as team progress, are also important to communicate and, as mentioned above, these points should be discussed as a regular part of each meeting. Key content for each meeting might look like this:

- The goals and objectives for the study. These are defined by your protocol once the study is designed. In the meantime, the goal is to get the study designed, as discussed in Chapter 6.
- Progress should be measured and reported from the timeline that the group will establish from the very first meeting (Table 4–2). Remember, this is flexible and should be readjusted according to the needs of the group.

As you begin to get your team organized, use Exercise 4–2 (page 72) to keep your project on track.

Communication Beyond the Team

The research team will not be available around the clock to communicate with other health care providers regarding the study. Myriad issues and questions often arise at unlikely times and the team must be prepared to answer these in an acceptable and timely manner so as not to delay enrollment into the study or compromise the care or progress of those patients already enrolled. A num-

Table 4–1	Key Points for a Meeting Agenda

Agenda	Discussion	Responsible Person
1. Timeline for the project and current standing:		
2. Patient enrollment update:		
3. Next steps: a. b. c. d. e.		
4. Other:		

ber of different ways to communicate study information could be used to inform those not directly involved with the project.

Staff Inservices

A verbal presentation of the study by someone directly involved should occur before the project starts, prior to enrollment of patients. This method affords an opportunity for questions and demonstrates commitment on the part of the research team to be responsive to the needs of the unit or patient care area. Inservices should cover the "nuts and bolts" of the study and specifically focus on why the study will be useful and what, if anything, other staff will be responsible for doing. Figure 4–2 (page 73) is an example of a "short sheet" or a summary of pertinent information about a particular study. This tool can be used

Table 4–2	Timeline for Monitoring the Plan and Progress of a Study											
	January				February				March			
Week :	1	2	3	4	1	2	3	4	1	2	3	4
**Team meetings												
Decide study question	✔	**										
Review literature		✔	**									
Research protocol development						✔						
Decide methods							✔					
Prepare forms									✔			
IRB submission												
Data collection											✔	✔
Statistical analysis												
Prepare publication												

to guide the speaker in covering important points during the inservice and can be given as a handout to participants as well.

> When to Use: Use at the kickoff of the study and again as needed. For example, if problems arise repeatedly with how data collection should be done.

Posters

One-page sheets of information or a large poster board displayed in the unit works well both for providing information and as a continual reminder of the project (Fig. 4–3, pages 74–75).

> When to Use: Post when the study begins, then update periodically with brief reports on the progress of patient enrollment.

Hospital Newsletters

Newsletters are an especially good mechanism when you have a creative writer on your team, or someone who is adept at word processing. Newsletters need not be complicated or long; however, they should be concise and catchy enough to draw the reader's attention (Fig. 4–4, page 76). Newsletters typically include study updates, interesting preliminary findings, or a staff question

▶ **Exercise 4-2**

Blank Timeline for Study Development and Completion

Month													
Week:	1	2	3	4	1	2	3	4	1	2	3	4
**Team meetings													
Decide study question													
Review literature													
Research protocol development													
Decide methods													
Prepare forms													
IRB submission													
Data collection													
Statistical analysis													
Prepare publication													

and answer section. Newsletter updates are also helpful for letting other nurses know you're still out there! There may be new nurses who are interested in joining your team or who are about to embark unknowingly on a similar study. Other means of communication similar to newsletters include unit bulletin boards and computer bulletin boards.

When to Use: Most are monthly or bimonthly and will typically print announcements of new studies as well as updates of ongoing research.

The Research Notebook

Having a notebook readily available for staff to use as a reference can be helpful for both investigators and noninvestigators who have questions related to the study. The notebook serves two primary purposes: (1) to provide structure and a sense of accomplishment for the progress of the team, and (2) to serve as a unit resource book for off shifts, visiting or new house staff, or float staff. A copy of the notebook should be kept on each area or unit participating in the study for easy access. Begun in the early stages of development of the research idea or question, and maintained throughout the project until completion of

Title: PAIN-CARE STUDY

Pain Assessment in Chest Tube Removal with EMLA cream

Principle Investigator / Contact Person: Pamela Boggs, RN
Page ID # 970-8267 for questions or help with patient enrollment!

Study Objective: To evaluate patient comfort during chest tube removal using a topical analgesic (EMLA cream) as compared to standard therapy.

Primary Endpoint: Perception of pain (as measured both subjectively and objectively)
Secondary Endpoints: Cost, time requirements for health care providers

STUDY DESIGN:

Design: Prospective, randomized trial

Inclusion Criteria	Exclusion Criteria
• CABG or CABG / Valve patients (32,33) • Awake and alert, able to give consent • < 3 chest tubes in place • Chest tube in place for < 8 hours • 18 years of age or older	• Chest tube in place > 48 hours • Sepsis • Off clinical pathway • Transplant patient • Known allergy to lidocaine or prilocaine

METHODOLOGY:

Patient Sample: 100 patients in Heart Center, units 3200 / 3300
Screening Process: Daily screening by care nurses and / or charge nurses on 3200 / 3300
Enrollment Process: Patients requiring chest tube removal and meeting inclusion criteria will be identified on a daily basis by the care nurse and / or charge nurse. Consent will be obtained and the nurse will pull the study packet from the research box, located by the HUC, on 3200. [NOTE: These envelopes are blinded and sequentially randomized, and should be used IN ORDER! Double check the randomization log in the research box to make sure you have the correct packet number]

Procedure: As outlined in detail in the study packet, once the patient is consented and randomized, the care nurse will negotiate a time for chest tube removal with the resident, treatment cream will be applied (see diagram in packet) to area surrounding chest tubes and covered with occlusive dressing at least one hour prior to CT removal time. Resident will be paged for CT removal. Pre-procedure, intra-procedure and post-procedure pain assessment tools will be completed by nurse and patient. All forms will be replaced in the study packet envelope and returned to the research box. One copy of consent form will be placed in the front of the patient chart for medical records.

Tools Used 1) One Modified McGill Pain Questionnaire, 2) BOD instrument, 3) demographic case report from
Follow Up Process: Data reviewed every 4 weeks by data safety and monitoring board (DSMB)

Study Timeline: Enrollment Start Date:

Figure 4–2. Example of a study "Short Sheet."

LIBRARY PROVIDES SUPPORT TO FAMILIES OF CARDIAC PATIENTS

Rebecca W. Johnson, RN, Gwynn B Sullivan, RN, MSN
Duke University Medical Center, Durham North Carolina

ABSTRACT

Supporting family members of patients is an integral part of health care. To increase this focus the Heart Center Patient Support Program performed a needs assessment to determine what could be done to improve the hospital experience for families of cardiac inpatients. Based on the results, a special room away from the main waiting areas was created and developed into an educational resource library. In the library, family members are able to read books, view video tapes and listen to audiocassettes with headphones, and use a computer with medline and web capabilities that will help them understand more about heart disease, risk factors, and treatment options. In addition, the library provides a comfortable room where families are able to have privacy for grieving, family conferences or counseling. The response of families for this alternative to traditional waiting areas has been overwhelmingly positive. Data will be presented which review utilization and outcomes of this supportive intervention for families of cardiac patients.

PROBLEMS

Distance frequently causes families of patients to be isolated from relatives and friends. Often family members spend their time at the hospital with limited support and few diversions other than television and the hospital cafeteria.

INTERVENTION

1) Needs assessment indicated desire for:
   - Additional space away from waiting room
   - Educational resources for varied literacy levels
   - Diversion from long hours in the waiting room

2) Develop plan:
   - Primary focus:
     - Library with educational resources
     - Material appropriate to literacy needs
     - Trained volunteers to provide assistance
   - Secondary focus:
     - 24 hour access by clinicians and chaplains for counseling and family conferences
     - A quiet place away from the main area

3) Design and implement plan:
   - Identify financial resources
   - Acquire physical space and design library
   - Compile library inventory:
     - Books on heart disease, stress management, humor and inspirational topics
     - Television, VCR, videos, headphones
     - Audiocassette players with headphones
     - Computer with medline and web capabilities
   - Procure furniture:
     - Comfortable seating, desk, utility cabinet
     - Bookshelves, magazine rack, bulletin board

4) Identify and train volunteers:
   - Train volunteers to identify resources to help families to cope with heart disease
   - Schedule volunteers to staff library

5) Advertise library:
   - Utilize flyers and the hospital newspaper
   - Place signs in lobby and / or waiting rooms

OUTCOMES

1) Provided a valuable service for families:
   - 100% of families surveyed felt the library and volunteers helped them cope with their family member's hospital stay.
   - 100% of families surveyed felt the library helped them understand their family member's heart problems.
   - 90% of families surveyed felt it was helpful to have additional space to wait while a family member was in the hospital.

2) 136.5 volunteer hours supplied during the first five months

3) 129 family members visited the library during the first five months

RECOMMENDATIONS

1) Perform a needs assessment of families

2) Assess available resources:
   - Space
   - Money
   - Coordinator
   - Personnel

3) Develop and implement an individualized plan

4) Periodical reevaluation of needs

Figure 4–3. Poster examples. A. Traditional poster

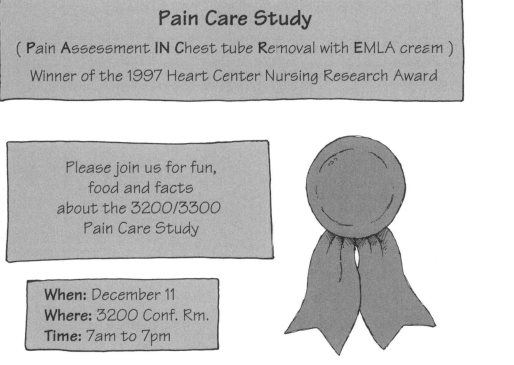

Figure 4–3. Poster Example, B. Fun Poster.

statistical analysis, the notebook contents easily translate into the initial manuscript draft. The notebook content should include the following:

- *Team members.* A list of contact numbers for team members and others who may have questions.
- *Research protocol.* A copy of the complete protocol should be available.
  - Purpose of the study: The protocol as well as the "short sheet" (Fig. 4–2) should have the purpose of the study clearly stated.
  - Review of the literature: A list of articles reviewed for the study should be available. Optimally an annotated bibliography, which is a brief summary of the articles or a copy of the abstract from key articles, should be included.
  - Methods: A written description of exactly what should occur for each step in data collection, from patient identification and consent through data collection and form completion, should be clearly spelled out.
- *Data collection forms.* A copy of the data collection form, and extra forms should be available in the notebook.

RESEARCH HAPPENINGS

A Critical Care / Heart, Lung & Blood Nursing Service Newsletter

Editors: Claiborne Davis (2J), Teresa Moroney (2J)   October, 1992
Managing Editor: Rick St. Germaine   Vol 1, No 2

Message From The Editors:

Many of our colleagues are extremely accomplished in the realm of nursing research. We have developed this newsletter in an effort to increase the communication about both nursing and Biomedical research within the CC/HL&B Nursing Service. Our primary focus is to communicate the results of these various studies as well as highlight the many accomplishments of our peers. We appreciate all the enthusiasm and effort the authors have contributed in making this newsletter a success.

Teresa & Claiborne

Research Committee News

7 East

The 7 East Research Committee has set the date for the second annual Nursing Research Forum. Mark your calendar for the afternoon of Thursday October 29th, 1:30PM to 3PM in the Medical Board Room. The program will focus on staff nurse involvement in nursing research on the Critical Care, Heart, Lung and Blood Nursing Service. Selected nurses will present research projects in various stages of development, as well as a summary of current nursing research on the service.

Newly Approved Protocols

Accuracy of coagulation studies obtained from heparinized, double-luman Hickman catheters.

PI: Donna Jo (DJ) Fleagle Mayo (Ambulatory Care)
AI: Eileen Diamond (Cancer Nursing)
     Annette Galossi (Cancer Nursing)
     Wendy Kramer (Clinical Pathology)

This study will determine what amount of blood withdrawal is required from a heparinized Hickman catheter in order to obtain accurate coagulation studies. Coag samples obtained from a Hickman catheter at various increments of blood withdrawal will be compared to simultaneously obtained venipuncture coag sample. Subjects for this study are outpatient cancer patients with Hickman catheter.

The effects of a preoperative orientation tour of the ICU environment on the stress level of family members.

PI: Terri Wakefield (BMT Unit)

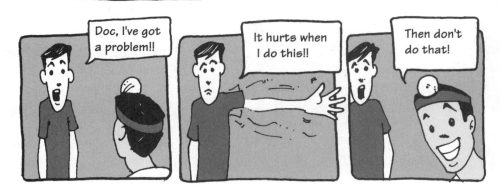

Figure 4–4. Example of a newsletter.

- Statistical analysis: A projected description of the selected analysis should be included, along with the rationale.

- IRB approval: A copy of the final IRB protocol with approval number should be included.

- *Data collection tips.* Include any suggestions that might simplify data collection for another staff member.

  - Key information that data collectors should know

  - Whom to contact with questions

  - Scripts for consent and survey administration if applicable

- *Minutes from meetings.* Include a section for minutes so that you can easily refer back to monitor progress and check accountability.

- *Timeline.* Keep a master sheet of the timeline and include any necessary modifications that would need to be communicated to others.

▶ MAINTAINING MOMENTUM

Another responsibility of the team is to maintain the momentum of the study. Though this activity may seem unimportant, it is critical that the team see progress during the long research process. Without recognition and celebration of accomplishment along the way, the team can prematurely lose steam and motivation. A number of strategies can and should be used to maintain momentum along the way, including seeking recognition from groups outside of the immediate study group and celebration of accomplishments within the group at various stages or turning points throughout the research process.

Maintaining Momentum through Recognition

A number of opportunities for recognition of studies in progress are available and, when taken advantage of, can serve to infuse energy and momentum into a study group. Consider whether any of the following might be helpful or applicable to your study:

- Giving presentations of the study and its progress, such as at a hospital conference or divisional meeting, or at a local chapter meeting of your professional nursing group.

- Submitting for small amounts of project money from hospital auxiliary groups, hospital grants, or seed money from professional groups.

- Acknowledging of team members through internal and external programs, such as hospital appreciation days, special nurse's week recognition for researchers, or local nursing newsletters put out by state ANA groups or specialty nursing organization groups.

Proposal Prepared	IRB Approved	Educational Inservices Begun	Enrollment! (Half-Way Point Reached)	Data Analysis	Publication!
Encourage the team with this sensational coffee cake for starters.	Cheese Board Party	Get your clinical area excited about your study with a great guacamole.	Semi-Chocolate Chips	Finally! Data collection is complete. Pass off to the statistician and serve "Data-Nut Bread"	Celebration Salsa
Coffee Cake for Starters	Pass the Review Board in style with a cheese board party!	Gung-Ho Guacamole	Keep momentum going with lots of sweet rewards!	Data-Nut Bread	Celebrate the chance to publish with a "hats off!" salsa party.

Data-Nut Bread

1 (8oz.) package chopped dates; 1/2 cup chopped pecans; 1 teaspoon baking soda; 1 cup hot water; 1/4 cup shortening; 2/3 cup sugar; 1 egg; 2 cups all purpose flour; 1/2 teaspoon salt; 1 teaspoon vanilla extract

(1) Stir dates, pecans, and soda into hot water; set aside to cool. (2) Cream shortening; gradually add sugar and beat well with mixer. (3) Add egg and beat well. Stir vanilla into this mix. (4) Combine flour and salt and gradually stir in date/pecan mixture and shortening mixture alternately until all ingredients are stirred together evenly. (5) Pour into 2 greased and floured loaf pans. Bake at 350 degrees F. for 1 hour. (6) Cool in pans for 10 minutes, then cool on wire rack.

Cinnamon Glazed Coffee Cake

3/4 cup firmly packed brown sugar; 1/2 cup chopped pecans; 1 teaspoon cinnamon; 1/2 cup butter; 1 cup sugar; 2 eggs; 2 cups all purpose flour; 1 teaspoon baking powder; 1 teaspoon baking soda; 1/2 teaspoon salt; 1 (8oz.)carton sour cream; 3/4 teaspoon almond extract; (extra 1/2 cup very finely chopped pecans)

Glaze

3/4 cup sifted powdered sugar; 1 tablespoon warm milk; 1/2 teaspoon almond extract

(1) Mix first three ingredients and set aside. (2) Cream butter and sugar; add eggs one at a time and beat well with mixer. (3) Combine all dry ingredients; add creamed mixture to dry ingredients alternately with sour cream until all ingredients are evenly stirred together. (4) Stir in almond extract. (5) Spoon 1/2 batter into greased and floured 10" bundt pan. Spoon cinnamon mixture on top and swirl partially through batter using the tip of a knife. Spoon rest of batter on top. Top with 1/2 cup very finely chopped pecans and bake at 350 degrees F. for 50 minutes. (6) Using mixer, beat all glaze ingredients together until smooth. Set aside. (7) Let cake cool in pan for 5 minutes; Invert onto plate and cool completely. (8) Drizzle with glaze.

Chocolate Chip Cookies

3/4 cup butter (softened); 1/4 cup shortening; 3/4 cup sugar; 3/4 cup firmly packed brown sugar; 2 eggs; 1 teaspoon vanilla; 2 3/4 cups all purpose flour; 1 teaspoon baking soda; 1/4 teaspoon salt; 1 (12 oz.) package semi-sweet chocolate chips

(1) Cream butter, shortening and sugars. (2) Beat eggs into creamed mixture one at a time; add in vanilla and mix well. (3) Combine dry ingredients and add gradually to creamed mixture. Mix well. (4) Stir in chips. (5) Drop by heaping teaspoons onto cookie sheet. (6) Bake at 375 degrees F. for 9–11 minutes. Cool on wire rack or paper towel.

Gung-Ho Guacamole!

Mix one 12 oz. jar salsa (mild, medium or hot) with one mashed avocado and juice of one lemon. Stir and serve with chips!

Celebration Salsa

2 (8oz.) cans diced peeled tomatoes (drained); 1/4 cup finely chopped onion; 12 sprigs chopped fresh cilantro or parsley; 2 cloves minced garlic; 2 fresh jalapeno pepper (finely chopped, or one 4 oz. can chopped); salt/pepper to taste

Mix all ingredients in food processor or blender and serve with chips.

Figure 4–5. Celebrating successes: **BIG** and small.

Maintaining Momentum through Celebration

Celebrations can come in a variety of shapes and sizes, and might include unit parties, a meeting at a restaurant, posters or banners placed in strategic spots in the unit, and/or announcements of study progress at staff or departmental meetings. Whatever the venue, the ability to formally acknowledge the team members' work and progress will provide that little extra energy needed to tackle the next phase of the project. Figure 4–5 addresses common intervals where celebration is important, and also suggests a few fast, fun foods to celebrate with!

▶ REFERENCES

Brinkman R, Kirschner R. Dealing With People You Can't Stand: How to Bring Out the Best in People at Their Worst. New York: McGraw-Hill, 1994.

Csokasy J. Building perioperative nursing research teams—Parts I & II. Association of Operating Room Nurses Journal 1997;65(2): 396–398, 400–401: 65(4):787–790.

International Committee of Medical Journal Editors. Uniform requirements for manuscripts submitted to biomedical journals. Journal of American Medical Association 1997;277(11):927–934.

Larson C, LeFasto F. Team Work: What Must Go Right, What Can Go Wrong. Newbury Park, CA: Sage, 1989.

Ludington-Hoe S, Swinth J. A successful long-distance research collaboration. Applied Nursing Research 1996;9(4):219–224.

Nelson B. 1001 Ways to Energize Employees. New York: Workman Publishing, 1998.

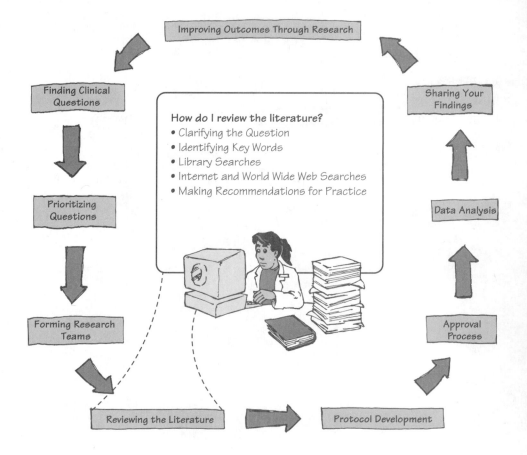

Improving Outcomes Through Research

Finding Clinical
Questions

Prioritizing
Questions

Forming Research
Teams

Reviewing the Literature

Protocol Development

Approval
Process

Data Analysis

Sharing Your
Findings

How _do_ I review the literature?
- Clarifying the Question
- Identifying Key Words
- Library Searches
- Internet and World Wide Web Searches
- Making Recommendations for Practice

Pragmatic Approaches to Reviewing the Literature

A good rule of thumb when reviewing the literature is to avoid doing more than is necessary to fulfill your purpose. "Your purpose" refers to what you will be using the information for, be it finding general information on a clinical subject, reviewing research to support a change in practice, developing a protocol, or preparing a final manuscript for publication. Regardless of the specific purpose, the review will be easier, less time consuming, and more focused if begun with a clear question in mind.

▶ CLARIFYING THE QUESTION

Narrowing a clinical problem to a single, specific question can be difficult. Examine your question and make it as specific and clear as possible by simply identifying any "fuzzy" areas in the question. For example, is normal saline helpful when instilled via endotracheal tube prior to suctioning? Answer the following questions before going to the literature: *Helpful* for what? Loosening secretions? Stimulating cough? Spreading bacteria down the bronchial tree? Or what? Clarifying "helpful" will force question specificity.

Consider another example: Are telemetry patches all the same? Answer the following questions before going to the literature: The *same* for what? Adhering in the shower? Transmitting a clear signal? Radiopacity? Arcing a current during a code? Clarifying "same" will answer what you really want to know, again, by forcing the exercise of question specificity. Using your question, complete Exercise 5–1.

▶ **Exercise 5–1**

"Question Specificity" Exercise

My question is: _____

_____

Potentially "fuzzy" areas of my question include: _____

_____

_____

What I *really* want to know is:

My secondary questions are:

_____

_____

You may wish to answer a number of questions about your topic at the same time. For example, using the normal saline example you may want to know about loosening secretions, stimulating cough, decreasing oxygenation, and implications for the spread of bacteria. You MAY look at a number of variables with a single research project; however, you must choose ONE variable as your "primary endpoint" or primary dependent variable. Pick the one that is most important to you. The other variables you are interested in become "secondary endpoints." Later when you calculate the sample size necessary to do your study, this calculation will need to be based on one single endpoint or dependent variable.

▶ LIBRARIES: WHERE DO I BEGIN?

A variety of resources are available to you in your library to access information on your research question. Some of these resources include published listings of journal articles, reference librarians, and computers designed to rapidly search the literature. Before beginning any review, key words from your research question must be identified to do a focused literature search.

Identifying Key Words

What are key words and how are the best key words identified? Key words are words, hopefully from within your question, that reflect the nature or bottom line of what you are trying to ask. Key words for your question were probably

► **Exercise 5–2**

Identifying Key Words

1. What is the frequency of bleeding in patients undergoing percutaneous translu-minal coronary angioplasty using a flexible sheath as compared to a standard sheath?

   Key words: bleeding, PTCA, percutaneous transluminal coronary angioplasty, flexible sheath, PTCA sheath

2. Does a structured communication plan improve families' needs to stay informed in the ICU setting?

   Key words: ICU families, family needs, communication needs, family satisfaction

3. Does organ donation increase in one community following a community educa-tion project?

   Key words: organ donation, donor organ(s), organ procurement, education

---

identified in Exercise 5–1. Key words are entered as the "topic" for your litera-ture review during the search. In each of the examples above, note how the key words are selected from within the question, and how synonyms for some words are also added to the list (Exercise 5–2). Using synonyms is helpful as one author may publish an article using the word "bypass" for "coronary artery bypass grafting" and another may use CABG. Complete Exercise 5–3 to iden-tify key words from your question.

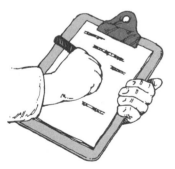

If you are having trouble identifying key words for your question:

• Find one article or research study that lists key words at the end of the abstract. Some journals require authors to list 4-5 key words at the end of an abstract or at the beginning of the article.

• Read several titles of articles that are related to your topic and choose words from those titles, or look up synonyms that are related to words in your own title.

Library Searches

Now that you have an idea of key words to use for doing the literature review, the next step is to begin! How, step by step, does one DO a literature review? The most efficient means of reviewing the literature will vary depending on the

► **Exercise 5–3**

Identifying Key Words

My question is: _____

_____

Key words derived from my question include: _____

_____

resources available to your unit or institution. Answer the following questions to identify your available resources:

1. Do you have a medical library at your institution? If not, identify the one closest to you.
2. Does the library have a copy of Medline and the Cummulative Index of Nursing and Allied Health (CINAHL) reference books? Because these are the most commonly used references for nursing studies, identify the closest source for these resources and continue with these questions.
3. Does the library have a Citation Index? This index is useful for locating all of the works done by a single author.
4. Is the library within walking distance from work? Specifically, could you go there for lunch or, alternatively, are there meeting rooms in close proximity you might reserve for staff to get to during a shift while being covered by a buddy?
5. If these resources aren't readily available, do you have a computer on your unit or in your institution that can access the library databases from a remote site? Having a computer with a modem will allow you to access library references regardless of your physical proximity to the library. Contact the library and ask about permission for computer access to their system. They should be able to assist you with connection from any location.

Once you have addressed each of these questions, you are ready to get started. Leave yourself at least an hour or two for your first trip to the library. Begin the review of the literature at the computer terminal or card catalogue in your library. Most libraries now have the catalogue on a computer. "Log on" or push "start" and follow the prompts for searching the Medline and CINAHL periodical literature by **topic.** Enter the key words that you identified in Exercise 5–3 and see how many references are identified (Fig. 5–1). You may need to narrow this list by combining key words, or "explode" the list by adding more general key words. Table 5–1 summarizes the issues you will need to address to get started once you get to the library.

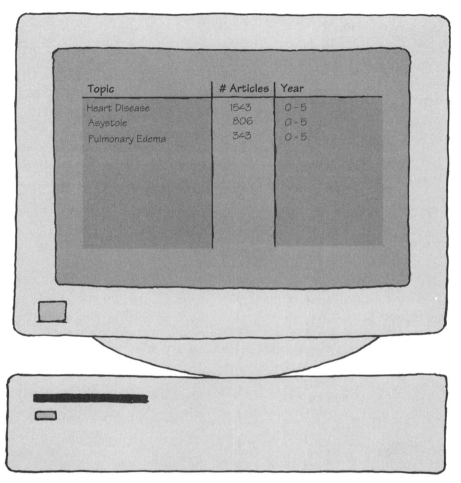

Topic	# Articles	Year
Heart Disease	1543	0 - 5
Asystole	806	0 - 5
Pulmonary Edema	343	0 - 5

Figure 5–1. Computer-generated literature review by topic.

Internet/Web Searches

A number of books are now available to facilitate searching for information on the World Wide Web (see reference list at end of chapter). In addition, there are a number of key sites on the Web that are frequent sources of information for nursing related topics (Table 5–2).

Searching by topic, using your key words. can also be done on the Web (Fig. 5–2). There are two main ways to do a literature search on the Web: (1) Enter the Web address for CINAHL and Medline and use these resources directly off of the Web, just as you would in the library. (2) Log onto the Internet and choose one of a number of search engines, such as Yahoo or Alta Vista, and enter your key word or "term." The second option will yield far more in-

Table 5–1	Cheat Sheet for the Library

The library closest to me is: _____

How to get there by computer: _____

Phone # / library hours are: _____

Cost / availability of faxed information from the library is: _____

The "log on" sequence for the computerized card catalogue is: _____

My key words I enter under "topic" are: _____

The time frame I am searching is (usually 0–5 years back): _____

Other important info: _____

_____

_____

_____

formation than simply listings from periodical journals. As you may be aware, topical searches on the Web will result in all sorts of information related to your word or topic, and the information may or may not be credible, published information. CINAHL and Medline can also be accessed through several sites on the World Wide Web (Table 5–2).

If using a search engine on the Web there are several ways to help narrow the search. The first is to choose "advanced search" rather than "simple"

Table 5–2	Helpful Sites on the World Wide Web

Another way to do a search using the Internet is to enter direct addresses. The following addresses may help you get information faster in some cases.

http://www.nlm.nih.gov (National Library of Medicine with access to **Medline** from the Web page)

http://www.healthfinder.gov (Department of Health and Human Services)

http://www.aacn.org (American Association of Critical Care Nurses with **CINAHL** available directly from home page)

http://www.nursingworld.org (American Nurses Association)

http://www.aha.org (American Heart Association with lots of patient education)

http://www.ama-assn.org (American Medical Association)

http://www.HELIX.com (Glaxo-Wellcome site with **Medline** access from the web page, as well as access to US Pharmacopeia Drug Information)

http://www.cinahl.com (Cinahl Information Systems)

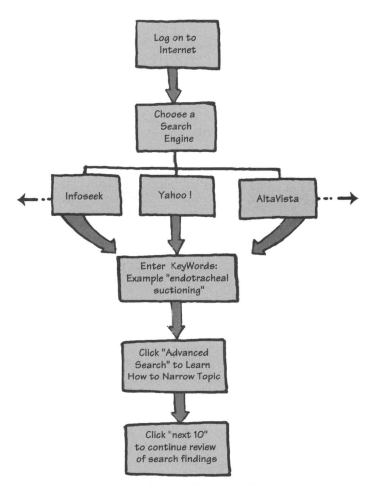

Figure 5–2. Internet algorithm for review of a topic.

search, and use word combinations. To use word combinations, enter your key words in brackets, using the word "and" between the brackets. For example [endotracheal]and[suctioning]. If you still find that the search results in non-applicable information, you may link "and not" to your list of words. For example [endotracheal]and[suctioning]and not[cancer]. The "and not" tool allows you to exclude topical information that does not apply to what you are interested in.

Another way to narrow your search on the Web is to use the Infoseek search engine. Infoseek may help you get closer to your key words because it allows an entire question to be asked, such as, should normal saline be used with endotracheal suctioning? The search engine identifies key words automatically and then gives you categories of information to choose from.

You may check the credibility of information found on the Web by looking for ".edu" in the site address, indicating that the information was posted from

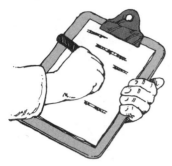

If your initial search yields way too much (more than several hundred articles):
• Further refine key words
• Combine key words
• Delete articles not specific to your patient population or age group
• Delete animal studies (select human only)
• Select " English only " articles (delete foreign languages)
If your initial search yields way too little (less than 25-30 articles):
• Re-evaluate key words and consider adding synonyms
• Conclude that not enough research has been done. Consider choosing another question or topic. Your question is valid, but may require more expertise than is advisable for a novice to embark on.

an educational institution. Other things to look for regarding credibility include information from a government site (.gov included in address), and information from a credible nursing or medical association such as the American Nurses Association (ANA), the American Medical Association (AMA), or the American Heart Association (AHA). Often sites offering health care information will include a bibliography or reference list as well.

When citing an online journal in a reference list, the citation should look like this: *Author, date.title.[on line]. Available at: http://www.address here* without a period at the end. Be sure not to put a period at the end because many readers may type that actual address, including the period, thereby creating an "unsearchable" Web address.

▶ WORKING WITH THE INITIAL REVIEW

Now that you have completed an initial review of the literature, you should have a large list of articles, including titles, authors, and the journal in which the article appears. You may also have printed the abstracts for a number of these articles. First, look for a recent review article that summarizes the critical studies on the topic. These articles will appear in your literature search as a "review article" or a "meta-analysis." The review of the literature articles is often listed in a separate section of Index Medicus/CINHAL or can be specifically requested in your computer search. This approach should allow you to quickly determine if previous research exists to answer your research question, or it will validate the need for more research.

A second helpful tool, particularly if a review article is not available, is a recently published chapter or book on your topic. Though a book chapter will give a good overall idea of the state of the science on a particular topic, it will not be as up to date as a current review article.

Once the initial review is complete, the next step is to read three to five of the articles most closely aligned with your topic. As you begin reading and critiquing the articles, you will want to organize and summarize each study for fu-

Table 5–3	Table for Organizing the Literature Review Articles			
Study Title	**Subjects**	**Study Comparisons**	**Results**	**Strengths and Weaknesses**

ture use. The tool in Table 5–3 is an example of one method for organizing your articles. At this point, attempting to read all the articles in your list will only add confusion. Create a table for the top three to five articles and save the rest of the list for future reference.

▶ GENERAL GUIDELINES FOR CRITIQUING RESEARCH ARTICLES

A number of articles and texts give easy-to-follow instructions on how to critique research (see references at end of chapter). The guideline in Table 5–4 is a short summary of a reasonable approach, and simply lists important points to consider when evaluating written research. Even if you have never evaluated written research before, try using this guide with your top three to five articles and see how comfortable you are with the material. You need not be a statistical expert or even an accomplished researcher to decide if the findings match the question asked by the researcher and if the methods used are logically derived and carried out. You may also think of ideas on your own that would improve the methods or that would work better in your specific patient population or setting. Keep notes of these ideas, either on the articles, on a note card, or in your table, while reading through the article.

▶ UNDERSTANDING HOW AND WHEN TO MAKE RECOMMENDATIONS FOR PRACTICE

At this point you will need to know how to differentiate the studies that will be very useful in answering your question from the studies that will be less useful. In general, research that is of a descriptive nature (case reports, observational studies, and descriptive studies) reflects the lowest level of research. Experimental design studies are at a higher level. There are two basic types of experi-

Table 5–4	Guide for How to Critique Research Studies

1. Read the study once to get the "gist" of the study before beginning the critique.
2. Keep notes, preferably on a small note card, on each of the studies. These notes will be used for summarizing the literature later. Include on the card information listed below.
3. After you have reviewed several studies, develop a table or grid like the one in Table 5–3 to keep track of the major studies and how they are similar to/different from one another.

Title of Study	Author Names and Journal Name, Volume, Issue, Date, Page #

Purpose of study

1. What is the researcher attempting to find out?
2. What are the hypotheses, if stated?
3. What are the specific variables?
   a. Independent: b. Dependent:

Significance of study

1. What importance does this study have to clinical practice?
2. How will the findings improve practice?
3. Does the review of the literature relate to the problem being studied?

Methods

Subjects

1. Who are the subjects who were studied (normal volunteers, hospitalized patients, similar physiologically to your projected sample)?
2. What were the inclusion and exclusion criteria?

Design

1. What is the independent variable: the "intervention" that is being tested or evaluated?
2. What is/are the dependent variable(s): the parameter that is being measured to determine if the intervention is effective?
3. Is the independent variable applied to all subjects in the same manner?
4. Are the dependent variables always obtained in the same manner for all subjects?
5. Is the study prospective or retrospective?
6. Is the study randomized or not randomized?
7. If the study is not randomized, what type of grouping or comparison strategy is used?

Procedures followed for the study

1. Is informed consent obtained?
2. List exact steps in how the independent variable/intervention was done.
3. List exact steps in how the data were collected.
4. How was consistency assured in data collection procedures?
5. List type of equipment used (if applicable).

Analysis

1. What type of analysis was done?

Results

1. What were the results of the study?
2. Do the graphs/figures make sense to you?
3. What was the authors' interpretation of the results?
4. What was your interpretation of the results?

Recommendations

1. Do you think the next study on this topic ought to be based on the findings of this study?
2. How would you improve on the methods of this study if you were to do a similar study?

mental designs, those that are simple, randomized intervention studies, and those that are done in the "gold standard" design of multicenter, double-blind, randomized, placebo trials. With experimental design studies, we can have more confidence that the results of the study would apply to similar patient care situations.

When is the information available in the literature enough to answer a question? In other words, when is the amount of existing data considered sufficient for decision making regarding a change in practice? Several standards or scales have been established for recommending changes in practice given the available evidence or research in a given area. These scales are based on the strength of the research design and the number of studies, if any, that are available. A common standard for making practice recommendations is the one used by the Agency for Health Care Policy and Research (AHCPR) in the AHCPR Guidelines (Table 5–5). As you try to summarize the research related to your question, be aware of the type and quality of research available. If few or no studies are in the highest level (multicenter, randomized, double-blind, placebo trials), additional research in this area is probably still needed. A large number of studies in the highest level, however, would cause one to reconsider whether additional research is necessary in this topic area (Fig. 5–3).

Determining whether or not existing data are "sound" and sufficient requires some work; however, if 50 people have concluded the same thing in the abstract that is available on Medline, then you probably don't need to look much further than the computer screen for an answer. In addition, if the majority of the articles you have identified indicate a high level of scientific merit, then you can be confident of the answer to your question with far fewer articles (as few as 5 to 15 studies), and without doing any further research. Remember, however, that the "state of the science" is constantly changing and additional information that will require practice changes may become available later. In summary, the best approach to deciding when "enough is enough" is to carefully evaluate the question being asked, taking into account the following considerations:

Table 5–5	AHCPR Guidelines for Making Practice Recommendations Based on Available Evidence		
	Strength of Evidence = A	**Strength of Evidence = B**	**Strength of Evidence = C**
Primary evidence	Randomized, controlled trials	Well-designed clinical studies	Panel consensus
Secondary evidence	Other clinical studies	Clinical studies related to topic, but not in the same patient population	Clinical studies related to topic but not in same patient population

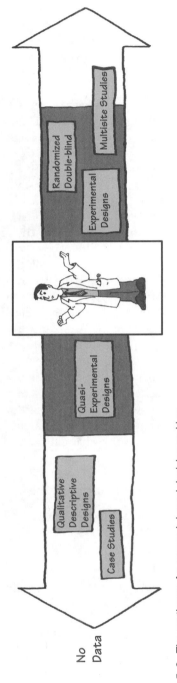

Figure 5–3. The continuum for research-based decision making.

1. Has a significant body of work been done on the topic?
2. Is there consensus among the experts regarding the answer to the question?
3. Is there a sizable body of work (5 to 15 articles) that ranks high in terms of scientific merit?

If it appears that enough information is available to answer your research question already, there is no reason to pursue a research study. You may then want to move forward toward changing practice at your institution. If it does not appear that enough research has been done on your subject, you may decide to pursue a research study. Remember, the answer to "when is enough, enough" is never black and white. You must carefully review the literature, and use your best judgment.

▶ CONTINUING THE REVIEW OF THE LITERATURE FOR A RESEARCH STUDY

Now that you have reviewed the literature, organized your articles, and have a clear (clear-er anyway) understanding of how valuable each article may be to your argument, the next question is how many articles from the overall list should you read at this point? Pursuing a research study requires a much more in-depth review of the literature than the preliminary review required. Think of reviewing the literature as a series of "rounds" that begins, in the first round, as a broad overview and progresses through three "rounds," gradually increasing in level of detail with each successive round. These three rounds, pictured in Fig. 5–4, build on one another in terms of content and amount of information yielded. Each round also takes an increasingly greater time commitment on the part of the researcher.

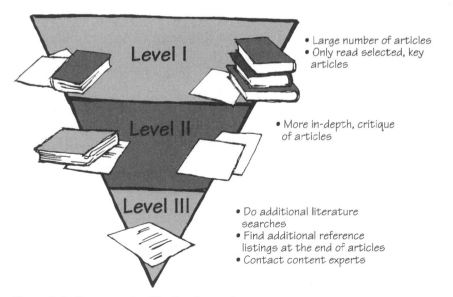

Level I
• Large number of articles
• Only read selected, key articles

Level II
• More in-depth, critique of articles

Level III
• Do additional literature searches
• Find additional reference listings at the end of articles
• Contact content experts

Figure 5–4. Three rounds of the literature review.

First Round

You have already completed first round by completing the general review of the literature and identifying any review articles and/or recent chapters written on your topic. You should be able to answer the following questions about your findings from the search:

1. How MUCH information exits? Are there 25 to 50 articles, or are there fewer? This will give you an idea about the question, how many other people are interested and how much has already been done.
2. Is there general CONSENSUS among the authors in answer to your question? It should be obvious from glancing at the abstracts whether or not general consensus has been reached. Are there differences in opinion among the experts as to the best approach or the best answer? If so, more research on the topic may be needed.

Second Round

The second round or level of detail in reviewing the literature is the evaluation of the quality and content of the literature that you found in the original list of articles. The second round of literature review will give you a greater level of detail about the existing literature related to your topic.

To do a second round review of the literature, use the long list of articles generated using your key words and read all of those that appear to be related to your topic or any of your dependent variables. Log each of these articles into the table that was started in Table 5–3. The table should be as long as necessary to comprehensively contain all of the current literature related to your topic. How far back to go (in years) in choosing articles to read will depend on the volume of articles available related to your topic. If several hundred seemingly relevant articles exist, read only the most recent few years. If fewer than 50 or so articles are available, then go back as far as five or even eight years. Remember, in many cases a "classic" study may be very old but should still be included in your review. You will recognize these types of articles because they will be referenced in a majority of other articles published on the topic.

At the end of the second round, you should be able to answer the following questions:

1. What will your study have to look like to make a meaningful contribution to existing literature?
2. What have you learned from existing studies about methodology?
3. What options do you have for measuring the dependent variable(s)?
4. What are possible intervening variables that you should and can control for?
5. What suggestions or recommendations from previous studies can you incorporate?

Third Round

This final round of literature review will help you identify any outstanding literature that may not have been uncovered in the initial review. Complete the following steps to uncover any newly published or ongoing research.

- Do another literature search using any new key words identified in round two. For example, you may have identified variables other than those in your research question that impact your study. Doing this exercise will also uncover any studies published while you have been busy on rounds one and two!

- You may want to call one or two experts in the field to validate your assessment of the literature and confirm areas of importance for study design. Experts may also be helpful for securing measurement tools for the dependent variable, such as surveys or questionnaires, that have established reliability and validity measures.

- Identify any additional articles from references listed at the end of key studies.

Each "round" of the literature review should reveal increasing levels of detailed information about your topic. These steps will hopefully help you to STOP where appropriate, without wasting excessive amounts of time and energy in overanalysis of any single article or in pursuit of older studies that may be less relevant to the design of your study. Figure 5–4 may help you progress to an appropriate level of detail when doing a literature search.

▶ REFERENCES

RESEARCH TEXTBOOK SUGGESTED READINGS

Polit D, Hungler B. Conceptual contexts for research problems: Literature reviews and theoretical frameworks. In: Essentials of Nursing Research: Methods, Appraisal, and Utilization, 4th ed. Philadelphia: Lippincott–Raven, 1997, pages 89–124.

OTHER SUGGESTED READINGS

Deets C. When is enough, enough? Journal of Professional Nursing, 1998, 14(4): 196.

Goode C, Wellendorf S, Cipperley J. Reading and Critiquing a Research Report (videotape). Horn Video Productions, 607 W. 2nd Street, Ida Grove, IA 51445, 1991.

Mayhew P. Evaluating research for use in practice. Medical Surgical Nursing 1993;2(6):496–498.

Mallet G, Martindale J, Hancock L. Medical Matrix: Premier Sites Handbook. SLACK Incorporated: Thorofare, NJ, 1998. (Available on the Internet at address: *hhtp://www.slackinc.com/matrix*)

Rankin M, Esteves M. How to assess a research study. American Journal of Nursing 1996;96(12):32–36.

Sparks S, Rizzolo MA. World Wide Web search tools. Image: Journal of Nursing Scholarship, 1998; 30(2): 167–171.

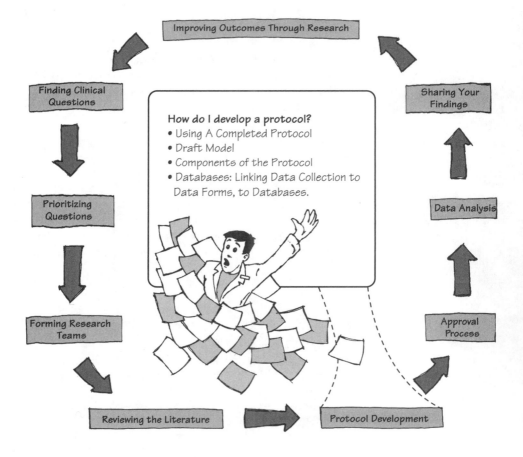

How do I develop a protocol?
- Using A Completed Protocol
- Draft Mode!
- Components of the Protocol
- Databases: Linking Data Collection to Data Forms, to Databases.

CHAPTER 6

Protocol Development: Keep-It-Simple Strategies for the Novice and Expert

One of the most important steps in protocol development is knowing what you want to be able to say about your question when the study is finished. The reason is that the design chosen for the protocol will dictate, to some extent, what can be said about the results. Poor planning up front can result in relative disasters in the end, such as insufficient sample size to demonstrate a significant difference between two things, inability to draw a conclusion for a desired patient population, or the inability to make assumptions or generalizations about your findings. To avoid some of these less savory outcomes, this chapter will help you anticipate and navigate roadblocks in protocol development.

▶ USING A COMPLETED PROTOCOL AS A TEMPLATE

The biggest roadblock in protocol development, almost without exception, is writing one for the first time. The best advice is to copy success. Using a previously accepted protocol from your institution, or one from the appendix of this book, replicate the section headers and wording style using your own research question.

The most fail-proof approach to completing a protocol for the first time is to write a replication of a well-constructed study. However, even if you are NOT replicating a study, using a completed protocol as a guide is still the easiest approach to getting started.

Replicating a Study

In a replication study *your* responsibility is simply to recreate the entire study and evaluate the similarities and/or differences in results. When replicating a study, your protocol should look like the original protocol; however, the original study's *protocol* is probably not available to you! Only the article is available to you. This should be good enough, assuming that the article is well written. The sections or subheaders in the article should mimic the headers required for your protocol. Likewise, the text under each section or subheader in the article should address the essential information necessary for you to replicate the study exactly.

Frequently the methods section does not elaborate on the "how, who, when, and where" details of the study. If critical information seems to be missing, you might try to contact the author or publisher for more information. Replicating a study is usually a compliment to the original author, and he or she should be more than willing to help by supplying additional information or tools for data collection.

Not Replicating a Study

Unfortunately, the first attempt at protocol development is not usually quite so straightforward as an exact replication study. Typically, even when doing a replication study, you will find a flaw or weakness in the original study that you wish to improve upon in your own study. More commonly, the articles found in the review of the literature do not *exactly* address the question that you are asking but are similar, or are good supporting evidence for the background of your study. These articles may be more helpful for justifying the need for your study. In this case it may seem as though you are starting from scratch, but you aren't really!

Regardless of major similarities or differences in your research question and the currently available literature, an existing protocol can still be used as a template to help you write your new protocol. The components or sections of all protocols should be similar. Using a protocol from your institution or the protocol templates located in the appendix of this book, see if you can draft your protocol by replicating the headings and borrowing wording, construction, or layout from the previously developed protocol or template. The exercises in this chapter will guide you through each section.

One word of caution is appropriate at this point. When requesting an example of a protocol from your IRB or from a colleague, be careful that you ask for a **short** protocol. "Short" means several paragraphs or so for each subheader, more for the background information and methods sections, less for most other sections. The examples included in the appendix of this book are considered "short."

The alternative to a short protocol is a long one! Examples of long protocols are those that are typically done for a master's thesis or doctoral dissertation, or those that are submitted for federal grant funding or major industry funding. These protocols are structurally no different, in that the components or subheaders are the same. The level of detail under each subheader, however, may vary considerably. Don't get overwhelmed! This level of detail is typically *not required* by most institutions. We do not recommend using a long protocol as a template or example for your protocol development. Your final protocol should be similar in length to those in the appendix of this book.

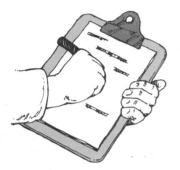

Don't waste too much time looking for a protocol from your own institution. If you know a friend or colleague that has had an approved protocol, ask to borrow a copy of theirs to help you get started. If you don't know of anyone off-hand, then ask the IRB office for a copy of an old protocol. They may be willing to give you a copy of an expired or blinded protocol. The advantage of getting one from your own institution is to replicate style, however, even within an institution style varies considerably from protocol to protocol, and the examples in this book generally represent all required content.

▶ DRAFT MODE: DON'T OVERWRITE!

Before embarking on your drafted protocol, remember when drafting the protocol for the first, or first *few* times, don't get hung up on any given section. Write down your thoughts and avoid "wordsmithing" too much with the first draft. If you get to a section that you don't understand or don't have enough information for, such as the data analysis section, skip it for now and go on! When the entire thing is drafted, then go back and fill in the blanks. This strategy prevents you from wasting time on any one section and gives you a sense of accomplishment for completing a draft, even if the final product still needs work.

There are any number of ways to begin drafting the protocol. Everybody has his or her own individual preference for writing, but one way to simplify the process is to break down the protocol into components. If you are working with a team, the components can be divided up among team members. The data analysis section should be "farmed out" to a statistical consultant or the expert identified to help with analysis (see Chapter 8, Data Analysis). Other components should be attacked by the team or author one component at a time.

▶ COMPONENTS OF THE PROTOCOL

Components of the protocol communicate to the reader or reviewer what you are planning to study, how you will study it, and why the study is an important contribution to patient care and to the literature. Components of the protocol typically include the abstract (not a necessary component of all protocols), statements addressing the significance or background of the problem, statement of the research question or hypothesis, a methods section that includes study design, sample or patient population, inclusion and exclusion criteria, setting, and a discussion of the tools or instruments to be used, and finally, a preliminary stab at the anticipated statistical analyses. In addition to these components that describe your study, there are also several "required" components that are standard for your institution's IRB. These components include statements related to patient risk, confidentiality, and patient reimbursement for participation in the study.

Begin by breaking the project into steps and take small bites. Work on one "bite" at a time, rather than allowing yourself to become overwhelmed by the whole project. The tendency or temptation to overwrite any given section should be overcome at all costs! Longer is not usually better (Table 6–1).

Protocol requirements may differ slightly from institution to institution; however, the general requirements for the protocol will be the same. Hospitals that require institutional review will always require as a minimum the standards set forth by the National Institutes of Health (NIH) for the protection of human subjects (see Chapter 7, Getting Through the Approval Process, and the Appendix, for more information). In this section we will discuss the "nuts and bolts" of each component of the protocol and give a few examples.

Abstract

The abstract, a 150 to 200 word summary of the project, is sometimes helpful to write initially for the purpose of getting thoughts in order and having a concise summary of the study. The abstract helps communicate the project to other staff

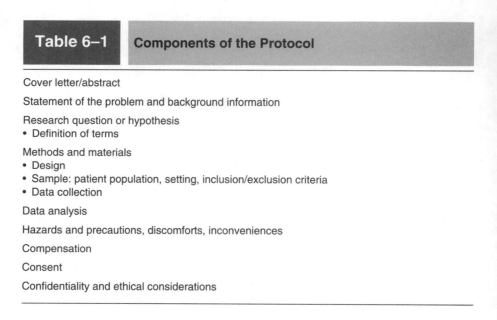

Table 6–1	Components of the Protocol

Cover letter/abstract

Statement of the problem and background information

Research question or hypothesis
• Definition of terms

Methods and materials
• Design
• Sample: patient population, setting, inclusion/exclusion criteria
• Data collection

Data analysis

Hazards and precautions, discomforts, inconveniences

Compensation

Consent

Confidentiality and ethical considerations

and co-workers in a short and concise manner. The purpose of the abstract is to summarize the need for the study and the plan for conducting the study.

Before drafting the abstract, it may help to draft the other components of the proposal first, and then come back to the abstract last. Although it is often the first item on the list of protocol components, it's often the last item drafted. Follow the template in Exercise 6–1 and create your own abstract when you are ready. The abstract typically includes the following key items:

- Statement of the problem and background information
- Statement of the specific research question or hypothesis
- Study methods:
  - Study design
  - Sample description (patient population and setting)
  - Data-collection process, including tools or instruments used
- Anticipated data analysis

If there are several components that you need more help with, simply skip those sentences and come back and fill them in later. After completing Exercise 6–1, have several friends or co-workers look at the abstract and validate its clarity. Do these informal reviewers have a clear understanding of the question and its significance? Do they feel the question adequately passes the "So What" test? If so, then the question is probably clear in your mind as well. If the question lacks merit in the eyes of your informal reviewers, this is a good time to "tune it up, or toss it out." Be specific about what you are really asking and then reexamine the relevance of your question. Validate for yourself again that you are on the right track.

Statement of the Problem and Background Information

The statement of the problem is broad and usually encompasses a global perspective of the issue to be studied. For example, "The incidence of (blank) is not well known," or, "The relationship between inpatient education and compliance in the outpatient setting in women with heart disease has not been well described in the literature." The broad problem statement is important for setting the stage and alerting the reader to the importance or significance of the proposed research. Exercise 6–2 demonstrates research problem statements and their role in establishing the argument or rationale for your study. Complete this exercise.

A discussion of background information typically follows the problem statement. This section varies in length from several paragraphs to several pages and includes information on the current "state of the science" about your topic area. This might include published statistics on the problem incidence, prior research, expert consensus reports/statements, and/or expert opinion on the topic. Create your paragraphs containing background information by choosing

▶ Exercise 6–1

Abstract Exercise

Use one or two sentences to describe each of the following components of your research project. Then merge the sentences together. The final product should be one paragraph, or about 150 to 200 words, and should resemble the example below.

1. Problem/background: _____

_____

2. Research question: _____

_____

3. Methods:

Design: _____

Sample: _____

Data collection process: _____

_____

4. Analysis: _____

Example: In the United States, the difficulty of early diagnosis of myocardial infarction has led to 1.6 million unnecessary hospital days and $600 million in hospital costs annually. In an attempt to expedite patient diagnosis and treatment and reduce unnecessary hospital charges, many institutions are experimenting with the use of early serum-enzyme markers. This study will compare sensitivity, specificity, and time to completed result, using one promising marker, Troponin-T, and the standard serum marker, CK-MB. Two hundred and fifty consecutive adult patients presenting to the emergency department in a large teaching hospital with complaints of chest pain will be asked to participate. Troponin levels will be drawn by the care nurse every 4 hours for 8 hours, and results will be compared with concomitantly drawn samples of the standard marker, CK-MB, in each of the patients. Functional study results and cardiac catheterization results will also be collected. Descriptive and inferential statistics will be used to analyze the relationship between Troponin-T and positive coronary artery disease.

the best articles from your literature review and briefly describing how they support your study. Use the protocols in the appendix as a guide for wording and length of this section.

Statement of the Research Question or Hypothesis

The statement of the research question is a sentence that clearly and concisely reflects the question you want your study to answer. For some types of research questions, you will replace your research questions with a declarative statement

▶ **Exercise 6–2**

Problem Statement Exercise

Note in the following list of problem statements how the information known about the problem is used for emphasizing the unknown. This technique helps establish the argument or need for doing the study.

1. Delayed extubation following coronary bypass surgery is a common problem, resulting in increased ICU costs and predisposing the patient to increased risk of further pulmonary and infectious complications; however, factors predicting late extubation have not been clearly defined.
2. Nosocomial bloodstream infection from central venous catheters is a serious complication known to frequently occur because of colonization, at the site of insertion. Specific parameters for site care that may decrease colonization, however, have not been well defined.
3. The experience of acute pain in critically ill patients is well documented; however, little is known about how nurses make decisions regarding the management of these patients.
4. The deleterious effects of malnutrition in the elderly are well documented; however, factors predicting early nutritional compromise are not well defined.

Now, create your own problem statement below:

_____
_____
_____
_____

in the form of a hypothesis. Research hypotheses are included in the protocol when research questions ask about relationships between two or more variables, or seek to compare one or more different approaches to care (interventions). Either way, the question or hypothesis summarizes in a succinct question or statement exactly what you will be studying. Look at some of the protocols included in the Appendix for examples of different research questions and hypotheses.

Before moving on to the next section of the protocol (Methods), compose your research question and complete the following steps to prepare for identifying the appropriate study design:

1. Clarify the variables you wish to study, dependent and independent.
2. Clarify the relationship between those variables that is of interest to you.

Table 6–2 lists examples of research questions "dissected" into these components. In Exercise 6–3 dissect your own research question. The wording of the research question is closely linked to design, in that the way the question is

Table 6–2	Identification of Study Variables and Relationships

Research Question	Variables		Relationship Between Variables	Population
	Dependent	*Independent*		
1. What factors predict hospital mortality in patients with acute MI, and what is the usefulness of two severity of illness indices?	a. Mortality b. Mortality, complications	a. The "factors" in patients with MI b. Severity of illness scale A versus B	a. **Identify** factors that seem to **predict** mortality in one group. b. **Compare** how well two tools accurately **predict**.	Adults with myocardial infarction who died in hospital
2. What are the differences in arterial pressure, pulmonary artery pressure, HR, Sao₂, and blood gas in ventilated CABG patients receiving manual hyperoxygenation during ETS as compared to ventilator-assisted hyperoxygenation during ETS?	MAP, PAP, HR, Sao₂, and ABG during ETS	Manual versus ventilator-assisted hyperoxygenation	**Compare** two groups	Adult coronary artery bypass graft (CABG) patients on ventilators
3. What are the structural and organizational characteristics of two ICUs with marked differences in risk-adjusted survival?	Structural and organizational characteristics	Hospital A vs. B risk-adjusted survival data	**Describe** characteristics along two parameters (structural and organizational) in two cases	Two ICUs with different survival rates
4. What are the physiologic effects of a bed bath on CABG patients?	Physiologic effects	Bed bath	**Describe** effects along one parameter (physiologic)	Adult CABG patients
5. Is there a difference in perceived quality of life before and after implantation of an internal cardioverter defibrillator?	QOL (before versus after)	Implantation of ICD	**Compare** one group at two different times.	Adult patients with an ICD device

► **Exercise 6-3**

Research Question Exercise

1. My research question is _____
    _____

2. The population I am studying is:
    Age: _____   Diagnosis: _____
    Gender:_____
    Other descriptor: _____

3. The variables in my research question are:
    Dependent: _____
    Independent:_____

4. The relationship I would like to demonstrate or explore between these variables is:
    ❏ descriptive
    ❏ comparative
    ❏ predictive
    ❏ causative

asked conveys information about how you will attempt to answer it. Design is the first component of the methods section.

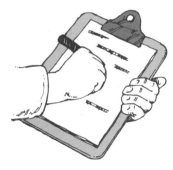

Dependent variable: The outcome variable of interest; the variable that is hypothesized to be caused by or depend on the intervention; the result or outcome of the intervention.

Independent variable: The variable that is believed to cause or influence the dependent variable; the manipulated or treatment variable; the intervention.

Methods

The methods section is a combination of several components, usually research design, population and setting, and the data-collection process. A description of tools or instruments used for the intervention is also presented here. This section is sometimes referred to as the "Methods and Materials" section. The methods section should answer the questions what, who, when, where, and how your study will be done. At the end of this section the reader should know **what** you intend to do, **who** will do it, **when** and **where** it will be done, and exactly **how** it will be done. If a stranger to your project can answer these questions after reading your methods section, then you have done a good job. Read the following details on design, sample, and data collection, and then draft your own methods section.

Design

The design is a description of how your study is set up to answer the question. It is the framework that defines how you will approach measuring the variables for your study. The purpose of design is to gain an optimal level of control over the variables being studied and by doing so, attain the most reliable or valid answer possible. This section answers the questions **what** data will be collected and **how**, or in what sequence. The simplest and safest way to go about deciding on a design is to follow three steps:

1. Start with your supporting literature to get an idea of how others have approached your topic. This should give you a preliminary design choice.
2. Double check the variables you wish to study and the relationships between those variables. Select a study design, using Table 6–3 for help if needed. Do you think you will be able to answer the question using the design you have chosen?
3. Use the expertise of a statistician, or one of the authors from a similar study, to validate that the chosen design will be able to answer your research question.

USE THE SUPPORTING LITERATURE. Using your literature review, get an idea of how similar studies have been designed. Look at recommendations from previous authors related to design. Frequently flaws or weaknesses in the design will be discussed in the "Discussion" section of the article. In this section the author may point out that data would have been easier to collect or more tightly controlled if the study had been set up differently. Design may also be discussed under "Limitations" in the article.

Design may not be discussed at all in the articles you have reviewed. In this case, evaluate your own clinical setting and patient population and determine what you *think* will be the best way to go about gathering data to answer your question. You might also want to call one or two authors of similar studies and discuss design. Ask why a particular design was selected and if the author recommends changes.

EXAMINE THE VARIABLES AND THEIR RELATIONSHIPS. When choosing a design, keep in mind the statements you would like to make about your results at the end of the study. These statements reflect the *relationships* between the variables and determine the type of study design that should be used to address your research question or hypothesis. Usually something is compared, described, iden-

Table 6–3	Research Designs

Experimental Studies

Design	Participants	Example
After-only	Two groups, one treatment and one control.	Does a dextrose-saline solution containing low-dose heparin prolong the use of infusion sites in children? (Wright, Hecker, & McDonald, 1995)
Before–after	Two groups, one treatment and one control.	What are the physiologic and psychological effects of a back rub in the institutionalized elderly? (Corley, Ferriter, Zeh, & Gifford, 1995)
Factorial	Four groups: one receiving each treatment, one with neither, one with both.	What is the effect of informational interventions on mothers' and children's ability to cope with an unplanned childhood hospitalization? (Melnyk, 1994)
Repeated measures	One group of participants receiving both treatment and control (standard) interventions in random order.	What is the effect of boomerang pillows on the respiratory capacity of hospitalized patients? (Roberts, Brittin, Cook, & deClifford, 1994)

Quasi-experimental and Preexperimental Studies

Design	Participants	Example
One group, before–after	One group participates.	Is a special educational program for nurses concerning causes of noise effective in decreasing noise levels in an intensive care unit for infants? (Elander & Hellstrom, 1995)
Nonequivalent control group, after-only	Four groups are compared.	How do four different methods of securing endotracheal tubes in orally intubated patients compare in terms of tube stability, facial skin integrity, and patient satisfaction? (Kaplow & Bookbinder, 1994)
Nonequivalent control group, before–after	Two groups, one participates and one does not.	Does participation in the Cardiovascular Health Education Program (CHEP) improve adolescents' cardiovascular health knowledge? (McDonald, 1995)
Time series	One group followed over a period of time and evaluated at intervals.	What is the effect of a dietary fiber and fluid intervention on the number of bowel movements and frequency of elimination among residents of a long-term care facility? (Rodrigues-Fisher, Bourguignon, & Good, 1993)

Nonexperimental Studies

Design	Participants	Example
Correlational–retrospective	Review of medical records.	What hospital workload factors are predictive of nurse medication errors? (Roseman & Booker, 1995)

(continued)

Table 6–3	Research Designs (continued)

	Nonexperimental Studies (continued)	
Design	*Participants*	*Example*
Correlational–prospective	One group questioned at a designated time after the intervention.	What factors best predict functional status after percutaneous transluminal coronary angioplasty (PTCA)? (Fitzgerald, Zlotnick, & Kolodner, 1996)
Case-control	One group selected (assaultive patients), and one group of normal control randomly selected.	Can assaultive patients be distinguished from nonassaultive patients on the basis of behavioral assessments or sociodemographic variables? (Lanza, Kayne, Pattison, Hicks, & Islam, 1996)
Descriptive	One group of participants questioned.	What factors do intensive care unit resident physicians and nurses perceive as influential in making decisions about level of aggressiveness of patient care? (Baggs & Schmidt, 1995)

Adapted from Polit D, Hungler B. Essentials of Nursing Research: Methods, Appraisal, and Utilization, 4th ed. Philadelphia: Lippincott–Raven, 1997, pages 163, 167, 171, 174, 177, with permission.

tified, predicted, or in some way evaluated. Table 6–3 lists common study designs and some examples of each one. Does your study question seem similar in design to any of these?

Remember that there are a number of possibilities for design. The reason for this is that design requires communication of how the independent variable will be controlled, how many groups (one or more) will be studied, what type of comparisons will be made between groups, and at what point(s) in time data will be collected during the study. Your exact combination of these factors may not be listed in the table. However, you should be able to glean whether or not you are close, even if the exact combination of groups, type of comparison, and time frames for intervention and data collection are different. Complete Exercise 6–4A and B.

If you would like to learn more about design selection, refer to some of the suggested references listed at the end of this chapter or any research theory textbook.

VALIDATE DESIGN CHOICE WITH AN EXPERT. Once you have made a "best guess" as to a research design, discuss your thoughts with a statistician or an author of a similar study to validate your choice (see Chapter 8, Data Analysis, for information obtaining statistical advice). Remember, data analysis is based on the relation-

▶ **Exercise 6–4A**

Describing Design

1. For this retrospective study we used a descriptive, comparative design to obtain information about ICD recipients' perceived QOL before implantation and their perceived QOL at the time of the study. Extraneous variables were accounted for through the collection of demographic data.

What:	
How:	

2. A within-subjects, repeated-measures design was used for this quasi-experimental investigation. Adult CABG patients in a medical/surgical ICU were studied to answer the research questions: (a) Does a 10-minute rest period after the bathing phase of a bedbath affect Svo_2 and heart rate in the immediate postoperative period? (b) What is the effect of the timing of a bedbath on Svo_2 and heart rate in the immediate postoperative period?

What:	
How:	

3. My sample description is: _____

_____

What:	
How:	

ships between your variables. The statistician cannot analyze data that you have not collected! Therefore, it is important to design data collection to reflect the correct or desired relationship between variables.

If at all possible, use the same expert in the beginning who will be helping you analyze the data in the end. Some details of design and analysis are based on individual preference, such as the selection of which statistical test to use for evaluating various relationships. The final analysis will be simpler if you can stick with one consistent statistical expert.

▶ **Exercise 6–4B**

Study Design Exercise

1. My research question is _____

_____

2. I have _____ (one, two, or more) groups.
3. Subjects in the groups are being compared:
   ❏ With themselves: Within subject
   ❏ With a different group(s): Between subject
4. The variables in my research question are:

   Dependent: _____

   Independent:_____
5. The time frame(s) for the treatment intervention (manipulation of the independent variable) are:
   ❏ Cross sectional: Single data-collection point.
   ❏ Longitudinal: Multiple data-collection points over time.
6. Data will be collected:
   ❏ Prospectively: Manipulation of the independent variable (treatment or intervention) and data collection are done in present or future time.
   ❏ Retrospectively: The thing being studied (dependent variable) is identified, and the research team looks back in time for causative or contributing factors. For example, chart review.
7. My design statement now reads as follows: _____

_____

Sample

This section should include a description of the population and setting you will be using for your study. It should also include a statement regarding how many subjects will be studied.

SAMPLE DESCRIPTION. Sample is the **who** and **where** of your study. For example, the patients or individuals you will be using for the study should be described as specifically as possible, including age, gender, diagnostic group, and any other information necessary to describe the specific subjects you are interested in. Often, when there are a number of qualifications for who will be admitted into your study, a listing of inclusion and/or exclusion criteria will be used. Several of the protocols included in the Appendix have used inclusion and exclusion criteria to succinctly describe individuals who will be studied.

The setting of the study, where the study will be conducted, may be described within the sentence describing the study subjects, or in an additional sentence. An example of a sample description might read as follows: "Adult patients being evaluated for radiation therapy of thyroid tumors in the outpatient oncology clinic will be asked to participate." This sentence provides information on the who and where of your study. Be as specific as possible and include enough detail that another researcher would be able to repeat your study if desired. In Exercise 6–5 read the examples and then describe your own sample.

SAMPLE SIZE. Another aspect of sample is determination of sample size. How *many* subjects are necessary to answer the question? The appropriate number of subjects for a study is based on a variety of factors, such as the type of research design, statistics and significance level, variables being measured, and how much of an effect you anticipate the study intervention will have on the dependent variables. Ideally, sample size determination should be done by a statistician or advanced researcher because it is typically beyond the expertise of new researchers. Several informational resources for sample size calculation are listed in the reference section at the end of this chapter and suggestions are provided in Chapter 8 for obtaining statistical assistance for data analysis and/or sample size calculations.

Data Collection

This section should answer the logistical questions **what, when,** and **how.** Describe for the reader exactly what data will be collected, when and how the data will be collected, and again, by whom. There are two "whos" that should be clearly addressed in the methods section: Who is doing the intervention and data collection, and on or to whom the intervention is being performed (sample description from above). The individual doing the intervention and data collection may be many people, for example staff nurses, or one individual. Be clear about these specifics.

Although many reviewing bodies do not require extensive detail in this section of the protocol, it will be to your advantage to be very thorough in describing the exact sequence of events, time relationships, and individuals involved during the data collection for your study. This level of detail will assist the team members to be practical in considering how data collection will actually be fit into the realities of the clinical environment.

BARRIERS TO DATA COLLECTION. The design and data-collection methods you have chosen have to be able to answer your research question, but they must also be feasible to accomplish given your geographic area, patient flow dynamics, and other realities of the clinical environment. Have you taken into account any logistical barriers specific to your situation that may slow or impede your ability to conduct data collection? Do the study methods enable ease of data collection given your setting, patient population, and normal patient care work pat-

▶ **Exercise 6-5**

Describing a Sample

Use the following examples of sample descriptions to describe your own sample.

1. Patients presenting to the emergency department with complaints of chest pain and no acute ECG changes will be asked to participate.

Who:	
Where:	

2. We studied 198 consecutive patients with gun shot wounds admitted to our ICU.

Who:	
Where:	

3. Patients admitted to the pediatric intensive care unit in acute asthmatic crisis will be enrolled.

Who:	
Where:	

4. All patients who died in the hospital following cardiopulmonary resuscitation (CPR) from January 1997 through January 1998 will be reviewed.

Who:	
Where:	

My sample description is: _____

_____

Who:	
Where:	

terns? Or have you set yourself up for the million mile march in terms of completing data collection?

Examples of logistical barriers that may interfere with study completion are unit routines, staffing patterns, patient flow patterns, communication patterns, and unit documentation processes or standards. For example, a three-group randomized design might work great in an area with a high volume of eligible patients, but if you only have access to a low volume of eligible patients, a three-group randomized design may not allow you to complete subject enrollment in a reasonable time frame.

Another example of a logistical barrier would be the case in which your data-collection procedures do not fit in well with normal patient care routines, and thus require additional staff to accomplish data collection. Finding the resources (personnel and/or grants) to support this type of data-collection requirement is difficult and could block your ability to complete the study (see Chapter 10, Finding Resources to Support Research, for additional information).

Examples of some common logistical barriers are listed in Table 6–4, but remember that other barriers specific to your situation may be lurking! The best way to avoid encountering barriers is to role-play your study methods when drafting the protocol. Walk through all the steps of your data collection, from patient identification, through consent, enrollment, data collection, and completion of data forms to see where any difficult (or impossible) steps may exist.

Read the examples in Exercise 6–6 and then draft a description of your own data collection. Ask a friend, a colleague or an objective reviewer to read your entire methods section. Ask that he or she check for missing steps or information, clarity, and logical flow of activities and for whether or not the methods are feasible given the realities of your clinical environment.

Data Analysis

This section should include preliminary plans for data analysis. While this section may change with the eventual completion of the study, a preliminary idea of the type of analysis planned is usually included here. For the protocol, very general ideas about analysis are acceptable (see sample protocol in the Appendix). For the institutional review board (IRB) even less detail is required. You may, in fact, simply say "descriptive and inferential statistics will be used after consultation with a statistician." This simply means that you will describe the sample characteristics and the relationships between variables in the study.

In spite of the relatively few "requirements" regarding data analysis for the protocol, the fact is that thinking all the way through the protocol, including a somewhat specific idea of the statistical tests that will be used, is helpful to do up front. This is primarily because identifying a specific statistical test forces you (or the statistician) to consider every piece of data that will be required. Frequently identifying a specific test points out data necessary for the analysis that have been left off of the data forms. This is an example of a very undesirable pitfall! It is unwise and unfortunate to go through an entire study and end up with missing information owing to a simple oversight in the beginning. For more details on data analysis, see Chapter 8.

▶ Exercise 6-6

Methods Exercise: The Data Collection Process

Case A	Case B
Methods: Survey packets containing a demographic data form, a modified version of the QLI:CV, and a consent form were mailed to 182 adult ICD recipients accrued from two hospitals in the mid- and south-Atlantic regions. Both hospitals had been performing ICD implants since 1987 and averaged four to five per month at study time; both sponsored a support group for ICD recipients, their families, and friends. One week after the mailing, reminders were sent to encourage potential participants to complete the surveys and return them to investigators (Bainger, E. M., & Fernsler, J. I., [1995]. *AJCC, 4* [1] 36–43.)	**Methods** In a prospective evaluation of ICU outcome and its relationship to unit management, we collected data in 42 ICUs at 40 US hospitals. Fourteen of the 40 hospitals were primarily university, tertiary care centers, and 26 were non-federal hospitals with 200 beds or more. Hospitals were selected using stratified random sampling criteria related to region, bed size, and teaching status. Demographic, clinical physiologic, and outcome data for an average of 415 ICU admissions at the 42 units were collected between May 1988 and February 1990. These data formed the basis for the APACHE III prognostic system, used to compare relative performance among the 42 ICUs in regard to risk-adjusted mortality, LOS, and case-mix adjusted use of treatment resources. While patient data were collected, we simultaneously obtained information on hospital and ICU structure and performed an organizational assessment based on questionnaire results at each study unit. (Zimmerman, J. et al, [1994]. Intensive care. *AJCC, 3* [2] 129–138).
What:	What:
When:	When:
How:	How:
Who:	Who:

Table 6–4	Logistical Barriers to Completion of Data Collection

Barrier	Example	Possible Solution
1. Unit routines • Data collection interferes with patient care • Collection of data for study purposes does not coincide with time patient care data are normally obtained	• Subjects' completion of a long research questionnaire during admission would cause hospital staff to wait to assess patient. • Temperatures for a comparison study of different devices not done when temperatures are needed for patient care purposes.	• Consider a shorter version of the questionnaire and/or change data collection times to occur after clinical care. • Redesign timing of data collection to coincide with usual activities.
2. Patient flow patterns • Low volume each month • Not available when data collectors available	• Study requires a sample size of 100 but only 6 patients eligible/month.	• Consider broadening the types of patients who would be eligible for the study to include other diagnoses. • Consider having other units and/or institutions participate in the study to increase the number of eligible patients. • Reconsider the feasibility of the study at this time.
	• Data collectors available only on day shift but data also need to be collected on pm/nights.	• Enlist some of the pm/night shift staff to join the study group.
3. Communication patterns	• Staff does not know when patients are eligible for, and/or subjects in, a study.	• Consider discussing on rounds and/or during the report which patients are likely candidates for which studies on the unit. • Assign an investigator each day to be responsible for identifying eligible subjects and to alert the staff. • Place some type of colorful, eye-catching sign or notation in the medical record and/or at the patient's bedside to alert staff that patient is a participant in a study.
4. Documentation patterns	• Patient needs to sign consent preoperatively but researchers don't see the patient until postoperatively.	• Enlist some of the staff on the admitting unit to join the study group so they can obtain consent.
5. Staffing patterns	• Not enough staff to do patient care and data collection at the same time. • Data collection complex, requiring 1–2 hours of time.	• Rethink staffing pattern. • Redesign and simplify data collection to be done during patient care routines or in brief 10-minute segments.

In summary, the components of the protocol should be viewed as building blocks that help construct a well-articulated, well-done study. These building blocks, approached one by one in a simple, straightforward fashion, are not as difficult as they may seem. Two tips to remember for simplifying the "building" process are (1) don't overwrite the protocol, and (2) use a completed protocol as a template to draft your own. For alternative or additional references on writing various components of the proposal, see the references at the end of this chapter.

Databases: Linking Data Collection to Data Forms and Databases

Simplicity is the key for getting data into a format that can be used for data analysis. More than likely, the statistician will want to have the data from your data forms transferred into a database. Databases are built, usually in a computer system, from the information on the demographic forms, surveys, questionnaires, and other instruments you use to gather and record data. Getting the data from your data-collection forms and into a database in a computer should be as well planned and streamlined as possible. The less transcription of data required, the fewer opportunities for error.

To check the simplicity factor, again role-play through your data-collection section. With each step ask yourself these three questions:

1. Is this piece of information necessary to collect?
2. Is this the most direct way to get the information?
3. Are the data easily transferable to a database that is familiar to the statistician?

Is the Information Necessary?

To answer whether or not the information is really necessary, ask yourself:

- Is it directly related to what I need to know to answer my question?
- Will it provide necessary supporting information for my question?

For example, if your question is about the incidence of nosocomial pneumonias with different types of ET tubes, you would obviously collect all information related to patient fever, infection, and death. These variables are directly related. You would also need to collect information on the underlying patient diagnosis, medications the patient was on, demographic information about the patient such as age and gender, and so on. These variables are supporting information in that they will enable you to describe the groups clearly. These variables may also help you to describe a relationship between various patient factors and the development of nosocomial pneumonia. Any factors that you think may contribute to your variable relationships should be collected.

Is This the Easiest Way to Get the Information?

To answer whether the plan for data collection is the easiest way to get the information, as yourself:

- Is computerized or scannable data entry being used whenever possible?
- Is direct download from a computerized medical record being used if possible?
- Are data configured correctly, meaning coded answers, for easy entry into a database?

For example, many clinical areas use computerized medical records. These systems can frequently be used to capture data. Variables such as vital signs, assessments, diagnosis, labwork, and many others, can be downloaded directly into a database software program. At the very least, they can usually be downloaded into a spreadsheet program, such as Microsoft Excel™, and then transferred into a database program, such as Microsoft Access™.

Another good option for close-to-direct data entry is the bubble sheet. Many clinical facilities have a scanner to read bubble sheets (blacken-the-circle-type answer sheets). Bubble sheets have the advantage of automating the entry of information directly into a database or spreadsheet, avoiding manual data entry. This benefit lessens the opportunity for errors in data entry, improving on the quality of your data for analysis. This approach also saves the team from spending valuable time doing data entry. Automated data entry systems are discussed in further depth in Chapter 8, Data Analysis.

Some researchers have succeeded in getting patients to enter data directly into the database. One example is a patient satisfaction study in which surveys are done in a clinic, directly on a computer workstation in the waiting room. Using a Windows format, the patients simply click on a selection box. The key is to streamline the number of steps necessary to get the data from the source into the database. Using your study, walk through the Methods section and see how many times data must change hands to get from the source into the database (Exercise 6–7).

Are the Data Transferrable to an Appropriate Database?

If your participants cannot enter data directly into a database, like the patient clinic example used above, is the data form in an easily transferrable format? To answer whether your data are transferrable to an appropriate database, ask yourself these questions:

- Are the data being entered into the database by the research team, and if so, is the database computer and software easily accessed by the research team?

► **Exercise 6–7**

Data . . . From Source to Finish

How many hands do your data pass through from source to database? (check all that apply)

1. Our data collection involves using:
   ❑ survey
   ❑ questionnaire
   ❑ interview
   ❑ written data form or case report form
2. The above is being completed by:
   ❑ care nurse
   ❑ research team member not doing direct patient care
   ❑ other
3. The person above passes data to _____ (#) people before it is ready for entry into database. These individuals are _____ and they (role with data).

   #1_____ / Role _____

   #2 _____/ Role _____

- Is the database accessible and familiar to the statistician who will be doing the analysis?

Many statisticians have specific preferences for the type of database programs they use for data analysis. Using the program that your statistician is familiar with when you do initial data entry will prevent having to transfer data or reenter data into another system for analysis. Spreadsheets are not the same

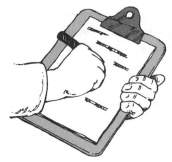

Spreadsheets versus database

Spreadsheets look just like the " Table " feature in a database. The difference is that databases allow you to query the columns on the page and draw relationships between the variables. Your statistician may have a preference.

as databases, but they can be used for the input of your data and to perform some computations. Later, the data file can be converted into a database management program for more advanced analysis. Check with your statistical expert before making a final decision about databases.

Data Forms

Good data forms make good databases, which makes for simpler analysis (Fig. 6–1). Once the study is designed and the logistical barriers have been thought through, you are ready to design the data forms. Data forms are sometimes referred to as case report forms or "CRFs." A "good" data form looks different for every study because of the differences in variables being collected; however, a good data form does have the following consistent characteristics regardless of the study:

- Logically, sequentially organized. The order in which data are recorded on the data collection form should be the same as the order in which the data collector will be obtaining data from the subject. Avoid requiring the data

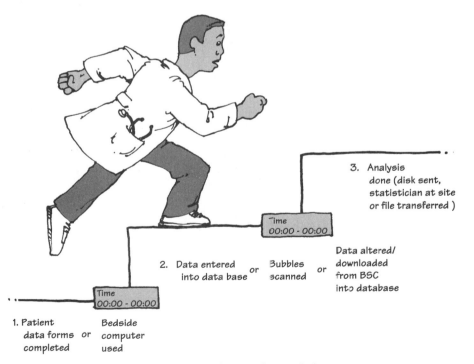

Figure 6–1. Data forms to data entry to database to data analysis.

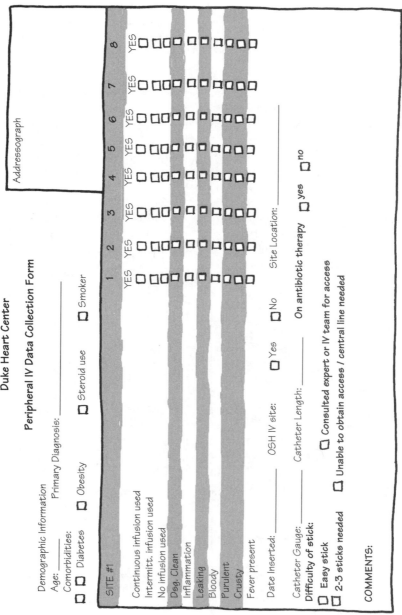

Duke Heart Center

Peripheral IV Data Collection Form

Addressograph

Demographic Information
Age: _____ Primary Diagnosis: _____
Comorbidities:
☐ ☐ Diabetes ☐ Obesity ☐ Steroid use ☐ Smoker

SITE #1

	1	2	3	4	5	6	7	8
	YES	YES	YES	YES	YES	YES	YES	YES
Continuous infusion used	☐	☐	☐	☐	☐	☐	☐	☐
Intermitt. infusion used	☐	☐	☐	☐	☐	☐	☐	☐
No infusion used	☐	☐	☐	☐	☐	☐	☐	☐
Dsg. Clean	☐	☐	☐	☐	☐	☐	☐	☐
Inflammation	☐	☐	☐	☐	☐	☐	☐	☐
Leaking	☐	☐	☐	☐	☐	☐	☐	☐
Bloody	☐	☐	☐	☐	☐	☐	☐	☐
Purulent	☐	☐	☐	☐	☐	☐	☐	☐
Crusty	☐	☐	☐	☐	☐	☐	☐	☐
Fever present	☐	☐	☐	☐	☐	☐	☐	☐

Date Inserted: _____   OSH IV site: ☐ Yes   ☐ No   Site Location: _____

Catheter Gauge: _____   Catheter Length: _____   On antibiotic therapy ☐ yes ☐ no
Difficulty of stick:
☐ Easy stick   ☐ Consulted expert or IV team for access
☐ 2-3 sticks needed ☐ Unable to obtain access / central line needed

COMMENTS:

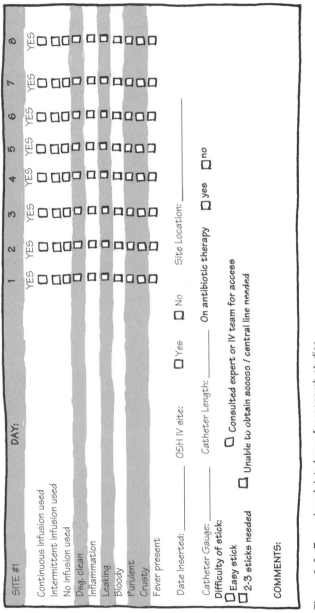

Figure 6-2. Examples of data forms for research studies.

collector to shuffle pages or skip around on the form to find out where the data should be entered.

- Coded. Analysis is easiest with coded data, so start off that way. "Coded" refers to designating numerical values for responses, so that those responses can be "tallied" or scored in the database and statistically analyzed. For example male = 1 and female = 2.

- Self-explanatory. The form should not require complex instructions. Anyone willing to help collect data should be able to pick up the form, read it, and use it. Test it on a colleague to validate.

- Clear, unambiguous definitions. The terms used in the questions should be clear. Remember, clear to you as a health care professional may not be clear to a patient or other user of the form. Even among health care professionals definitions differ. Use a key with terms specifically defined if necessary.

- Objective data points. The data form should ask for as little subjective data as possible. Even patient perception of pain, possibly one of *the most* subjective variables, can be objectively quantified on a variety of valid pain scales. Use objective, previously tested, valid, and reliable scales whenever possible.

Each of these characteristics is represented in the data forms in Fig. 6–2. Other examples of data forms can also be found in Chapter 8, Data Analysis, and in the Appendix. Give thoughtful consideration to these characteristics when developing data forms.

Other considerations regarding data forms are less related to development and more pertinent to the *use* of forms. Data forms used at the bedside, or sent in the mail, or downloaded from a computerized medical record system should be entered into the database as received. There is no advantage to saving all the forms until the last subject has been enrolled and then beginning data entry. Sometimes deficits in data collection are identified early on by beginning data entry into the database. In this case corrections can be made before data collection gets too far along.

Another point to remember regarding use of forms is that forms that are not directly downloaded into a database have approximately a 5% to 15% error rate when manually entered. For this reason, it is important to double-check that data entered are correct. Although a tedious and time-consuming task, this is a critical step to ensure data accuracy for analysis.

▶ **REFERENCES**

RESEARCH TEXTBOOKS SUGGESTED READINGS

Polit DF. Data Analysis and Statistics for Nursing Research. Stamford, CT: Appleton & Lange, 1996.

Polit D, Hungler B. Essentials of Nursing Research: Methods, Appraisal, and Utilization, 4th ed. Philadelphia: Lippincott–Raven, 1997.

OTHER SUGGESTED READINGS

Cobb E. Planning research studies: An alternative to power analysis. Nursing Research 1985;34(6):386–388.

Fields W, Siroky K. Converting data into information. Journal of Nursing Care Quality 1994;8(3):1–11.

Geitgey D, Metz E. A brief guide to designing research proposals. Nursing Research 1969;18(4):339–343.

Haynes R, Mulrow C, Huth E, Altman D, Gardner M. More informative abstracts revisited. Annals of Internal Medicine 1990;113(1):69–76.

Rudy E, Kerr M. Unraveling the mystique of power analysis. Heart and Lung 1991;20:517–522.

Tournquist E. From Proposal To Publication: An Informal Guide to Writing about Nursing Research. 1986 Addison-Wesley Publishing Company, Inc. Menlo Park, CA.

Yarandi H. Planning sample sizes: Comparison of factor level means. Nursing Research 1991;40(1):57–58.

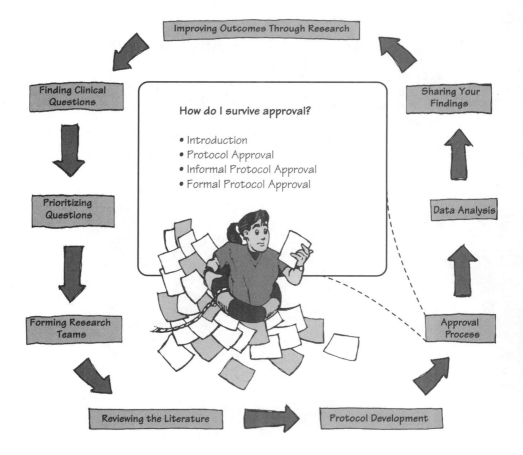

Improving Outcomes Through Research

Finding Clinical Questions

Prioritizing Questions

Forming Research Teams

Reviewing the Literature

Protocol Development

Approval Process

Data Analysis

Sharing Your Findings

How do I survive approval?

- Introduction
- Protocol Approval
- Informal Protocol Approval
- Formal Protocol Approval

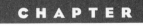
Getting Through
The Approval Process

Once the protocol is written, one last step must be taken prior to beginning data collection. Approval! Not every project will require formal approval; however, *every* project requires informal approval, or "buy-in." The support and participation of peers and unit leadership will be invaluable to the success of your study. Peer support serves to speed the project's completion and also contributes to enthusiasm and general buy-in for the study. Administrative support is equally valuable and may impact the degree to which the study ultimately influences practice in your institution. In this chapter we walk step by step through the approval process and explore tips for identifying and building key supportive relationships.

▶ PROTOCOL APPROVAL

The approval process can be traumatic as individuals begin to review your protocol; however, it need not be. The primary reason for frustration at this point in the process is that now you are opening up your ideas and plans to others for feedback and constructive criticism. Whether formal or informal, written or verbal, feedback from reviewers may not be what you wanted to hear. Try to step back from the proposal and be objective when receiving reviewer comments. Should initial feedback hit you the wrong way, consider the following reasons why and try again to "hear" the feedback.

- The reviewers are not as familiar with the subject matter as you are, and are therefore prone to question issues that may seem obvious to you. Address any unclear areas and resubmit.

- Reviewers may contradict one another, causing you to make changes repeatedly on a single issue, first to please one group, then reversing the change to please another. When resubmitting the proposal with incorporated changes, always return the original comments to the reviewer and clearly justify any suggestions that you chose not to incorporate.
- The reviewers may be from different backgrounds or clinical areas. Questions may be raised because of a lack of background information on the topic. Again, be as clear as possible and if you feel some suggestions should not be incorporated, then explain why.

These trouble spots are to be expected; however, the resulting delays can be easily avoided if one is prepared for potential setbacks before they occur. The goal in the approval process is to go in with as much preparation and organization as possible, having the background and the supporting documentation for your clinical question well in order. By doing so, one can convey enough subject authority and clinical expertise to convince readers that the study is indeed warranted. In short, have your ducks in a row and put your best foot forward!

The algorithm in Fig. 7–1 depicts an overview of the approval process. The approval process involves two basic "phases," the *informal phase* and the *formal phase*. The informal phase consists of protocol review by individuals in the organization that could be impacted by your protocol plans. The formal phase consists of protocol review by various committees in the organization to receive official permission to conduct the stated research.

▶ INFORMAL APPROVAL PROCESS

Although the informal phase may not be clearly delineated as a required step at your institution, a wise investigator will do it anyway. This step helps clarify details of the study in your own mind through discussion with others. It also generally helps avoid trouble down the line by enlisting buy-in from key individuals in your work area.

Identifying Key Stakeholders

Begin by identifying the key "stakeholders." Who is a "stakeholder"? This is an individual or a group who will be affected by the study but possibly not directly involved in the development or data collection for the study. These individuals or groups of individuals may share a patient population, a staffing pool that will be involved in data collection, or an interest in the outcome of the patients being studied or may simply have a vested interest in the question. Examples of stakeholders include the nursing and ancillary staff in the unit, the nurse manager of the unit in which the study will be conducted, the physician group caring for your particular patient population, and other multidisciplinary health care team members such as respiratory therapists, physical therapists, or pharmacists involved in the care of the identified patient population.

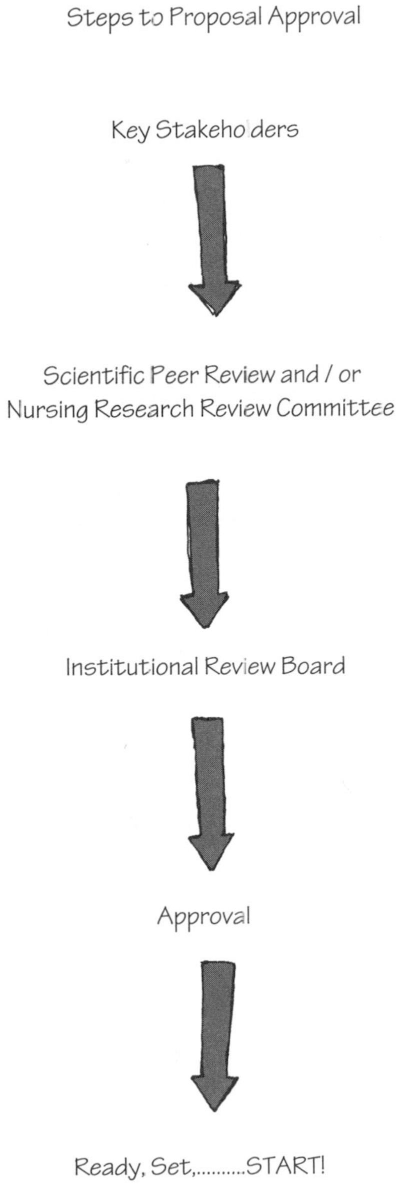

Steps to Proposal Approval

Key Stakeholders

Scientific Peer Review and / or
Nursing Research Review Committee

Institutional Review Board

Approval

Ready, Set,..........START!

Figure 7–1. Algorithm—steps to approval.

Of the many stakeholders out there, the two most critical in the approval process include the management group in the clinical area in which you will be working and your colleagues who will be immediately affected by the data-collection process. All of these individuals should be identified early in the proposal process.

Early Feedback

Once the key stakeholder groups or individuals have been identified, the next step is to get feedback from them early in the proposal process. Early, informal feedback helps avoid major setbacks later. For example, will the nurse manager support the study being done during staff work time? Will the staff agree to collect pieces of the data, or will you need a core group of staff designated as data collectors? Will the physicians involved with your patient group agree to this particular intervention, or will you need to find a way around or through this issue?

Ask the key stakeholders to review a draft of your proposal early on. While the proposal need not be perfect or even entirely complete, be sure there is enough detail so the reviewer gets a clear picture of your proposed study. Simply submit the cover letter in Fig. 7–2 along with a copy of the protocol to these identified individuals, asking for input or feedback. Some of these same individuals may be tapped later on to give a more formal review for scientific merit, but for now you are only concerned with buy-in.

Potential barriers in the informal phase of approval are easily overcome. The difficulty lies in identifying where the issues exist, if in fact they do, and whom to approach for the best shot at a successful resolution. Table 7–1 gives examples of issues that commonly arise and lists several possible solutions and strategies.

DEPARTMENT OF NURSING MEMORANDUM

TO: (Name of key stakeholder)

FROM: (names and titles of investigators)

DATE:

RE: PROPOSAL REVIEW

We would appreciate your feedback on the feasibility of the proposed study in the enclosed protocol, (insert title of protocol here). The proposal has been preliminarily drafted at this time. We would appreciate your input regarding the study question or any concerns you may have about the study before we move forward for IRB approval.

If you have any questions, please don't hesitate to call me. Thanks again for your timely review of this project.

Attachments:
   Protocol
   IRB forms

Figure 7–2. Cover letter for review of a protocol.

Table 7–1	Problems and Solutions for the Informal Approval Process

Potential Barrier	Possible Solution
1. Leadership buy-in	• Have a meeting to discuss protocol • Highlight the significance of the question being addressed, benefit to patients, and any financial issues that may surface as a result of the study
2. Physician participation—particularly regarding access to patients	• Have a meeting to discuss protocol • Highlight the significance of the question being addressed, benefit to patients, and possible changes in practice that may come as a result of the study
3. Staff participation	• Communicate!!! • Have frequent, small staff inservices or educational sessions regarding the significance of the study question and the possible impact on practice • Highlight the impact on patient care and the patient benefit

Clarifying the Commitment of Stakeholders

In addition to obtaining feedback on the protocol from the key stakeholders, another important point to clarify early on is their commitment to the project. Although the necessary level of commitment will vary among the stakeholders in your particular project, whatever that level of commitment is should be clarified from the start. For example, if the nurse manager of the emergency department agrees to allow a study of tympanic thermometers to be conducted by the staff on the unit, that nurse manager should not also mandate a change in thermometer devices for budgetary reasons midway through data collection for the tympanic study. Likewise, if your unit is conducting a study on the rate of infection when using long-term indwelling central line catheters, the physician(s) in that unit should not alter the unit stock by ordering a sulfur-coated central line catheter midway through data collection. Either of these examples would significantly hinder the progress and affect the outcome of the study.

Contracts and Agreements

How formal should the informal phase be? In other words, is a verbal agreement all that is necessary at this stage? Are discussion of the study and a general "OK" enough, or should some form of written contract be established?

The answer to these questions is dependent upon the individuals involved. If the number of key stakeholders is relatively limited, and the relationship of the research team with those individuals is a good one, then a verbal agreement is probably sufficient. If, however, the people with whom you are negotiating are not typically working closely with you, or are spatially removed from your clinical area and therefore likely to forget about a verbal agreement, then some form of written acknowledgment of the agreement may prove useful.

Another time that written agreement might be recommended is for documentation of administrative approval. Documented administrative approval may be required by your Institutional Review Board (IRB) or by a funding source, if you are seeking funding. Though this is not always a requirement, it is nice to have on reserve in the event that you need it. Figures 7–3 and 7–4 are examples of a cover letter and review form for seeking administrative approval.

Another example in which written agreement may be helpful is for holding researchers accountable. If a number of studies are being conducted in a given patient care area, each researcher should be aware of the potential burden this places on staff and patients. A written agreement regarding the communication of information and the expected time commitment for staff, is often helpful. Figure 7–5 is one example of this type of written agreement.

▶ FORMAL APPROVAL PROCESS

The formal approval process is begun once the proposal is completed and informal arrangements discussed above have all been cleared. As depicted in Fig. 7–1, the formal process generally begins with scientific peer review followed by

---

DEPARTMENT OF NURSING
MEMORANDUM

DATE:

TO:

FROM:

RE: ADMINISTRATIVE REVIEW OF A NURSING RESEARCH STUDY

The enclosed nursing research study has been submitted for approval. I would appreciate your review of this proposal by (insert date here) to determine if the study has administrative support. Please don't hesitate to call me if you have any questions about the proposed study.

Figure 7–3. Cover letter for administrative approval.

ADMINISTRATIVE APPROVAL OF NURSING RESEARCH PROPOSAL

Title of Protocol:

1. Nurse Manager Approval (if appropriate)

The results of this study have the potential to address clinical situations of:

High priority to the hospital _____

Medium priority to the hospital _____

Low priority to the hospital _____

Hospital resources (personnel, supplies, clinical practice routine changes) required to support this study are minimal or are justified by the potential benefit(s) to the hospital or patient outcomes
Yes _____   No _____

_____ I administratively approve the proposal for submission to the Institutional Review Board.

_____ I approve the proposal for submission with the stipulations specified below:

_____ I disapprove of administrative support for this proposal for the following reason(s):

Signature: _____

Date: _____

2. Division or Service Line Director

_____ I administratively approve the proposal for submission to the Institutional Review Board.

_____ I approve the proposal for submission with the stipulations specified below:

_____ I disapprove of administrative support for this proposal for the following reason(s):

_____ Approval of funds to support study (see separate budget for details).

_____ No additional funds required to support study.

Signature: _____

Date: _____

3. Physician Unit or Service Director

_____ I administratively approve the proposal for submission to the Institutional Review Board.

_____ I approve the proposal for submission with the stipulations specified below:

_____ I disapprove of administrative support for this proposal for the following reason(s):

Signature: _____

Date: _____

Figure 7–4. Template for administrative approval.

an IRB approval process. Most institutions have an IRB, as well as some type of formalized departmental peer review, such as a Nursing Research Review Committee (NRRC). The purpose of these formal boards is to monitor the research being conducted throughout the institution and to ensure content validity as well as legal, ethical, and scientific standards.

RESEARCH APPROVAL FORM
(Hospital) Cardiac Care Unit

Due to the volume of research in the CCU, the following criteria have been established as a means of ensuring adequate time for provision of quality medical and nursing care and to protect our commitment to timely, accurate data collection from the nurses and house staff.

Name of Project: _____ IRB # _____

Name of PI: _____ ID #: _____ Phone: _____

❏ The name and ID number of the primary investigator or research nurse must be available for further information or questions.

❏ A dated copy of the protocol and guidelines should be available on the unit (in the research notebook).

❏ A monthly enrollment update should be provided to the CCU Research Committee by the 30th of each month (for inclusion in the monthly Clinical Trials Enrollment Summary located in the research notebook).

❏ The responsibilities for completion of the case report form should be clearly spelled out and should not consume excessive time on the part of the patient, nurse, or house staff.

❏ Any RN or house staff participating in data collection will have access to updates of study progress and results and will be given credit for participation in the study.

❏ The following signatures should be obtained prior to initiating the study to ensure awareness of leadership group.

_____ (Medical Director, CCU)
_____ (Nurse Manager, CCU)
_____ (CCU Research Committee Chair)

Date: _____

Thank you for your involvement in our clinical research efforts!

Figure 7–5. Contracts and agreements for research.

Nursing Research Review Committee

Role

Nursing research review is a review of your proposal by other nurses within your institution. Some institutions, primarily academic ones, have a formalized NRRC in place. The primary purpose of departmental review is to review the proposal for feasibility and scientific merit, and to ensure the proposal is complete prior to submission to the IRB. Research committees at the departmental level can serve a number of other purposes and should complement the work done in the unit level by the work group (Table 7–2). Depending on the needs of the organization and stage of development, nursing research committees may be responsible for one or two functions, or all of them. It is im-

Table 7–2	Common Purposes or Functions of Nursing Research Committees at the Unit and Departmental Level	
Unit-Based Research Committee	**Departmental Nursing Research Committee**	
Identify clinically relevant areas for research studies	Review and approve nursing research studies	
Facilitate/ensure the integration of current research findings into clinical practice	Develop departmental guidelines for research studies	
Coordinate data-collection requirements at the unit level for research studies	Identify organizational priorities for research	
Assist with quality improvement activities	Liaison with schools of nursing to facilitate research supportive of organizational initiatives	

portant to be clear on what the intended purpose or function of the departmental review is in your institution since purpose and function will vary from place to place.

Peer review examines the importance of the study to clinical practice and the appropriateness of the research materials and methods to the study objectives. There are two basic approaches to scientific review. The most common is for the NRRC members themselves to review each study and evaluate its scientific merit using standardized guidelines. A second approach is to delegate scientific review to experts. Given the complexity and diversity of patient care today, some research committees are delegating the primary scientific review to two or three experts within the specialty area that the study addresses.

In the second approach, the same standardized guidelines are used and expert clinicians from nursing or other disciplines independently review the study for scientific merit (Figs. 7–6 and 7–7). Results of these evaluations are then

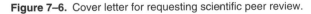

DEPARTMENT OF NURSING MEMORANDUM

DATE:

TO:

FROM:

RE: SCIENTIFIC REVIEW OF A NURSING RESEARCH STUDY

The enclosed nursing research study has been submitted for approval. I would appreciate your review of this proposal by (insert date here) to determine if the study has scientific merit. A form is included to guide your review of this proposal. If you are unable at this time to complete the review, please call me so we can arrange to have someone else perform the review.

Thank you in advance for your support of nursing research at our facility.

Figure 7–6. Cover letter for requesting scientific peer review.

SCIENTIFIC REVIEW OF NURSING RESEARCH PROPOSALS

Title:

Principal Investigator:

Associate Investigators:

	YES	NO	COMMENTS
I. Purpose and Scientific Justification			
A. The purpose of the study is clearly stated			
B. The literature review substantiates:			
1. familiarity with related and current literature			
2. accurate interpretation of literature			
3. implications for nursing practice			
C. The research questions or hypotheses are clearly stated			
II. Methods A. Subject selection includes:			
1. criteria for subject selection			
2. sample size and justification			
B. Research design is appropriate to research question			
C. Research procedures are clearly stated and justified			
D. Procedures for data collection are appropriate			
III. Data Analysis			
A. Validity and reliability issues of measurement tools are addressed			
B. Statistical procedures are appropriate to the research questions			
IV. Hazards, precautions, discomforts, inconveniences are discussed			
V. Ethical considerations			
A. Written informed consent required			
B. If no, reason for not requiring written informed consent stated			
VI. Impact of study implementation on use of hospital resources (personnel, supplies, routines) described adequately			

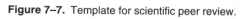

Figure 7–7. Template for scientific peer review.

VII. Briefly list areas of the proposal that require additional information/clarification or changes from
     the PI:

VIII. Additional Comments:

I have reviewed the Nursing Research Proposal cited using the attached guidelines and:

_____ Recommend it for submission to the Institutional Review Board.

_____ Recommend it for submission to the Institutional Review Board upon completion of the attached
        stipulations.

_____ Recommend revision and resubmission for a second scientific endorsement review (suggested revi-
        sions attached).

_____ Do not recommend it for submission (see attached).

Reviewer: _____
Title / Position: _____
Date: _____

Figure 7–7. (Continued)

submitted to the committee. The committee as a whole then uses these evaluations to form the basis of their summarized recommendations to the author.
This type of approach assures that each study being reviewed is critically evaluated by several individuals with specific expertise in the research area, rather
than relying on the clinical composition of the committee to cover all the potential clinical areas for which research might be submitted. A table such as the
one depicted in Table 7–3 can be used to keep track of the responses from reviewers.

Often nursing research has never been conducted before at an institution,
and nursing research guidelines are not available. Guidelines for medical research can usually be substituted to guide research being conducted by any discipline. The process for answering a clinical question and the rules applied to
that process are in place for patient protection and should be consistent regardless of who or what discipline is attempting to answer that question.

Who Is on a Nursing Research Review Committee?

The NRRC is generally comprised of nurses with a variety of clinical experience and academic background. If your institution is affiliated with a school of
nursing, members of the faculty are generally reviewers in addition to experts
from the clinical area.

What Does the NRRC Need From Me?

The NRRC may have special guidelines or instructions for proposal preparation
that are in addition to those required by the IRB. As will be discussed further
in the next section, some of the IRB standards are requirements for all human

Table 7–3	Peer Review Worksheet

Protocol:

Reviewers	Date Sent	Date Returned	Status
Scientific Peer Review A. B. C.			
Administrative Review A. Nurse manager B. Director C. Physician director/liaison			
IRB Submission			

research. Some of the standards to which you may be held may be requirements of your institution only, and are not federally or nationally mandated, but must be adhered to all the same. Either way, these guidelines can be obtained by contacting the department and IRB review office, or the IRB chairperson.

Usually, the NRRC requires a copy of your proposal, complete with all appendices and references. Other questions to clarify with the departmental review committee include:

- When they meet, especially in relation to when the IRB meets, so that you have time to make any changes to the proposal prior to the IRB submission deadline.

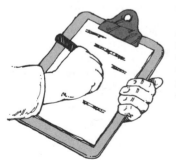

Commonly, the investigator is not expected or invited to be present during the review of the proposal. In this case identify who your department IRB representative is and discuss your proposal with this individual prior to the review date. This can help prepare your representative to be a better advocate during the review process.
If you are allowed to be present for the review remember the following tips:
- Dress professionally
- Arrive on time for the meeting
- Bring a copy of the proposal and all appendices, including any supporting information that may be helpful in defending the purpose or methods chosen.
- Be prepared to give a brief description of your study if requested

- Whether or not you are expected to be present during the review, and if so, what is the usual format for presentation.
- How early you must submit a copy of the proposal to them prior to the meeting date.
- How many copies of the proposal to submit, and whether they should be blinded.

As a final reminder, the role of the NRRC is to facilitate your IRB review. Take advantage of this opportunity if available, recognizing that this group will want more content detail and background information than that which will be required for the final IRB proposal form. See Table 7–4 for a checklist of things to complete prior to submitting your proposal to the NRRC for review.

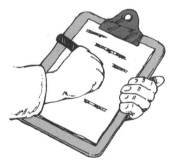

What is "Blinded"?

A "blinded" copy of a proposal or abstract has the authors' names and any other identifying information removed from the final copy of the document. Usually this is done by simply covering the names with sticky note paper and photocopying the document the requested number of times. The original (with names) is then submitted along with the requested number of blinded copies.

Institutional Review Board

Role

The purpose of this review board is to protect the rights of human subjects who will be enrolled in the study and to evaluate and resolve any ethical issues that may arise in the course of the study. As previously mentioned, most of the standards for ethical conduct of research on human subjects are developed at a national level by the National Institute of Health (NIH) and are required for all approved research. Your institution may add to the national criteria, requirements that are pertinent to your institution only and are not federally or nationally mandated, but must be adhered to all the same. Guidelines specific to your institution can be obtained from the IRB office or chairman. If you cannot locate the office responsible for disseminating institutional guidelines for research, call a nurse administrator for help.

Table 7–4	Checklist for Proposal Completion

✔	Proposal Content Required for Review

☐	1. Abstract
	    a. Usually one paragraph or less than 500 words
	    b. Brief statement of problem, proposed intervention/methodology, proposed analysis

☐	2. Purpose or problem statement
☐	3. Background information supporting significance of study

☐	4. Methodology:
	    ☐ a. Patient population defined (patient type and number sought)
	    ☐ b. Setting defined (type/size hospital, unit, or patient care area defined)
	    ☐ c. Data-collection process defined step by step (who does what, when)
	    ☐ d. Instruments or tools to be used defined and described (also an example of your tool or survey attached as an appendix or appendices)
	    ☐ e. Follow-up procedure, if any, defined, including time frames for follow-up (if the follow-up is a phone call or survey, include copy as an appendix)

☐	5. Statistical analysis (proposed; general—need not specify exact tests to be used)
☐	6. References (refer to the preferred reference style of *your* IRB; APA is typically not required)

☐	7. Appendices:
	    ☐ a. Informed consent form
	    ☐ b. Instruments or tools used (surveys, questionnaires, or other tools)
	    ☐ c. Instruments or tools used for follow-up
	    ☐ d. Any other forms or tables integral to the study, such as conversion tables for medication administration or pain scales or visual analogue
	    ☐ e. Details necessary to carry out certain procedures for the study (standard protocols or procedures used for aspects of the study)

☐	8. Statement regarding possible risks to the patient/subjects (see example in appendix)
☐	9. Statement regarding confidentiality (see example in appendix)

Who Is on the IRB?

IRB members generally include clinical experts, nurses, physicians, ethicists, clergy, social workers, lawyers, risk-management representatives, and non-health care members of the community. Because of the variety of individuals and the range of expertise and experiences represented, one must be prepared to address a wide range of questions and concerns. For this reason, the more *clearly* and *simply* the proposal is written for the IRB, the better.

What Needs Approval?

The IRB must review and approve all research on human subjects, both patient and staff research, conducted in the institution prior to the beginning of data collection. Research, as defined by the IRB, is "any activity designed to test an hypothesis, permit conclusions to be drawn, and thereby to develop or contribute to generalizable knowledge."[1]

Several situations exist in health care institutions that are not usually considered by IRBs to be "research" and therefore do not need IRB review and approval. Information or data that are collected for the purposes of quality improvement activities and/or program evaluations are not likely to be classified as "research" by most IRBs. For example, doing patient satisfaction surveys after discharge to identify areas for practice improvements would be unlikely to be called research by most IRBs. Another example would be data collection to track complication rates and patient outcomes of usual nursing or medical care.

The interpretation of what constitutes human subjects research, and therefore what requires IRB review and approval, varies with each institution. When it is not clear if IRB review is required or not, consult with the IRB chair and follow his/her guidance. The motto, "when in doubt, submit it to the IRB," would always be a prudent approach to follow!

If your protocol does require review, you may still be able to qualify for expedited review. In expedited review, the protocol may be quickly reviewed by the IRB chair or his/her designee, without being reviewed by the entire IRB committee. To undergo expedited review, the protocol must involve no more than minimal risk and only involvement of human subjects that fits into one or more of the following categories:

- Collection of: hair and nail clippings in a nondisfiguring manner; deciduous teeth; and permanent teeth, if patient care indicates a need for extraction.

- Collection of excreta and external secretions including sweat, uncannulated saliva, placenta removed at delivery, and amniotic fluid at the time of rupture of the membrane prior to or during labor.

- Recording of data from subjects 18 years of age or older using noninvasive procedures routinely employed in clinical practice. This includes the use of physical sensors that are applied either to the surface of the body or at a distance and does not involve input of matter or significant amounts of energy into the subject or an invasion of the subject's privacy. It also includes such procedures as weighing, testing sensory acuity, electrocardiography, radioactivity, diagnostics, echography, and electroretinography. It does not include exposure to electromagnetic radiation outside the visible range (for example, x-rays, microwaves).

- Collection of blood samples by venipuncture, in amounts not exceeding 450 mL in an 8-week period and no more often than two times per week,

---

[1]Belmont Report: Ethical Principles and Guidelines for the Protection of Human Subjects of Research, OPRR Reports. Washington, DC: US Government Printing Office, April 18, 1979, page 3.

from subjects 18 years of age or older and who are in good health and not pregnant.

- Collection of both supra- and subgingival dental plaque and calculus provided the procedure is not more invasive than routine prophylactic scaling of the teeth and the process is accomplished in accordance with accepted prophylactic techniques.
- Voice recordings made for research purposes such as investigations of speech defects.
- Moderate exercise by healthy volunteers.
- The study of existing data, documents, records, pathologic specimens, or diagnostic specimens.
- Research on individual or group behavior or characteristics of individuals, such as studies of perception, cognition, game theory, or test development, where the investigator does not manipulate subjects' behavior and the research will not involve stress to subjects.
- Research on drugs or devices for which an investigational new drug exemption or an investigational device exemption is not required.
- Research oriented to surveys of hospital personnel.[2]

If you do qualify for expedited review, it may be helpful to include a cover letter to the IRB chair when you submit your protocol that suggests expedited review of the protocol (Fig. 7–8).

What Does the IRB Need from Me?

The IRB meets at designated times throughout the year for proposal review. These dates should be included in the information you receive with your packet of guidelines for research. Specific requirements for submission of a research proposal will be outlined in the guidelines for your institution. These instructions should be followed closely, and all forms should be completed as exactly as possible. Your attendance at the meeting for questions and/or a brief presentation of your proposal may be required by the IRB. If required, check with the chair or a member of the IRB for direction on what needs to be presented.

IRB review is usually a time when less is better. If the guidelines don't ask, or a certain piece of information is not central to the main message that you are trying to convey, *don't put it in*! It may only serve to confuse the issue for the reviewers and increase review time for the protocol.

Specific protocol requirements for your institution can be found by calling the IRB office or chairman. Again, every institution does not have an IRB, in

---

[2]Federal Register Number 46.110 of 45 CFR Part 46. Washington, DC: US Government Printing Office. January 26, 1981.

MEMORANDUM

TO: (Insert name), Chairman
         Institutional Review Board (IRB)

FROM: (Insert name and title)

DATE:

RE: REQUEST FOR EXPEDITED PROPOSAL REVIEW

The enclosed protocol, (insert name), (name, RN, principal investigator) is submitted for review by the IRB committee. The proposal has received scientific peer review within the Nursing Department at (name) Hospital. We would appreciate your consideration of this protocol for expedited review since the study activities meet the IRB's criteria for expedited review. Also, please note that this study is proposing a verbal consenting process only (no written consent documentation) owing to the nature of the study. The criteria for exception to the written consenting process (Section 46.117, item c of the Code of Federal Regulations for the Protection of Human Subjects, 45 CFR 46) are applicable to the design and methods of this study. There are no risks associated with this study and the use of the intervention would not normally require consent outside the research process. All patients eligible for the study will have the study thoroughly explained to them and will be given the opportunity to voluntarily participate in the project.

Attachments:
 Protocol
 IRB forms

Figure 7–8. Request for expedited review of a proposal.

which case one would simply refer to the Ethics Review Board (ERB), the Divisional Director or Nursing Director, or the Hospital Ethics Committee. A statement or description of each of the following is generally required by all hospital review boards:

- Research purpose and rationale of study
- Study procedure or methodology
- Benefits of participating
- Risks or possible discomfort incurred due to participation
- Alternative treatments, therapies, or options if one does not participate
- Procedures to ensure confidentiality
- Research related injury clause (ie, responsibility for, and course of action in the event of)
- Statement guaranteeing voluntary participation
- Consent for participation

Examples of several completed IRB proposals can be found in the Appendices. Several sections of these examples can easily be adapted for use in other studies since the concepts change little from one study to another.

► **Exercise 7-1**

Final Checklist for Submitting for Formal Approval

❑ Cover letter to the IRB chair seeking approval for the project
❑ Letter of support or approval from appropriate individuals (ie, nurse manager, divisional director, and/or physician director) for the conduct of research in the unit and/or institution where data will be collected.
❑ Letter of support validating scientific merit (NRRC or peer reviewer comments)
❑ Proposal
  ❑ Abstract
  ❑ Purpose of the study
  ❑ Background information supporting the significance of the study
  ❑ Methodology (see detail in Table 7–4)
  ❑ Statistical analysis (proposed)
  ❑ References
  ❑ Informed consent
  ❑ Appendices (see details in Table 7–4)
❑ Timeline
❑ Copies of entire packet (usually three copies; blinded if requested by your IRB)

Strategies to Speed the Approval Process

There are a number of tips to help speed the approval process. When preparing for review, remember the following:

- Follow the guidelines as exactly as possible.
- Include all appendices (ie, tools, surveys, questionnaires, consent forms) in the proposal and make sure they are well labeled and referenced in the text.
- Know the review date for your proposal. Don't wait around for someone to call you. You should be notified by the IRB office soon after the meeting/review date. If you do not hear from them as to the status of your proposal within one to two weeks following the meeting, call the office or the individual from whom you obtained the guidelines, and ask.

Complete the checklist in Exercise 7–1 to determine how prepared you are for the approval process.

► **REFERENCES**

RESEARCH TEXTBOOK SUGGESTED READINGS

Polit D, Hungler B. The ethical context of nursing research. In: Essentials of Nursing Research: Methods, Appraisal, and Utilization, 4th ed. Philadelphia: Lippincott-Raven, 1997, pages 65–88.

OTHER SUGGESTED READINGS

American Nurses Association. Human Rights Guidelines for Nurses in Clinical and Other Research. Washington, DC: American Nurses Association, 1975.

National Commission for the Protection of Human Subjects of Biomedical and Behavioral Research. Belmont Report: Ethical Principles and Guidelines for Research Involving Human Subjects. Washington, DC: US Government Printing Office, 1978.

Protection of Human Subjects. Federal Register Number 46.110 of 45 CFR Part 46. Washington, DC: US Government Printing Office, January 26, 1981.

Tetting DW. Preparing for human subjects review. Critical Care Nursing Quarterly 1990;12(4):10–16.

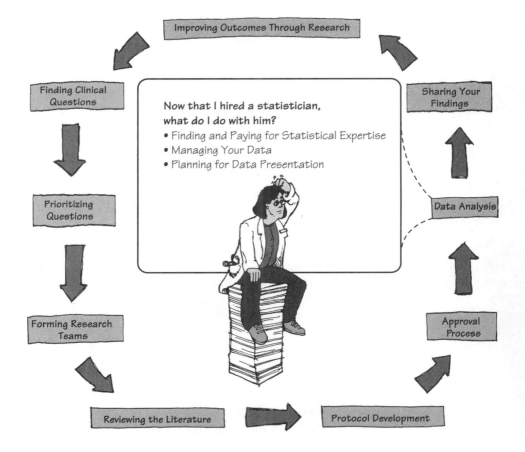

Data Analysis

Lack of statistical help and guidance during the research process is often perceived as a major roadblock to successful project completion. Even individuals who have had statistic courses in graduate programs feel intimidated by this aspect of the research process! The reality is that you don't have to do this phase of research by yourself—there are resources to assist with data analysis. In this chapter we will share with you some tips for making the "data analysis woes" a thing of the past.

▶ FINDING STATISTICAL EXPERTISE

The assistance of a statistician is needed *before* you collect your data, not when you are ready to analyze the data. The reason for this is quite simple: The statistician's role is primarily to advise the researchers on issues relating to the statistical design of the study (sample size calculation, statistical tests, data-collection tools). This needs to be done during the protocol development phase, not after data collection.

Unless you work in a university teaching hospital, it is unlikely that you will have ready access to statisticians at your facility. So where do you find these experts? A couple of suggestions include:

- Schools of nursing that use your facility for clinical placements. While the faculty members themselves may not have the specific expertise you need, they usually have an extensive network of local statisticians who support their research.

- Statistics departments at local universities. This may be a separate department or included in the mathematics department.

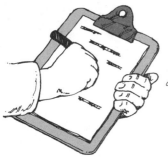

Get a statistician's advice early in your proposal development process!

- Find out where other researchers in the community get support for their studies. You may also be able to tap into those resources.
- Consult with researchers who have expertise in the area that your research addresses. They may have enough statistical experience to guide you in this area. This is particularly true if you are doing a replication study, in which similar data analysis techniques would likely be used.

▶ PAYING FOR STATISTICAL EXPERTISE

Once you've located someone with statistical expertise to consult on your study, the next question becomes, "How will we pay him/her?" Typically, money for statistical consultation is just not present in most nursing department budgets.

First and foremost you must be clear on the essential services you will require from the statistician (Table 8–1). His/her unique expertise is needed to review your draft protocol and recommend the statistical procedures you will use to analyze your data. In addition, he/she can assist in identifying the number of subjects that will be required to address your research question. These are activities that would be very difficult, if not impossible, for most clinicians to accomplish independently. This type of consultation is probably in the neighborhood of three to five hours of consultation from a statistician with expertise in your particular type of research design.

With the advent of new software programs for personal computers, other types of support for data analysis, such as transferring the data into the computer and actually performing the analyses, can usually be done by the investigators themselves. Though one could pay a statistician to perform this function, it is not necessary and doing so will dramatically increase the cost of data analysis.

After clearly defining what services you need from the statistician, you need to negotiate his/her payment. It is not uncommon for typical consulting fees for statisticians to range from $25 to $100 an hour. If you are request-

Table 8–1	Areas for Statistician Assistance

Essential Services

- Protocol review
- Recommendations on statistical analysis
- Sample size calculations

Other Services

- Database management
- Statistical analysis of data

ing a limited three- to five-hour consultation, you may find him/her agreeable to being listed as a co-author on the publication in lieu of a fee payment. Another approach would be to consider having a graduate student in the statistics department be the consultant. In this situation, the student may be able to use your consultation to meet some course objectives, and co-authorship on the resulting publications may be a real benefit.

As your institution negotiates contracts with schools of nursing for student's clinical placements for the year, it may be reasonable to ask for support for some of your statistical needs through department resources. As the partnerships become stronger between the academic and service setting, there should be many opportunities to support each other's pursuits of research-based practice.

Another source of financial support for statistical consultation is to apply for a research grant. Most grant budgets allow for some of the monies to be spent on statistical support. If statistical support, though, is the only aspect of the research study for which you need funds, we would strongly recommend that you seek support using one of the aforementioned mechanisms for statistical, consultative support. It is probably an unrealistic expectation to hope for funding of your first one or two research projects (see Chapter 10, Finding Resources to Support Research).

▶ MANAGING YOUR DATA

Assuming that you do not have the luxury of having money to hire someone to manage your study data, you will need to plan for how data will be entered into a spreadsheet or database and how the statistical analysis will be done.

Statistical Programs

Although many researchers pay statisticians to do data entry into the computer, as well as running the analyses, given the user-friendly statistical software packages on the market today, this is really an unnecessary expense. Table 8–2 lists some products currently available for Macintosh and DOS-based personal computers. Gone are the days of having to spend days and weeks learning complex computer commands to be able to "talk" with large, mainframe computers to do your data analysis. With just a little time spent learning the software program for statistical analysis on the personal computer, data entry and analysis can be a relatively painless experience.

Of primary concern when deciding which program to use is to determine what type of computer you will potentially have easy access to for data entry. If your facility uses predominantly DOS-based computer systems, then choosing a Macintosh statistical package would severely limit your potential access to computers. Another consideration would be what types of statistical programs are already in use at your facility. Oftentimes the nursing department or administrative or finance offices have various spreadsheet-type programs (eg, Excel™, Access™, SPSS™) that may be suitable for the types of data analysis you will be performing. By doing a little investigating into what your facility currently uses for number crunching, you may be able to avoid purchasing software (typically a $500 to $1500 per program). This approach ensures that you will have experienced users available who can guide you in the basics of learning the program.

The best approach to entering data in your spreadsheet/database is to avoid waiting until you have completed data collection on a large number of subjects, but enter data after you complete every two or three subjects. And it's best to have each investigator participate in data entry. That way, each individual be-

Table 8–2	Common Software Programs for Data Entry, Summary, and Statistical Analysis on Personal Computers
Program Name	**Software Company**
Excel	Microsoft Corporation, Redwood, CA
dBase	Ashton Tate, Inc, Torrance, CA
Lotus 1-2-3	Lotus Development Corporation, Cambridge, MA
SAS	SAS, Research Triangle Park, NC
SPSS and New View	SPSS Inc, Chicago, IL
Statview	Abacus Concepts, Berkeley CA
Super Anova	Abacus Concepts, Berkeley, CA
Access	Microsoft Corporation, Redwood, CA
Paradox	Borland International, Inc, Scotts Valley, CA

comes *very* familiar with what his/her data look like, where the missing values are occurring, and if there is any pattern to data-collection problems. Another advantage is that no one person has to endure the tedious process of entering data for hours at a time. Thirty minutes spent entering data once a week will not be an overburdening task for members of the research team.

If the only computers available with the statistical program you'll be using are far from the clinical area, find out whether computers in or near your unit may have programs on them that would allow you to enter your data on a simple spreadsheet that can be imported into the statistical program when it is time to analyze your data. This would greatly simplify data entry and avoid your purchasing the software for your area computer. For example, you might enter your data on the unit's computer that has Excel and then analyze the data later by importing the file into Stat View on the nursing administration's computer. There are endless possibilities. If you are not a computer guru, find someone in your organization who has computer expertise to advise you on possible approaches that would allow for easy computer access for frequent data entry.

Organizing Data Entry Spreadsheets

Data entry can be simplified by setting up the columns of your spreadsheet to coincide with how the data are organized on your data-collection tool. Fewer mistakes in data entry will be made if the person inputting the data does not have to jump around on the data-collection tool to locate what goes next on the spreadsheet. Another tip is if each subject has repeated measurements on one or more variables (eg, blood pressure before, during, and after the intervention), put your one-time demographic variables at the end of the repeated measures columns. Table 8–3 is an example of a data-collection form that was organized to facilitate bedside data collection and Table 8–4 is the layout used for the spreadsheet for computer data entry. Notice that the demographic data were the first items collected on the bedside collection tool, but the last items entered during computer data input. This will cut down on the number of "entries" made on each record.

Automated Data Entry Systems

Several different methods are now available that can transfer data from your data-collection sheets directly into the data analysis spreadsheets or databases (Table 8–5, page 154). These types of computer programs can virtually eliminate the need for manual data entry.

Although each automated data entry system works differently, purchase of the computer software program and a scanning device is typically all that is necessary. The automated data entry program is used to create the data-collection tool for the study (Fig. 8–1). These scannable forms are then used

Table 8–3	PAP Study Data Collection Sheet

Name: _____   Study ID #: _____   Date: _____

Sex: _____ (1=male, 2=female)   Cath Data: PAS _____ PAD _____ PCW _____

Racial Origin: _____ (1=Asian, 2=African American, 3=Caucasian, 4=Hispanic, 5=other)

Vent Settings:
   Mode: ____ (1=AC, 2=IMV, 3=PS, 4=other)
   Rate:_____ breaths/min
   O_2: _____
   PEEP: _____ cm H_2O

ECG Rhythm: _____ (1=NSR, 2=ST, 3=Afib, 4=Aflutter, 5=other)

Heart Rate: _____ beats/min

LOC: _____ (1=awake, 2=unresponsive)

	HOB 0°		HOB 20°		HOB 30°		HOB 45°		HOB 0°	
	G	*M*	*G*	*M*	*G*	*M*	*G*	*M*	*G*	*M*
RA										
PAS										
PAD										
PCW										
MAP										
CI										

G=graphic recording M=monitor dispaly

for data collection by filling in the appropriate "bubble" or entering alphanumeric data in special boxes. The completed data form is then scanned into the software program with a scanner or via a fax/modem connection. Data on the form is then "read" by the software program and automatically transferred into the designated database file.

While these automated data entry software programs are not inexpensive ($1500 to $5000), depending on the type and volume of your research projects, it may be a fiscally advantageous approach to data input. Your institution may already have such a scanner device that is used for patient or employee surveys, or schools of nursing in your area may have one for automated test grading. Negotiating to use one of these preexisting de-

Table 8–4 Computer Spreadsheet Used for Data Entry From the Pulmonary Artery Pressure Measurement Study

Name	ID	Vent Mode	Vent Rate	Vent O₂	Vent PEEP	Cardiac Rhythm	Heart Rate	Consc.	Graphic 0° HOB						Monitor 0° HOB		
									RA	PAS	PAD	PCW	MAP	CI	RA	PAS	PAD
Jones	001	3	10	50	10	1	90	1	10	25	14	12	78	3.5	12	27	12
King	002	2	13	40	5	2	58	2	15	35	14	17	65	2.1	18	39	20
Ranger	005	4		40	10	5	110	1	8	19	6	6	70	4.0	14	25	12
Smith	010	1	16	55	15	3	120	2	20	45	25	27	50	1.5	20	50	35

Employee Opinion Survey
Clinical Associate
Program

Date:

☐ / ☐☐ / ☐☐

Position prior to becoming a Clinical Associate:

○ NT I   ○ NT II   ○ Respiratory Therapy   ○ Phlebotomy

Last Name

First Name

Survey: ● Pre-implementation
○ Post-implementation

Work Activities

Comments

1. Considering all aspects of your job, do you like your job in general?   ○ Yes   ○ No

2. Have you received enough training to do your job properly?   ○ Yes   ○ No

3. Does your job make good use of your skills and abilities?   ○ Yes   ○ No

4. Do the departmental in-service programs meet your needs?   ○ Yes   ○ No

5. Is the work you do interesting to you?   ○ Yes   ○ No

6. Is the work distributed fairly among you and your work group?   ○ Yes   ○ No

7. Are you able to set priorities among tasks?   ○ Yes   ○ No

8. Are you performing the skills you were trained for?   ○ Yes   ○ No

Figure 8–1. Example of a research study data-collection tool designed with an automated data entry software program (Teleform, Cardiff Software).

Work Conditions

10. Is the equipment you work with in satisfactory condition?
    O Yes   O No

11. Is there adequate equipment to do your job?
    O Yes   O No

12. Are you satisfied with the safety practices in your work environment?
    O Yes   O No

13. Are there adequate supplies in order to do your job?
    O Yes   O No

14. Do you have adequate time to perform your job responsibilities effectively? For example, have we given you too many jobs to do?
    O Yes   O No

RN Supervision Skills

15. Do the RNs provide instruction and coaching to help you do your job well?
    O Yes   O No

16. Do the RNs provide you with regular feedback on how well you are doing your job?
    O Yes   O No

17. Do the RNs have an adequate understanding of the job skills required to do your job?
    O Yes   O No

18. Do the RNs work closely with you and other personnel on your unit to promote a team approach to patient care?
    O Yes   O No

Figure 8–1. (continued)

Table 8–5	Examples of Automated Data Entry Systems for Personal Computers
Program Name	**Company Location**
Teleform	Cardiff Software 1782 LaCosta Meadows Drive San Marcos, CA 92609 1-800-659-8755 http//www.cardiffsw.com
NCS Viewpoint	National Computer Systems, Inc. 4401 West 76th Street Edina, MN 55435 1-800-447-3269 http//www.ncs.com

vices may be possible, particularly if it is for a limited number of research studies.

▶ PLANNING FOR DATA PRESENTATION

One of the best bits of advice on how to analyze and present your data is to start your study with the end in mind. Before you finish writing the protocol and start collecting data, you should envision what the data might look like and how to graph the findings. This allows you to think more clearly about a simple approach to presenting the findings before you are overwhelmed with the actual results from your study. Typically, neophyte researchers become confused with the reams of information that can be generated by statistical calculations from even a simple research study. They seem to lose sight of what the original research questions or hypotheses were for their study.

For example, in the pulmonary artery study presented in Tables 8–3 and 8–4, the researchers original hypotheses were:

- H1: There will be no differences in pulmonary artery pressure measurements obtained in different levels of backrest elevation (0°, 20°, 30°).

- H2: There will be no difference in pulmonary artery pressure measurements obtained with the graphic or monitor method.

Though a typical computer analysis of the study data will generate lots of descriptive statistics on this data set (eg, the range and average of all the demographic data [age, sex, ethnic origin]), all of which can be easily displayed in a

Table 8–6	Sample Presentation of Demographic Data in Table Format From the Pulmonary Artery Pressure Study

Table 1. Demographic and Medical Diagnosis for 71 Subjects From Three Critical Care Units

Unit	N
Cardiovascular ICU ($N = 26$)	
Valve replacement	10
Coronary artery bypass graft (CABG)	9
Valve replacement & CABG	3
Left ventricular myotomy & myectomy	3
Other	1
Surgical ICU ($N = 26$)	
Immunotherapy treatment	
Renal cell carcinoma	7
Melanoma	2
Abdominal resection	11
Thoracotomy	2
Endocrine	1
Other	3
Medical ICU ($N = 19$)	
Lymphoma	6
Multisystem failure	3
AIDS	1
Hematologic disorder	1
Neurologic disorder	1
Carcinoma	5
Other	2

table (see Table 8–6 for an example), the data of primary interest from the hypotheses will compare pulmonary artery pressures in each of the three backrest positions and then compare the pressures obtained with the graphic and monitor method. A simple approach would be to use a bar graph to present each of those concepts (Figs. 8–2 and 8–3). These "planned graphs" were actually mocked up during the final completion of the protocol, before data collection had ever begun, and helped the investigators envision how their data might look at the end of the study.

By preparing graphs before you consult with the statistician, it will also help him/her understand what you want to accomplish with data analysis. And it will make it easy for you when your study is completed and it's time for data analysis—all you have to do is plug in the data from the study!

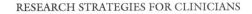

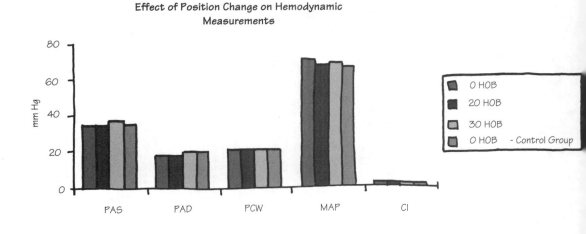

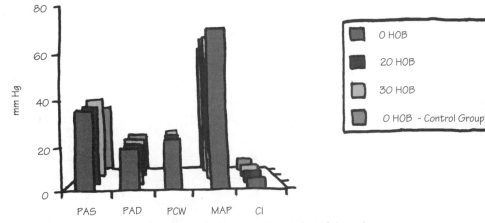

Figure 8–2A & B. Two possible approaches to the presentation of the pulmonary artery pressure study results relating to backrest position.

▶ REFERENCES

RESEARCH TEXTBOOK SUGGESTED READINGS

Polit D. Data Analysis and Statistics for Nursing Research. Stamford, CT: Appleton & Lange, 1996.

Polit D, Hungler B. Part V: Analysis of research data. In: Essentials of Nursing Research: Methods, Appraisal, and Utilization, 4th ed. Philadelphia: Lippincott–Raven, 1997, pages 315–398.

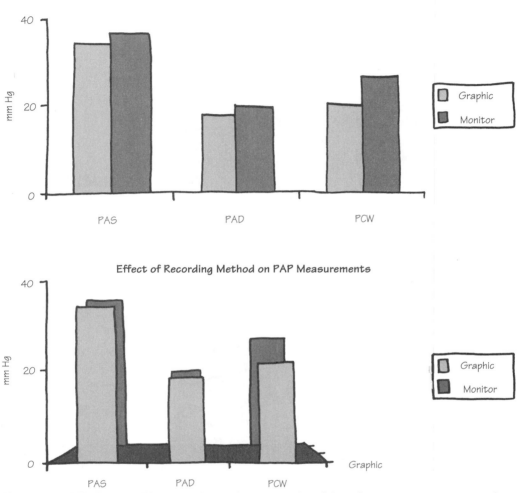

Figure 8–3A & B. Two possible approaches to the presentation of the pulmonary artery pressure study results relating to graphic or monitor measurement.

OTHER SUGGESTED READINGS

Davidson L, Clochesy J, Rohay J, et al. Automated data entry. Nursing Research 1996;45:30–34.

Dennis K. Managing questionnaire data through optical scanning technology. Nursing Research 1994;43(6):376–378.

Iwane M, Palensky J, Plante K. As user's review of commercial sample size software for design of biomedical studies using survival data. Control Clinical Trials 1997; 18(1):65–83.

Rudy E, Kerr M. Unraveling the mystique of power analysis. Heart and Lung 1991;20:517–522.

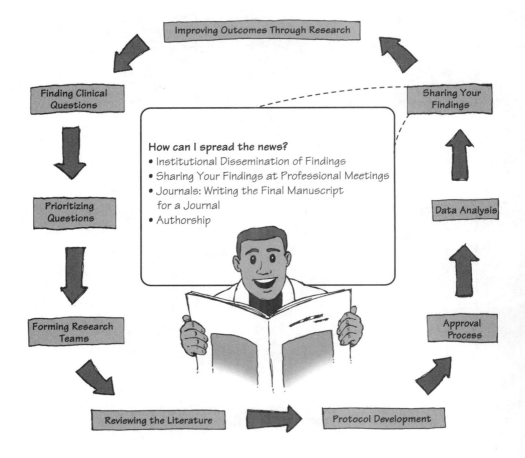

How can I spread the news?
- Institutional Dissemination of Findings
- Sharing Your Findings at Professional Meetings
- Journals: Writing the Final Manuscript for a Journal
- Authorship

Improving Outcomes Through Research

Finding Clinical Questions

Sharing Your Findings

Prioritizing Questions

Data Analysis

Forming Research Teams

Approval Process

Reviewing the Literature

Protocol Development

CHAPTER 9

Sharing Your Findings

If no one knows about your research, why did you do it? Chances are, if you had a clinical issue worthy of research, a number of other clinicians or patients probably have the same question. Not sharing the answers you found, or equally important, those that you didn't find, defeats the purpose of doing clinical research. If patients and others cannot benefit from your work, you have served only yourself. In this chapter we will present quick tips for helping get your "pen to paper." The rest is up to you. We feel it is imperative that you "just do it"!

▶ INSTITUTIONAL DISSEMINATION

The first level at which findings should be shared is within your own unit and institution. These are the individuals and groups who, we hope, have supported the process of your study and have possibly participated in one way or another to bring the study to fruition. Feedback to these individuals and peer groups should be done as soon as possible. A punctual, well-organized presentation of findings is a fitting way to say "thank you" for your help, even if it was nothing more than moral support. Suggestions for how to go about institutional dissemination are listed in Table 9–1. A good place to start in-house dissemination is in-house publications and forums such as:

- Newsletter
- Inservice
- Staff meeting presentation
- Poster
- Hospital or unit open forum

Further detail on some of these suggestions can be found in Chapter 4.

Table 9–1	Vehicles for Institutional Dissemination			
Institutional Vehicle	**Editor/Contact Person**	**Phone/Fax**	**Submission Deadline**	**Meeting Date**
Hospital newspaper				
Divisional newsletter				
Unit newsletter				
Divisional open forum				
Unit inservice				
Staff meeting				
Poster—in unit or other area				
Other				

▶ **PROFESSIONAL MEETINGS AND PRESENTATIONS**

Professional meetings are a second avenue for sharing findings. They offer a wonderful opportunity to get the word out to a peer group outside of your own institution. These forums and opportunities range from local chapter meetings of your professional nursing or specialty group to national and international meetings of nursing and other specialty organizations. If you are a first-time presenter it may be wise to start small and work up. Some researchers prefer to start big, and this approach is fine too! Figure 9–1 is an example of various levels of professional organizational meetings. You may have to do a little leg work to identify meetings of your own specialty organization or interest group. Completing Exercise 9–1 may help you identify opportunities specific to your own interests or work area.

Typically, presentation at a professional forum requires submission and acceptance of an abstract or summary of your work. If the abstract is accepted for presentation, you will be asked to present a poster or do an oral presentation of your project. This section will address how to write a convincing abstract, and how to pull together a poster or oral presentation should your abstract be accepted.

When submitting an abstract for professional presentation:
- Write formally. No slang or sentence fragments.
- Follow instructions for the abstract guidelines carefully.
- Don't leave out critical information:
  - Research question
  - Methods
  - Results
  - Implications for practice

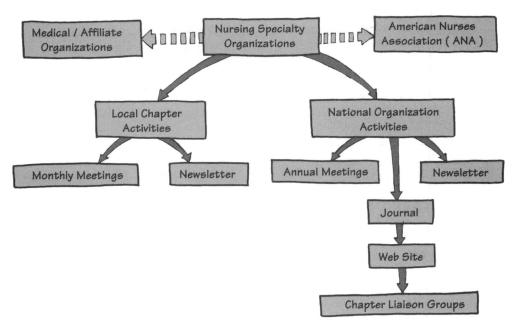

Figure 9–1. Levels of professional organizational meetings.

▶ Exercise 9–1

Tapping into Professional Meetings

1. My specialty nursing organization is _____ .
2. My local chapter is _____ , and meetings are held _____ .
3. The programs chair is / is not interested in my topic for presentation at this time.
4. After scanning the back of my favorite journals for upcoming conferences, some possibilities listing calls for abstracts are:

Conference	Contact Person	Deadline for Abstract Receipt:	Phone Number	Contact Made Yes	No

5. Nonnursing organizations that may also be interested in my project include:

_____

_____

_____

Taking the Pain Out of Abstract Submission

The abstract is a short summary of the project. "Short" is generally *one paragraph* or 100 to 200 words. The abstract and should include one or two sentences addressing each of each of the following:

- Purpose or problem
- Research question
- Research methods
- Summary of results
- Implications for practice

A completed abstract should read similar to either of those in Figs. 9–2 and 9–3. Though this book primarily addresses research, be aware that often pro-

2:15

Use of Diagnostic Tools in a Chest Pain Evaluation Unit:
Value of Troponin T Testing

L.K. Newby, E.M. Ohman, B.B. Granger, T. Sawyer, F. Sedor, C.M. Holleman, R.M. Califf. Duke University Medical Center, Durham, NC, USA

Chest Pain Units (CPU) are increasingly used for evaluating patients with possible acute coronary ischemia. Most use serial enzyme and EKG analysis over 9–12 hours for risk stratification. To evaluate troponin T (TnT) as a risk marker in CPU patients, we compared evaluation by TnT drawn at 0, 4, and 8 hours with a standard 12-hour protocol of q4 hour EKG and CK-MB analysis in 208 consecutive patients assigned to our CPU over a 4-month period. Diagnostic work-up was left to the attending cardiologist.

25 patients (12.0%) were TnT (+) (≥0.1 ng/mL); 1 patient (0.5%) was CK-MB (+) (>9 ng/mL). No TnT (−) (< 0.1 ng/mL) patients were later CK-MB (+). 68 patients had no further work-up due to low-risk atypical features, life-limiting co-morbidities, or alternative or established diagnoses; 9 (4%) were TnT (+), 59 (28%) were TnT (−). The remaining 140 had diagnostic cath (50, 24%) or stress test (98, 47%). The table reviews diagnostic test results.

	TnT (+) (n = 16)	TnT (−) (n = 124)	p value
CAD by cath	8/10 (80%)	15/40 (38%)	0.016
Positive stress test	3/8 (38%)	11/90 (12%)	0.050

False (+) TnT by cath results occurred once in hypertensive urgency and once in chronic renal failure.
Conclusion: In the CPU setting, TnT identified more patients with active CAD than did CK-MB. Use of TnT in this group could facilitate diagnosis and risk stratification.

Figure 9–2. Sample research abstract. (From Newby, LK, et al. *JACC, 29* [2]. Supp. A. February 1997, p. 211A. Reprinted with permission.)

fessional associations are also interested in abstracts that address creative solutions to clinical problems. Sometimes these ideas and solutions may not require research. Sometimes they are the results of a quality improvement or process improvement project. For example, solutions may include a new way to organize patient care delivery, new ideas for successful development of patient education tools, or new strategies for self-government. Any new idea that was successful for solving a problem in your workplace should be shared, either in a poster presentation or in a journal. The abstract for a creative solution project is similar to, but not exactly the same as, the abstract submitted for a research project.

Figure 9–2 presents an example of an abstract for a research project. Figure 9–3 presents an example of an abstract for a creative solution project. The differences lie in the type of information presented. A problem and an intervention are presented with both types and results are discussed with both types, albeit one presents results of the research and the other presents results of the implementation of the creative solution.

The abstracts discussed here differ from those discussed in Chapter 6 in that these are examples of abstracts written *after* the project is complete. The pur-

START PROGRAM IMPROVES CRITICAL CARE RESEARCH
Granger, B, Fullwood, J, Bride, W, Mostaghimi, Z, Turner, B. Duke University Medical Center, Durham, NC.

Nursing research was recognized at our institution as being critical to the ongoing improvement of clinical practice. Nurses were frequently stymied by the time consumed for patient screening and enrollment. In addition, no centralized mechanism existed to expedite data entry or to create and distribute monthly progress reports. As a result, overall enrollment in nursing research projects was slow and it was difficult for staff to maintain enthusiasm through the duration of a project or study with little or no ongoing feedback. The START (Strategies To Accelerate Research Teams) project was initiated to resolve these logistical barriers and enable staff to participate in the entire process of unit based research. The four step process simplifies patient screening and enrollment using plastic "hot files" which are hung in each unit. These folders contain all necessary materials for patient enrollment into studies in progress on that unit. An example of a completed form is attached to the outside of the folder. Completed enrollment forms are collected daily from the hot file and entered into a database by a designated rotating RN. A monthly report is then generated for each unit, as well as each division, which highlights enrollment status of ongoing studies. The new model has succeeded in increasing staff involvement in research, increasing patient enrollment, and providing consistent feedback to the staff.

Figure 9–3. Sample creative solutions abstract.

pose of these abstracts is to present a summary of the research study and findings. The abstract developed in Chapter 6 as part of the protocol is developed before the study is actually done, and therefore when results are not available. The primary purpose of the abstract in Chapter 6 is to summarize what the study will address and how the study will be done.

▶ Exercise 9–2

Create Your Own Abstract

For each of the following lead-in statements, insert your own research study components.

_____(*Problem*) has been widely documented in the literature; however, little is known about _____(*specific area of your problem*).
We investigated _____(*research question*) in _____
(*sample description*). A _____ design was used to test
_____ (*variables tested*). (*Describe data collection process here. For example, we compared, or we observed, or we surveyed . . .*).

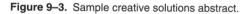

_____

(*Follow the sentences addressing methods with a statement of statistical findings.*)
These findings suggest _____

_____(*Conclusions/implications for practice*).

Complete Exercise 9–2 and draft an abstract for professional presentation using your own research question, methods, and results. Remember, this abstract is typically submitted to a journal or professional organization to win permission for presentation or publication. Be convincing about the importance and relevance of your problem statement and the significance of your findings. Sell your study!

Parts of the Perfect Poster

The perfect poster for professional presentation has six basic components, with the methods section requiring three subsections (design, sample, data collection) (Table 9–2). A poster is similar to an abstract in that *every word counts*. Space is at a premium; therefore, be as succinct as possible without eliminating

Table 9–2	Content for Research Posters	
Poster Components[a]	**Other Ways to Say (Almost) the Same Thing[b]**	**Content**
Title Board	• Label • Heading	Title of study, authors' names, and institution should be on a separate title board, top and center on the poster.
1. Abstract	• Summary	1. A summary of the entire project, including analysis strategy, results, and implications for practice.
2. Background	• Review of the literature	2. Summarizes the purpose for doing the project. Discusses the research problem and relevant prior research, as well as the reasons, aims, or objectives for pursuing the research question.
3. Research Question or Hypothesis	• Problem statement • Hypothesis	3. One or two sentences stating the specific research question or hypothesis tested.
4. Methods	• Intervention	4. Within the Methods include: • **Design** description • **Sample** description (population and setting) • **Data Collection** description
5. Results	• Outcomes	5. Results should report the statistical analysis. Graphs and tables are often used to summarize data.
6. Conclusions	• Evaluation • Recommendations • Implications for practice	6. A discussion of the benefits of the project to nursing practice or patient care. Recommendations for others who may be interested in doing a similar project are included.

[a]Title boards for each section heading are bold.
[b]Note that research terms are not always consistent, but usually synonymous, across publications.

any key information. The content for each of the six parts is very much like the abstract with two exceptions: a little bit more detail should be added to the methods and results sections, and recommendations or implications for practice should be included. The following information should be included as key content for each component of the poster.

- Abstract
- Background of the problem
- Research question or hypothesis
- Research methods
  - Design
  - Sample description
  - Data collection
- Results (statistical analysis)
- Conclusions or implications for practice

Figures 9–4 and 9–5 are examples of completed posters, one research poster and one that presents results of a creative solution to a clinical problem. As with abstracts, posters communicating a creative solution to a clinical issue do not generally require the same components as a research poster. For example, if you developed a plan for orienting new nurses that was superior in content and efficiency, presenting the benefits of that plan would not require statistical analysis. A poster communicating your work would therefore not require a statistical analysis section. Posters communicating a new solution to a clinical issue in which research was not necessary, such as process improvement initiatives, use the FADE method (Focus, Analyze, Develop, Execute and Evaluate) or nursing process (Problem, Goal, Intervention, Evaluation) to define the section content of the poster (Table 9–3, page 169).

Regardless of the information being presented—research results, QI data, or creative solutions to clinical problems—posters offer an opportunity to be colorful, creative, and concise in the presentation of information. General guidelines for poster composition, such as font size, headers, and layout, are listed in Table 9–4 (page 170).

Effective Oral Presentations for First-time Presenters

Oral presentations come in two basic configurations, short and long. The short version is a simple, brief presentation of the study and your results. This type is generally only 10 to 15 minutes in length and is not much more than a spoken rendition of the posters described in Table 9–2, and Figs. 9–4 and 9–5. Frequently, professional associations want to showcase a number of different research studies, and therefore the 10- to 15-minute presentation offers an opportunity for many people to present. These forums are for the purpose of sharing information and ideas. There isn't time to bore the audience; however,

EARLY CARDIAC ENZYME MARKERS:
TRANSITIONING INTO A NEW ERA FOR ACUTE ISCHEMIC HEART FAILURE

Bradi Granger, RN, MSN, Kristin Newby, MD, Tenita Sawyer, RN, BSN, Monica Harper, RN

Duke University Medical Center, Durham North Carolina

ABSTRACT

In the United States the difficulty of early diagnosis of MI has led to 1.6 million unnecessary hospital days and $600 million in hospital costs annually. In an attempt to expedite patient diagnosis and treatment and reduce unnecessary hospital charges many institutions are experimenting with the use of early serum enzyme markers. Troponin T, one of the most promising early cardiac markers, was evaluated in this trial. Two hundred and fifty patients who presented to the Chest Pain Program with complaints of low to moderate chest pain were evaluated. Troponin T levels were compared with concomitant samples of the standard cardiac enzyme marker, CK-MB. Functional study results and cardiac catheterization results were also collected. Preliminary analysis of these data suggest a strong correlation between positive Troponin T and positive coronary artery disease as measured by functional study (p=0.050) and cardiac catheterization (p=0.016).

OBJECTIVE

To determine the value of Troponin T testing in a low-moderate risk chest pain population, we evaluated the use of Troponin T and CK-MB in 439 consecutive patients assigned to our Chest Pain Unit during a nine month period.

METHODS

Sample:

Convenience sample, patient presenting to the ED with:

- Low-risk or atypical chest pain
- Negative ECG
- Negative CXR
- Negative initial total CK enzymes

METHODS cont.

Settings:

- Four dedicated beds on a cardiac telemetry unit
- Monitored beds, telemetry, pulse oximetry and O2
- Staffed by RN's

Design:

Single group, self used as control:

- Serial CK/CK-MB at 0, 4, 8, 12 hours
- Serial ECG testing at 0, 4, 8, 12 hours
- Troponin T testing at 0, 4, 8 hours
- Diagnostic testing and management at the discretion of cardiologist after rule-out MI protocol complete.

RESULTS

	Outcomes		
	Cardiac Catheterization		
	TnT + (n=19)	TnT - (n=72)	p = 0.003
CAD by cath	17 (89.5)	31 (43.1)	
0 vessel	2 (10.5)	41 (56.9)	
1 vessel	5 (26.3)	12 (16.7)	
2-3 vessel	12 (63.2)	19 (26.4)	

values are n (%)

False positive TnT by cath:

-hypertensive crisis; ESRD

OUTCOMES

- In a low moderate risk Chest Pain Unit population, Troponin T identified more patients with AMI and multivessel CAD than CK-MB.
- Use of Troponin T in the Chest Pain Unit could facilitate diagnosis, risk stratification and patient management.
- A positive Troponin T indicates a higher likelihood of underlying coronary artery disease.
- Further evaluation of the effect of Troponin T testing alone or in combination with other cardiac markers on patient management and outcomes, resource use and costs of care in Chest Pain Unit patients is warranted.

Concordance of Enzyme Marker Results

396 Patients — Concordance

CK-MB- N: 389 → TnT + N: 33 — 8.3%

TnT - N: 356 — 363 — 91.7%

CK-MB + N: 7 → TnT + N: 7 — 0%

TnT - N: 0

Figure 9-4. Sample research poster.

LIBRARY PROVIDES SUPPORT TO FAMILIES OF CARDIAC PATIENTS

Rebecca W. Johnson, RN, Gwynn B Sullivan, RN, MSN
Duke University Medical Center, Durham North Carolina

ABSTRACT

Supporting family members of patients is an integral part of health care. To increase this focus the Heart Center Patient Support Program performed a needs assessment to determine what could be done to improve the hospital experience for families of cardiac inpatients. Based on the results, a special room away from the main waiting areas was created and developed into an educational resource library. In the library, family members are able to read books, view video tapes and listen to audiocassettes with headphones, and use a computer with medline and web capabilities that will help them understand more about heart disease, risk factors, and treatment options. In addition, the library provides a comfortable room where families are able to have privacy for grieving, family conferences or counseling. The response of families for this alternative to traditional waiting areas has been overwhelmingly positive. Data will be presented which review utilization and outcomes of this supportive intervention for families of cardiac patients.

PROBLEMS

Distance frequently causes families of patients to be isolated from relatives and friends. Often family members spend their time at the hospital with limited support and few diversions other than television and the hospital cafeteria.

INTERVENTION

1) Needs assessment indicated desire for:
   Additional space away from waiting room
   Educational resources for varied literacy levels
   Diversion from long hours in the waiting room
2) Develop plan:
   Primary focus:
   - Library with educational resources
     - Material appropriate to literacy needs
     - Trained volunteers to provide assistance
   Secondary focus:
   - 24 hour access by clinicians and chaplains for counseling and family conferences
   - A quiet place away from the main area
3) Design and implement plan:
   Identify financial resources
   Acquire physical space and design library
   Compile library inventory:
   - Books on heart disease, stress management, humor and inspirational topics
   - Television, VCR, videos, headphones
   - Audiocassette players with headphones
   - Computer with medline and web capabilities
   Procure furniture:
   - Comfortable seating, desk, utility cabinet
   - Bookshelves, magazine rack, bulletin board
4) Identify and train volunteers:
   Train volunteers to identify resources to help families to cope with heart disease
   Schedule volunteers to staff library
5) Advertise library:
   Utilize flyers and the hospital newspaper
   Place signs in lobby and / or waiting rooms

OUTCOMES

1) Provided a valuable service for families:
   - 100% of families surveyed felt the library and volunteers helped them cope with their family member's hospital stay.
   - 100% of families surveyed felt the library helped them understand their family member's heart problems.
   - 90% of families surveyed felt it was helpful to have additional space to wait while a family member was in the hospital.
2) 136.5 volunteer hours supplied during the first five months
3) 129 family members visited the library during the first five months

RECOMMENDATIONS

1) Perform a needs assessment of families
2) Assess available resources:
   Space
   Money
   Coordinator
   Personnel
3) Develop and implement an individualized plan
4) Periodical reevaluation of needs

Figure 9–5. Sample creative solution poster.

Table 9–3	Content for Creative Solution Posters[a]		

| | Other Ways to Say the Same Thing | | |
Poster Component[b]	FADE[c]	Nursing Process	Creative Solution Content
1. Abstract			1. An 8½ × 11 inch copy of the abstract in 12-point type.
2. Problem statement	Focus	Problem	2. One or two sentences stating main problem or purpose of the project.
3. Background (traditional practice or past solutions, if any)	Analyze current situation	Goal as compared to current practice	3. Summarizes the purpose for doing the project.
4. Intervention or Methods	Develop	Intervention	4. This section may contain a bulleted sequence of intervention steps, then mounted copies of tools or instruments used.
5. Results or Outcomes of the intervention	Execute—results of execution	Results of intervention	5. Results of a creative solution project don't usually require statistical analysis. They simply describe behavior or practice pre- and postimplementation of the project. Graphs of % are often used.
6. Evaluation, Conclusion, Recommendations or Implications for practice.	Evaluate	Evaluation	6. A discussion of the benefits of the project to nursing practice or patient care. Recommendations for others who may be interested in doing a similar project are included.

[a]Refer to Fig. 9–4 for example of completed creative solution poster.
[b]Title boards for each section heading are bold.
[c]FADE is an acronym refering to a process for quality improvement or process improvement initiatives commonly used in business and healthcare organizations.

there is plenty of time to leave them feeling confused. The risk of talking too long about one thing and not long enough about a more important point is great! Keep the presentation very focused.

The first point of emphasis should be on presenting a clear and concise account of the research question (or hypothesis), methods (intervention) and results. The second point of emphasis saves approximately 15% to 25% of allocated time for discussing implications for practice. This discussion is very valuable to the listener and will leave a lasting impression of the study's significance.

As a general rule, time is *not* wisely spent discussing the details of the statistical analysis. Other than to state the tests that were preformed, nurses are gen-

Table 9–4	Typographic Guidelines for Posters

Typographic Guidelines for Posters

1. Avoid abbreviations, acronyms, and slang terms.

2. Type should be readable from at least four (4) feet.

3. A type font size of 24-point is desirable for easy reading at a distance of four (4) feet.

4. Use sentence case (Headline) lettering for ease of reading. ALL CAPITAL LETTERS IS DIFFICULT TO READ.

5. Use a consistent, clear, simple type style throughout.

6. Contrasting colors may be useful for emphasis and readability. The best six color combinations are:
   • Green on White
   • Red on White
   • Black on White
   • Blue on White
   • White on Blue
   • White on Black

7. Layout should flow naturally and logically for easy reading (left to right, or down columns).

8. Use color, figures, and tables to help clarify interventions and/or results. Make these graphics clear, with brief, self-explanatory legends.

9. On a standard 4 × 8 foot poster, the title board should be approximately 10 inches high with 2-inch lettering for the title and 1 inch for authors.

Adapted from the American Association of Critical Care Nurses (AACN) Guidelines for Poster Presentations, unpublished paper, Aliso Viejo, CA.

erally not conversant in "statistic-ese" and will not likely value the time spent discussing these details.

An extended version of the short presentation is the long one. "Long" is generally 30 to 50 minutes in length, and the expectation is for much more detail to be presented regarding methods, analysis, and results (Table 9–5). Long presentations offer the luxury of more time for each of these sections, but also pose a risk of getting both the presenter and the listener lost in superfluous information. Remember, stay on track!

Long presentations, like short ones, are greatly improved by including a solid discussion of implications for practice. If you can, stick with the 15% to 25% rule and give your audience a good dose of "What does this mean for me and my patients?"

The content that should be included in short and long oral presentations is similar to the content of a poster. When preparing for an oral presentation of your project, however, *don't stop with content!* Even a very intriguing study can be lost on an audience if the presentation style is boring or confusing. Likewise, a less interesting or negative study can be made far *more* interesting if well

Table 9–5	Content for Oral Presentations		
Short Presentations		**Long Presentations**	
Time	Content	Time	Content
00:00	Overview of the problem	00:00	Overview of the problem
00:02	(Brief background)	00:10	(Background—more detail)
00:03	Research Question	00:11	Research Question
00:08	Methods: • Design • Sample (population and setting) • Data Collection	00:26	Methods: • Design • Sample (population and setting) • Data Collection
00:12	Results	00:40	Results
00:15	Conclusions	00:50	Conclusions

Remember, as a general rule of thumb, one minute = one slide!

presented. Information that is well presented is more likely to be incorporated into clinical practice and may stimulate further research in the topic area.

Regardless of the length of your presentation, the most important points to remember when giving an oral presentation are (1) don't bore the audience and (2) practice, practice, practice!! Many an excellent research project has been misunderstood or misapplied because of poor presentation. The following section includes tips and suggestions originally intended for the folk art of story-telling. When used for preparing an oral presentation of research, a boring presentation of numbers and statistics can be transformed into an exciting drama—one that focuses the listener on the patient, the problem, and the application and implications of your work in practice.

Mastering the Story

The first step in an exciting presentation is mastery of the content so that you can talk about your experience like a story. There are two steps to mastery of the story: (1) defining the aim or purpose of the story, in this case, your research purpose, and (2) integration of the components of the story (research project), including how each component contributed to the final result or overall significance of the project.

DEFINING THE PURPOSE. Have a clear concept of the meaning you wish to convey with your story before beginning. Decide for yourself what the main point is that you wish the listener to walk away with. If there are areas of the research that are vague to you, there will be a corresponding loss of force when you relate the research to others. This means that you must have a firm grasp on the difficult details of your presentation, including understanding the analysis as well as the implications that can be derived from it. Even if the details of the analysis are not discussed, having a good understanding of how the analysis was derived will give you confidence when presenting the results.

INTEGRATION OF PROJECT COMPONENTS. Become thoroughly familiar with each component of the study. DON'T memorize your presentation, because this technique results in loss of spontaneity; however, DO have a thorough grasp of the study as a whole. This means understand clearly how the methods, design, and data-collection process contributed to decisions regarding analysis. And then be able to clearly articulate how all of these components together impact practice.

Also have a clear appreciation of the feelings that are to be stirred in the listener. In other words, review the key points and decide the tone your research carries. Were the results exciting? Were the implications for practice surprising? New or different? Was the process grueling and arduous because your team bit off more than they could chew? If so this may be valuable insight to the listener. Without being negative, convey your honest, sincere emotions when presenting the research experience.

ANALYZE THE STORY INTO ITS ELEMENTS. Once you have summarized the study as a whole, then work backward and identify the individual elements of the research experience. Decide what forms the climax of the presentation of the study, what events are necessary to pave the way for the climax, and decide on the order in which the events can be most effectively presented. Begin this process with an outline and identify the following:

- The beginning—to rouse interest
- The succession of events—must be orderly and complete
- The climax—to form the story's point
- The conclusion—"should leave the mind at rest"

Once the outline of these critical components is laid out, decide how the "story" or presentation of the study can be ended without detracting from the force of the climax. Likewise, decide how it can be begun in such a way as to arouse immediate interest without giving the climax away.

Giving the Story Form

Once the framework has been developed and the points of emphasis and interest identified, begin the practice phase. Write or tell the research experience to a friend with as much elaboration of the bare outline as is desirable. The purpose of this step is to test mastery of the content and to prepare the way for refinement and enrichment of both content and form.

Expansion for Emotional Effect

Next carefully delete any unessential information and then elaborate on essential features of the study. Improve the emotional effect of your presentation by adding touches of description, adding details of key points, telling anecdotes (if applicable), and adding any other details that will enhance effectiveness without obscuring the main point.

Visual Support

Once you decide on the verbal content, it's time to identify the content for slides or overhead transparencies. These visual aids should serve to emphasize the key messages of your presentation. General rules of thumb on the number of slides to use during an oral presentation are 1 slide for every 1 minute of your talk. Slides with a large amount of detail (for example, data or graphs) usually require more time for the audience to digest than a simple text slide.

The content of each slide or transparency should mirror your spoken words, following the general headings or components used in a research poster presentation (Table 9–2). Your institution's AV department can then translate your slide or transparency ideas into a professional-looking product.

Developing Presentation Skill

The final step prior to presentation is practice! Practice for familiarity with the study by telling the story of your research experience again and again. As one gains familiarity with the story, there is less self-consciousness evidenced in the presentation of the experience. Record yourself telling the story, then replay for self-evaluation. Time the length of your practice sessions to make sure you have not exceeded your time limits for the presentation.

Practice for improvement through reaction *to* the audience. One learns through practice to give oneself wholly to the story and *to the audience*. If you are less conscious of yourself, you are free to be more conscious of the response of the audience and can respond better to them. Practice *making it your own*. Personalize the research experience for effectiveness. The value of following such a plan is immeasurable and cannot be underestimated.

Tips for practicing presentations:
- Clearly define purpose for doing the study
- Present each component of the research as succinctly as possible
- Elaborate on essential features of the research selectively, for impact
- Discuss implications for practice for at least 25% of the allocated speaking time.
- Practice, practice, practice!!

Remember: " If motives are to be stirred....one can afford to honor his art and take such time and pains as are necessary to perfect his technique. Skill is nothing more than the possession of correct habits of procedure "

Edward Porter St. John

▶ JOURNALS: WRITING THE FINAL MANUSCRIPT

While writing the final paper can be an arduous process, it is extremely rewarding and is also one of the highest contributions one can make to his or her profession. A contribution to professional literature is lasting, widely available to peers, and efficient in terms of a comprehensive presentation of your work. A summary of steps for getting your work into print is depicted in Fig. 9–6. Getting started is frequently the most difficult step of all.

Ready, Set, . . . GO!

For many authors getting something on paper is not easy. There are a number of strategies for overcoming this initial barrier, but everyone is different and what works for someone else may not be helpful for you. Use whatever tricks work for you to get the initial paper rolling.

One tip is to use the proposal you wrote at the beginning of the research process as your starting block and work from there. Take each section of the proposal one by one and edit sections that need more detail or description. Remember, the reader will be uninitiated to much of the background informa-

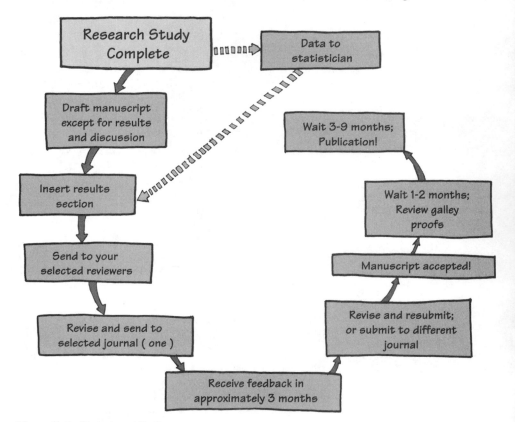

Figure 9–6. Steps to publication.

tion that led you to developing the study, so you'll probably need more detail in that section. As you are editing the protocol into a manuscript, change your major section heading titles to match the terms used in the journal to which you will be submitting. For example, in the protocol your "Materials and Methods" heading may need to be changed to "Study Procedures" if that is the title the journal uses for the section on how the study was done. Another editing tip is to change all the future tense verbs of the protocol to the past tense for the journal article.

A second method for getting started on your first draft is to talk out loud to yourself or to a friend, record the conversation, and later transcribe the spoken word into your word processor. Begin with discussing your rationale for doing the study, your methodology, the results, and implications for practice. There may be a few "holes" in your dictation, for example, if you are unable to thoroughly discuss the analysis. That's OK. Continue taping the entire "story," and when it is transferred to paper the holes can be filled in.

A third strategy for getting started with writing the final paper is to write the first and last sentence, then come back and fill in the middle. By getting the beginning ("why" you did it), and the end ("what" happened) on paper, it is then easier to work through the "how," which goes in the middle. Using this strategy can also make the task seem less lengthy, because the "end is in sight" so to speak.

Another strategy for getting started is to sit down at a word processor or with a pad of paper and simply start writing everything that comes to mind about the project. This method results in a regurgitation of your thoughts about the project that may or may not be in logical order. That is OK! You can come back later and organize the thoughts into logical order from beginning to end of the process. It is much easier to edit previously written content than to work with a blank page. Another suggestion is to always stop a working session in the middle of a thought. The concept of stopping in the middle of a thought makes re-starting much easier. Always jot down the thought that you stopped in the middle of so that the thought is not forgotten. Then when starting up again, simply jump back into that thought and go!

No matter which strategy you use, it's helpful to begin your writing on a word processor, if possible. Using a word processor from the outset saves much time when editing and rearranging content pieces. It also saves time in translating from paper to disk for final submission to the journal, as most journals require a disk copy eventually. It's also a good idea to follow the guidelines for manuscript preparation from the journal to which you will submit the manuscript from the beginning of your writing efforts.

Editing

Editing the initial draft will take several go-rounds by yourself and/or various members of your team. It is not uncommon to have 5 to 10 drafts prior to the manuscript being ready for submission to a journal. Before submission, at least one review by an "outside" reviewer, someone familiar with the topic but not a part of your specific project, is helpful to identify areas that need further editing. All editing by the authorship group should be complete prior to asking an outside reviewer to spend time reading the paper.

What exactly should you look for when editing? The following is a list of tips and suggestions to use when editing.[1] Refer to the list of references at the end of this chapter for more information on these and other tips for writing and editing your manuscript.

- Use the active voice. For example,

  "Patients rarely participate in self-care," in place of

  "Patients were not used to participate in self-care."

  Or

  "We assessed patient temperature by oral, rectal, tympanic, or core means," in place of,

  "In the ICU, patient temperature could be taken one of several ways, orally, rectally, tympanically or core."

- Don't use more words than necessary. Omit unnecessary or extra words such as "it is" or "there are" or "there is."

- Avoid empty phrases such as "on account of the fact that" or "in the event that."

- Avoid unnecessary adverbs and adjectives. These descriptors may be clutter.

- Avoid qualifiers such as "pretty" or "little" or "rather" or "quite."

- Use definite, specific, concrete language that calls up pictures in the reader's mind. For example, rather than "a period of unfavorable weather set in," write "it rained for four days straight."

- Use examples, anecdotes, analogies. Case studies use good descriptive prose.

- Avoid exaggeration. The reader won't believe you anyway.

- Use familiar, simple, concrete words and prefer the shorter word over the longer word.

- Avoid "nounification." For example, "The nurse provided assistance to the patient" should be changed to "The nurse assisted the patient."

- Avoid personification. For example, "the hospital provided" or "the hospital said." Remember that inanimate objects don't talk or act.

- Put statements in the positive form. Avoid *not*.

---

[1]Adapted from Elizabeth H. Winslow's presentation entitled "Effective writing: A key to advancement," 1997 National Teaching Institutue and Critical Care Exposition, Orlando, FL, May 1997.

- Have one central controlling idea in the paper and stick with it throughout; don't wander.

- Use first person.

- Write about something you know and are passionate about.

- Use a hook sentence. The first and most important sentence should be the best one and should draw the reader in.

- The ending is the second most important sentence. The last sentence should take the reader by surprise if possible. Though this is not always realistic with research manuscripts, it is a refreshing finale to a scientific paper! Consider creative ways to jazz up the implications for practice based on your own research experience.

Timeliness and Expectations

When beginning the writing process don't make the mistake of setting unreasonable expectations, for either yourself or the publisher. In any manuscript submission process a number of small steps must occur before the final product is ready for publication. As noted in Fig. 9–6, even after the manuscript is written and reviewed on your end, it must still be formally reviewed by reviewers selected by the journal editors. When an editor receives the manuscript it generally takes 2 weeks before it is sent out to reviewers. These reviewers are then given 6 to 10 weeks to submit comments back to the editor, at which point the editor must compile and collate comments from all reviewers and send those comments back to you. As you can see, 3 to 4 months is not unreasonable for a manuscript to be "in review" with a given journal.

Table 9–6	The Most Common Reasons for Manuscript Rejection

- Poorly written—most common
- Poorly developed idea
- Term paper style
- Not consistent with purpose of journal
- Method problems
- Content undocumented
- Content inaccurate
- Content not important
- Clinically not applicable

Adapted from Elizabeth H. Winslow's presentation entitled "Effective writing: A key to advancement," 1997 National Teaching Institutue and Critical Care Exposition, Orlando, FL, May 1997.

When you *finally* receive comments back from the editor, the ball is again in your court. At this point you may be so discouraged with the task of revising that it will take a while to get started. This is common! Even if the recommended changes are relatively minor, you most likely worked hard to get the manuscript "perfect" and you may feel offended at the thought of changing it. Recognize that it is rare *not* to receive recommendations for changes; then jump in!

The most common reasons for rejection of a manuscript are listed in Table 9–6. Note that the most common reason for rejection is poor writing. Refer back to the tips for editing above and make sure that all bases have been covered in terms of stylistic accuracy. Give yourself a deadline for completing revisions. A more exciting trick might be to "reward" yourself once the changes have been made and the revised manuscript has been resubmitted. Choose any reward, but choose something valuable enough to make you work! Once the final product is in print, you and your readers will be glad you persevered.

▶ AUTHORSHIP

As has been discussed a number of times in previous chapters, authorship can be an opportunity for recognition and reward, or an area for potential conflict. Manuscripts, posters, and oral presentations should be seen as an opportunity to acknowledge and reward all the members of the working group. Though all participants can't be first author on everything, the following strategies should be employed to recognize everyone:

- Rotate the spotlight by presenting at various meetings and allowing different people a turn at presentation.
- Include a section on the poster, or first or last slide of a presentation, that lists all team members or contributors.
- Publish several papers from one project, each focusing on a different aspect or outcome of the study.

See Chapter 4 for other suggestions on authorship and recognition of contributors to the project.

▶ REFERENCES

You may want to contact your specialty nursing organizations for any unpublished documents they may have to assist with abstract writing and manuscript publication.

Linquist R, Beecroft P. Writing Research Abstracts Successfully, 2nd ed. Aliso Viejo, CA: American Association of Critical-Care Nurses, 1992.

Lippman D, Ponton D. Designing a research poster with impact. Western Journal of Nursing Research 1989;11(4):477–485.

Rempusheski V. Resources necessary to prepare a poster for presentation. Applied Nursing Research 1990;3:134–137.

Sexton D. Presentation of research findings: The poster session. Nursing Research 1984;33:374–375.

Strunk W, White E. The Elements of Style, 3rd ed. New York: Macmillan, 1979.

Tournquist E, Funk S, Champagne M. Writing research reports for clinical audiences. Western Journal of Nursing Research 1989;11(5):576–582.

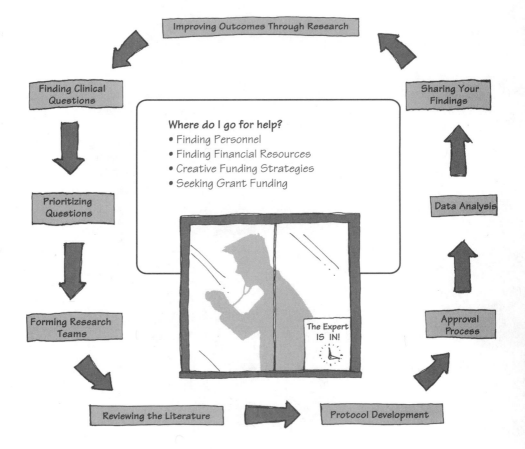

Improving Outcomes Through Research

Finding Clinical Questions

Sharing Your Findings

Where do I go for help?
- Finding Personnel
- Finding Financial Resources
- Creative Funding Strategies
- Seeking Grant Funding

Prioritizing Questions

Data Analysis

Forming Research Teams

The Expert IS IN!

Approval Process

Reviewing the Literature

Protocol Development

10

Finding Resources
to Support Research

Critical to your success with nursing research will be your ability to identify and secure essential resources to support the research process. Two major types of resources will likely be required by you at some time during your study: personnel and/or financial resources.

▶ FINDING PERSONNEL RESOURCES TO SUPPORT RESEARCH

No one can know *everything* about how to do research. Even experienced researchers need assistance in various phases of their research projects. And the neophyte researcher will also probably need a mentor to guide her/him through the research maze. What if you don't have a "research expert" at your facility to advise you along the way? Where will you find these folks to help on your research studies?

First, it's important to determine what type of assistance you need (Table 10–1). If you have never done research before, you'll probably need an individual who can provide guidance or mentoring through the entire research process. This research mentor would be someone who could help you organize the approach to the project, anticipate problems, suggest experts to assist you in specific areas, and in general help with problem solving during the entire process. The research mentor should have prior research experience and be willing to provide long-term guidance.

Regardless of your level of research expertise, you will also need assistance in specific aspects of the research process (Table 10–1). Unlike the research mentor, this individual provides focused, time-limited consultation on an area in which he/she is a content expert. For example, help from a statistician may be

Table 10–1	Sources of Research Expertise	
Type of Assistance	**Individuals to Contact**
Research Mentors	Nurses in your facility with research experience (Clinical Nurse Specialist [CNS], educator, manager, staff)
	Nurses with research experience at other local facilities
	Faculty in schools of nursing who have worked with you in the past
	Other professionals with research experience (physicians, pharmacists, etc)
	Content experts outside your local area (authors of previous studies or articles on topic, or experts from your nursing organization)
Specific Research Expertise	
Selection of research questions	CNS with clinical expertise in the content area of your study
	Experts in content area
Research methods and proposal development	CNS or faculty in school of nursing
Sample size calculations	Statistician or simple computer programs for calculating sample sizes
Statistics	Statistician or faculty in school of nursing
Investigational review process	Guidelines from your institutional review board
	Member of nursing research committee
	Nursing administrator
Data entry and analysis	Quality assurance/Continuous quality improvement specialist in your facility
	Faculty in school of nursing
	Finance office personnel
	Nursing administration personnel
Preparation of final report, manuscripts, and presentations	Colleagues with presentation/publishing experience
	Faculty in school of nursing
	Physicians

required to determine the sample size of the study. Or you may need assistance getting the manuscript prepared for publication. These individuals should have expertise in that specific area and be willing to provide consultation on a one-time, short-duration project.

Although having individuals who either work in your facility or live in your local area would be ideal, it is also possible to tap into the expertise of those who live far away. Much of the consultation that you need could actually be done very efficiently by telephone, mail, and/or electronic file transfer. In fact, sometimes you may find that the advantages of working with someone who is an expert in your particular research area far outweigh the disadvantages of distance. Finding these "experts" at first may seem overwhelming, but use your local contacts and ask, "Who do you know either locally or nationally who is an expert in this?" or call one of the authors of a previous research study. You may find that authors would be happy to share their expertise with you or may be able to suggest other experts in the area for you to contact.

Another approach to finding research expertise is to collaborate with colleagues at other institutions to do a multisite study. This will increase the options you have for gaining research expertise and improve your networking opportunities. For example, if you are interested in researching chemotherapy-induced nausea and vomiting, oncology nurses at other local institutions could be contacted to determine their interest in participating in a nausea/vomiting research project. You might also contact your local or national specialty nursing organization to determine if other individuals or institutions might be interested in a collaborating relationship.

▶ GUIDELINES FOR ESTABLISHING EXPECTATIONS WITH OTHERS

To avoid misunderstandings later, it is a good idea to clearly spell out expectations that you have of the individuals with whom you will be working early in your relationship (Table 10–2). Whether expectations are clarified in writing and/or verbally will vary with the type of groups or individuals with whom you work. Key, though, will be to establish what everyone's expectations are and to set some ground rules on handling any issues or concerns that may develop in the future.

To begin with, it is important to clearly delineate the role that you want the individual to play in your project. What is the specific contribution the individ-

Table 10–2	Guidelines for Establishing Expectations With Others

Discuss each of the following aspects of project involvement:
- Role of individual in project (specific task to be completed, time commitment)

- Process to be used for decision making

- Reason for individual's involvement in project and what she/he would like to get out of involvement

- Authorship of articles and presentation of findings at meetings

- Process to use for ongoing communication of issues and concerns

ual will make to the project and what, if any, are the boundaries or limitations of his/her participation? What are the time commitments related to the project, both in terms of deadlines and time estimates for completion of their portion of the project? For example, the statistician may be asked to provide information on two items: the sample size calculation and suggestion for data analysis. You estimate that it will involve four hours of his/her time and would expect the information within one month of your providing him/her with the draft protocol. For a research mentor, you may want to consult approximately once a month for one hour plus whenever any unusual situations arise. In addition, you would like them to review the protocol two or three times prior to submission for approval at your facility.

It is also important to discuss what processes will be used to make decisions about the project. Will the individual have any decision-making power in the research project or be primarily a consultant, with other individuals making final decisions? Will final decisions be made by one individual after input from group members or will decisions be made by group consensus?

Another area that is crucial to discuss is what others want to achieve from their participation in the group. Everyone has different driving forces for getting involved in various projects and activities. Asking what participants hope to achieve by participating in this project will do a lot to avoid any potential disappointments later if those expectations are unrealistic. Some individuals agree to participate to meet a job expectation, say to meet a clinical ladder requirement or for faculty tenure. Others may get involved out of professional interest and commitment to the particular area of research.

No matter what the level of participation in the research project, it is imperative to discuss expectations surrounding publication authorship and presentation of research findings with everyone at the beginning. For many individuals, particularly faculty members, the ability to co-author publications may be an extremely important outcome of their involvement in the project. Be clear on whether that is a realistic expectation or not. Also, you may want to discuss where, in the ordering of authors, you anticipate the placement of their name and to what journal you anticipate submitting the manuscript. It is best to have authorship discussions with each member of your project at the beginning of the project, not at the time the manuscript is being drafted. Similar discussion should also take place about presenting the study results at national or local professional meetings. Discussions should focus on how decisions will be made about where data will be presented and by whom. What involvement, if any, do you anticipate each participant will have in data presentations?

Once you've discussed individual expectations, it's often a good idea to put the agreements in writing, for example in meeting minutes. That way if conflicts arise later about one of the agreements, for example authorship, the written record will help everyone's fuzzy memory on the discussion that may have taken place 6 to 12 months earlier.

▶ FINDING FINANCIAL RESOURCES FOR RESEARCH

The availability of research funds, at both the national and local level, is so limited at the present time that it behooves researchers to carefully consider the issue of research funds right from the beginning of the project. It is not uncommon for at least 20 to 30 grant applications to be submitted for every grant that receives funding. Given those odds, it's only prudent to consider that the likelihood you will be funded to do research is quite low, even if you have a very good research study. Those odds are further reduced if you've had limited, or no, experience with the grant applications process or have never done research before.

The best approach to the issue of finding funding for research is to design a study that does not require additional funds. That way, you won't have to spend the time and energy applying for research funds and risk not being able to do the study if you do not receive funding.

You might ask, though, how can I do research without research funds? First, the issue of funding should be considered during the time you are considering the feasibility of a particular research project. If the proposed study will require funds to support it, you may want to chose a different research topic. Or you might be able to redesign the study so that it does not require funds.

Typically, research funds are required for one or more of the following items: purchase of equipment; salary of data collectors; statistical consultation; photocopying and mailing of surveys; salary of typists or data entry personnel. The key to avoiding the need for research funds is to design your protocol so you don't need money for these items. This can be accomplished by using creative financing strategies! Here are just a couple of suggestions of ways to avoid the need to obtain research funds:

Equipment

- Design your protocol to use equipment currently used in patient care or that can be borrowed from other departments. For example, you might be able to borrow or use a water bath from the chemistry laboratory or the biomedical engineering department if your study requires that to verify thermometer accuracy. Or if you need to measure skin resistance for a study examining ECG signal quality for different types of ECG electrodes, the biomedical engineers may have a device that could be used rather than purchasing a device.

- Ask the company that makes the required equipment if they have a special program for short-term lending for research or clinical trial situations. Many manufacturers will be happy to lend a device to support your study if there is a possibility that your institution may purchase the equipment if the results support long-term use.

- Consider renting the equipment you need if it can't be borrowed. This is usually a cheaper approach for short-term studies. Investigate whether there are any companies in your area that specialize in medical equipment rental.

Salary for Personnel

- Design your procedures for data collection so they can fit into your normal clinical practice routines. Then staff on the unit can actually be collecting data at the same time they are doing their usual patient care. For example, if vital signs are normally obtained every 2 to 4 hours, design your data-collection times for blood pressure measurements at the same interval.

- Streamline your data-collection procedures so it can be done in a 10- to 20-minute block of time. That way, staff who are collecting data for the study can get coverage from another team member for their patient care responsibilities while they do data-collection. If staff cover each other for breaks, meals, and other meetings, why not use the same process for data collection?

- Use a spreadsheet or database software program for data entry that is easy to use and can be loaded on a computer that the investigators have easy access to. This will eliminate having to pay someone to input data. If data input is done throughout the data-collection period, much of the pain of data entry can be alleviated.

- Consider use of an automated data-entry process if that technology exists in your institution (see Chapter 8, Data Analysis, Automated Data Entry Systems).

Statistical Consultation

- Talk with individuals in the mathematics or statistics department or the school of nursing (faculty or graduate students) about the feasibility of trading services: their statistical expertise for inclusion in any final publications and/or associate investigator status on the study (see also Chapter 8, Data Analysis, Finding Statistical Expertise).

Miscellaneous Creative Funding Strategies

- Hospital volunteer programs might have money to donate for the purchase of specific equipment or services.

- Administrative support of the research study as a CQI project may be available if the study addresses methods to potentially improve patient outcomes and/or costs. For example, a research study that compares two different methods for femoral sheath removal after cardiac catheterization (the current technique and a new approach) may have the potential to decrease length of stay and costs associated with sheath removal. The administrative group may be very willing to provide monies for study support if there is a potential of cost savings to the organization.

- Solicit support from community resources, such as businesses or churches, that have a strong connection to the hospital. The support may be in the form of money to buy equipment or the lending of equipment, for example a computer and software, to help support your study.

- Ask hospital departments to provide any laboratory tests you need without charge to support the study. By including members of that department on your research team from the beginning, gaining support from the department will really not be very difficult. Another approach is just to discuss the study and its importance to the head of the department and request that all research specimens be processed without charge. For example, if arterial blood gases are needed for a study, the respiratory therapy department could be approached early in the study development to become co-investigators. The issue of getting support for required blood gases will not seem so daunting with respiratory therapy department buy-in for the study.

- Solicit schools of nursing at local universities to donate faculty expertise and/or statistical support for the project. Given the tremendous clinical site support given by many service agencies to academic programs in nursing today, it would seem that some type of arrangement would be negotiated for a sharing of resources.

▶ TIPS FOR SEEKING FUNDING FROM GRANTS

As previously discussed, seeking grant monies is far from a sure-bet method of ensuring financial support for your research study. Sources of grants for clinical research are numerous and include federal agencies, national foundations, and professional associations (Table 10–3). If you do decide, though, to pursue this approach, the following are some helpful suggestions or tips to maximize your chances of success:

- Get someone with grant-writing expertise to assist you in the grant-application process.

- Gain some insight into the types of studies that have been previously funded by the granting agency and why. By talking to individuals at the granting agency or members of previous review groups, you can gain valuable information to assist in your decision of whether your study is well suited to the grant purpose.

- Clearly identify in your grant proposal the match between your research

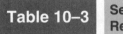

Table 10–3	Selected Sources of Grant Funding for Clinical Research Studies

Federal Government

- National Institutes of Health, Department of Health and Human Services, particularly the National Institute of Nursing Research

- Agency for Health Care Policy and Research, Department of Health and Human Services

- National Institutes of Health, Guide for Grants and Contracts, Office of Extramural Research and Training, Bldg. 1, Room 111, NIH, Bethesda, MD 20892

National Organizations/Foundations

- Professional organizations (particularly specialty nursing organizations)

- Sigma Theta Tau International, Indianapolis, IN

- National Guide to Foundation Funding in Health, published by The Foundation Center (800-424-9836)

- Directory of Biomedical and Health Care Grants, The Orxyz Press, 2214 N. Central at Encanto, Phoeniz, AZ 85004

- Grantsmanship Center, 1091 South Grant Avenue, Los Angeles, CA 90015

Local Groups

- State nursing associations and specialty nursing organizations

- Businesses in your local community

- Local universities

topic and the objectives or purpose of the grant for which you are applying. Example: a study on nursing interventions to decrease chemotherapy-induced nausea and vomiting would be well targeted for an Oncology Nursing Society grant rather than a grant from the American Association of Critical-Care Nurses.

- Follow the guidelines for proposal submission carefully. Do not improvise or submit proposals in formats used for other purposes (ie, your IRB). If the guidelines say five pages, single-spaced with Courier font no smaller than 10 point, keep to those instructions. If the reviewer guidelines are included in your grant application information, have a colleague rate your study using those criteria before you submit the study and make necessary changes to the proposal.

- Succinctly present your proposal. This is not the time to write an extensive review of the literature! Try to synthesize as much of that information as possible so the proposal can be quickly read by a reviewer. There should be a logical flow of ideas/thoughts so that the reviewer with limited experience in that content area will be able to comprehend the importance of the study and its design. The most important aspect of your grant proposal is a methodologically sound research study.

- If you have minimal experience writing grants, plan four to six revisions of your proposal before submitting it to the funding agency. Be sure to have informal critiques periodically by your colleagues and experts in the content area.

Once a grant application is submitted, it may be 6 to 9 months before you are advised about whether your proposal was funded. And if the study is not funded, then another grant application will need to be written and submitted, which could mean an addition 6 to 12 months' delay. Though this length of time may be typical, you need to consider that members of the research group may lose interest in the project during the waiting period. This is particularly true if you have designed a study that cannot be done without funding from an outside group. Group members must carefully consider this potential negative impact prior to selecting a topic for research. As was discussed in Chapter 3, Prioritizing Clinical Questions, whether additional funding is required should be taken into consideration in the ranking of potential research questions.

▶ REFERENCES

Campbell G, Chulay M. Establishing a clinical nursing research program. In: Spicer J, Robinson MA, eds. Environmental Management in Critical Care Nursing. Baltimore: Williams & Wilkins, 1990, pages 52–60.

Coeling H. Limiting the indirect cost of research in healthcare institutions. Applied Nursing Research 1993;6(2):92–97.

Holland P. A model research grant proposal. Gastroenterology Nursing 1990;13(2): 17S–22S.

Ludington-Hoe S, Swinth J. A successful long-distance research collaboration. Applied Nursing Research 1996;9(4):219–924.

Martin P. Clinical settings need organizational support for research. Applied Nursing Research 1993;6(2):103–104.

Redeker N. Critical care nursing research: Opportunities and resources. American Journal of Critical Care 1994;3(2):139–144.

Winkler V, Hirtzel-Trexler B. Tips from consultants . . . monies to support a nursing research program in service settings. Journal of Nursing Administration 1994;24(4):4.

Wujcik D. Foundation grants provide important funds for new and experienced researchers' work: Oncology Nursing Foundation. Oncology Nursing Society News 1993;8(11):9.

Protocol Examples

Clinical Evaluation of ECG Electrode Performance Over Time

Principal Investigator

Becky McBurney, RN, BSN

Associate Investigators

Kay Anderson, RN, BSN   Ok Sook Heath, RN, BSN
April Bower, RN, BSN   Robyn Lance, RN, BSN
Noreen Giganti, RN, BSN   Patti Magno, RN, BSN
Cindy Gottschalk, RN

PRECIS

ECG monitoring is commonly used to assess cardiac response to various disease processes and medical therapies. A clear ECG signal is essential to correctly identify dysrhythmias and ensure therapeutic management. The purpose of this study is to evaluate the signal quality of different ECG electrodes over a 72-hour period. Adults who require ECG monitoring with continuous visual observation will be monitored with five different, randomly assigned ECG electrodes. ECG signal quality, skin integrity, cost, and patient comfort will be evaluated at intervals over a 72-hour period. Data will be summarized with descriptive statistics and analyzed with multivariate techniques.

SCIENTIFIC JUSTIFICATION

Previous studies on ECG signal quality have focused on different skin preparation techniques but not on different types of electrodes. Though individual manufacturers claim improved performance with their brand of electrodes, no data have been published to support this claim. Because the cost of electrodes does vary greatly, evaluation of electrode performance is important to justify product selection for clinical use.

Despite the frequency of ECG monitoring, very few studies have been done examining the clarity of the ECG signal. To date, five studies have evaluated the impact of different skin-preparation techniques prior to ECG electrode placement on signal quality.[1-5] Two of the studies compared alcohol to two different types of commercial skin-preparation products, using abrasive and nonabrasive techniques.[1,4] These studies were conducted in normal volunteers and used the forearms for electrode placement. Measurements of offset potential were obtained shortly after electrode placement. Minimal differences in offset potential were found betweeen the three skin-preparation techniques. Limitations of these studies included inappropriate statistical analysis, lack of an adequate control group (offset potential with no skin preparation), inadequate duration of electrode placement prior to offset potential measurement, and ECG sites that are not consistent with clinical practice.

One study examined the use of a sandpaper-like abrasive substance and compared different amounts of skin sanding (from 10 to 100 strokes).[3] Skin impedance was said to decrease with the use of an abrasive, reaching maximal reductions at 20 strokes. Some skin irritation was noted with the abrasive technique. Limitations of this study included poor description of methods and lack of control of the independent variable.

Previous studies of ECG electrode performance have examined only one aspect of ECG signal quality (offset potential) and have not considered other variables that have impact on performance. Factors such as patient comfort and skin integrity also need to be evaluated. ECG electrodes that cause discomfort or disrupt skin integrity may result in increased motion artifact during monitoring. This can impede dysrhythmia identification and/or cause false alarms. Another area that has not been evaluated is ECG electrode performance over time. Though ECG performance may be adequate immediately after application, monitoring for dysrhythmias usually continues over a 24- to 72-hour period. As electrode duration increases, there is a deterioration of adhesive qualities, conductive media efficiency, and skin integrity, which may decrease ECG signal quality. Finally, the initial cost of various electrodes and time expenditure in applying and replacing electrodes need to be considered when evaluating ECG performance. Our study proposes to evaluate several different types of ECG electrodes, incorporating all the ECG monitoring variables of importance for clinical practice.

Research Hypotheses. In patients who require continuous ECG monitoring:

1. There will be a significant difference in ECG signal quality over time among different types of ECG electrodes.
2. There will be a significant difference in patient comfort over time among different types of ECG electrodes.
3. There will be a significant difference in skin integrity over time among different types of ECG electrodes.
4. There will be a significant difference in cost over time among different types of ECG electrodes.

Definition of Terms. The following terms serve to define the variables of this study:

1. ECG Electrodes. ECG electrodes provide the electrical interface between

the patient's skin surface and the ECG monitoring system. Features of the electrode, such as adhesive, connector, shape, and conduction medium, differ based on the manufacturer's specifications. For the purposes of this study, the following five types of electrodes will be evaluated:

Type A: A carbon-based ECG electrode (Carbo Cone M-55, Lynn Medical Instrument Co, Bloomfield Hills, MI)

Type B: A silver chloride–based ECG electrode (Clear Trace 1710-001, Medronics Andover Medical, Haverhill, MA)

Type C: A silver chloride–based ECG electrode (Conmed 111-3864, Conmed Corp, Utica, NY)

Type D: A silver chloride–based ECG electrode (Blue Sensor R-00-5, Medicotest, Lynchburg, NY)

Type E: A silver chloride–based ECG electrode (Meditrace 3601, Buffalo, NY)

2. Signal Quality. Signal quality is the clarity of the graphic tracing of the ECG. For the purposes of this study, signal quality will be defined as the offset potential (mV) across an electrode pair as measured by a digital multimeter (Appendix A). In addition, signal quality will be defined as the signal-to-noise ratio on a graphic ECG tracing (Appendix B).

3. Patient Comfort. Patient comfort is a state of mind and body with freedom from pain and anxiety. For the purposes of this study, patient comfort will be evaluated with a visual analog scale (Appendix C).[6]

4. Skin Integrity. Skin integrity is the condition of the body's protective barrier. For the purposes of this study, skin integrity will be the description of skin condition at the contact site of the ECG electrode (Appendix D).

MATERIALS AND METHODS

Study Design.   This is an experimental, comparative study examining different types of ECG electrodes over time. The independent variable for this study is the types of ECG electrodes. Dependent variables include ECG signal quality, skin integrity, cost, and patient comfort. Five types of ECG electrodes will be randomly assigned to one of five positions on the chest wall.

Sample Selection.   The target population is patients requiring continuous ECG monitoring. The sample for this study will consist of 40 adult patients under the age of 65 years who require continuous ECG monitoring. Criteria for exclusion from the study include the following:

1. Altered skin integrity at the ECG electrode placement site.
2. Hair at the electrode placement sites.
3. Allergy or sensitivity to adhesives.
4. Application of creams or lotions to the chest wall within the last 8 hours.

Sample size was determined using power analysis for ANOVA with $\alpha = 0.05$, $1 - \beta = 0.80$, effect size of 0.25 and 5 groups.[7]

Data Collection. The following procedures will be carried out for all adult patients who meet the study criteria:

1. Eligible subjects will be approached to participate in the study, and informed consent will be obtained by one of the investigators.
2. Obtain demographic data (Appendix E).
3. A computer-generated randomization scheme will assign the five types of electrodes to the electrode locations on the chest wall.
4. Measure skin integrity and patient comfort at electrode sites prior to placement.
5. Apply ECG monitor electrodes using a standardized electrode placement technique (Appendix F). Connect the ECG cable with alligator clips to the electrodes.
6. Measurements of offset potential, signal-to-noise ratio, and patient comfort will be made 5 minutes after electrode application and every 12 hours thereafter using standardized techniques (Appendix A through D) for 72 hours. During the measurement of offset potential and signal-to-noise ratio the monitoring ECG cable will be removed.
7. At the end of the 72 hours, electrodes will be removed and skin at that site will be assessed with the skin integrity scale (Appendix E). If early removal of electrode is required, skin at that site will be assessed using the skin integrity scale at that time.
8. At the completion of the study, a new set of electrodes will be reapplied for routine monitoring purposes.

DATA ANALYSIS

Data will be analyzed for all subjects with 24 hours or more of continuous ECG monitoring. Data will be summarized with descriptive statistics. Analysis of variance (ANOVA) for repeated measures will be used to determine if there is a difference in ECG signal quality, skin irritation, and patient comfort between each of the ECG electrode types. Scheffe's multiple comparison test will be used to identify specific group differences. The level of significance for all tests will be $p < 0.05$.

HAZARDS AND PRECAUTIONS, DISCOMFORTS, INCONVENIENCES

ECG monitoring represents the standard and practice for inpatients undergoing cardiac evaluation. Some patients experience discomfort from electrodes placed on skin for cardiac monitoring. Concurrent placement of a second set of electrodes for study purposes may cause additional discomfort. Participation in this study may cause inconvenience due to increased time spent on data collection. Patients will receive no direct benefit from participation in this study.

ETHICAL CONSIDERATIONS AND PROVISIONS/INFORMED CONSENT

No dose or therapeutic modification will occur because of participation in this study. Confidentiality of the patient will be assured and informed consent will be obtained based on NIH guidelines for the Protection of Human Subjects (Appendix G).

REFERENCES

1. Medina V, Clochesy JM, Omery A. Comparison of electrode site preparation the techniques. Heart & Lung 1989;18:456–460.
2. Thakor NV, Webster JG. Electrode studies for the long-term ambulatory ECG. Medical & Biological Engineering & Computing 1985;23:116–121.
3. Patterson RP. The electrical characteristics of some commercial ECG electrodes. Journal of Electrocardiology 1978;11:23–26.
4. Clochesy JM, Cifani L, Howe K. Electrode site preparation techniques: A follow-up study. Heart & Lung 1991;20:27–30.
5. Tam HW, Webster JG. Minimizing motion artifact by skin abrasion. IEEE Transactions on Biomedical Engineering 1977;24:134–139.
6. Lee KA, Kieckhefer GM. Technical notes measuring human response using visual analogue scales. Western Journal of Nursing Research 1989;11:128–132.
7. Cohen J. Statistical Power Analysis for the Behavioral Sciences. New York: Academic Press, 1977.

APPENDIX A
Offset Potential

Offset potential across each of the electrode pairs will be measured with a digital multimeter.

1. Disconnect one of the monitor lead wires from the patient's primary electrode.
2. Connect the positive multimeter lead wire to the primary electrode and the multimeter lead wire to the reference electrode.
3. Record the digital display of the multimeter during a period of stability.
4. Remove the multimeter lead wires and reconnect the monitor lead wire to the patient's primary electrode.
5. Repeat steps 1 to 4 for each pair of the five pairs of electrodes.
6. Repeat offset potential measurement procedure every 12 hours for 72 hours.

APPENDIX B
Signal-to-Noise Ratio

1. Position the patient supine with the head of the bed at a 20 to 30 degree angle.
2. Remove the monitor lead wires from the primary electrodes and connect to the reference electrodes.
3. Using the Page Writer™ 12 Lead ECG machine, connect the limb leads according to manufacturer's instructions.
4. Attach the chest leads (V_{1-5}) to the study electrodes in the following order:
   - V_1 Right arm electrode
   - V_2 Left arm electrode
   - V_3 Right leg electrode
   - V_4 Left leg electrode
   - V_5 MCL_1 electrode
5. Obtain the 12 Lead ECG analysis following manufacturer's instructions during a period when the patient is immobile.
6. Reconnect the monitor lead wires to the primary electrodes from the reference electrodes.
7. On the ECG printout, label each of the V leads with its corresponding ECG electrode type.
8. Calculations of the signal-to-noise ratio will be made by two independent observers. The two results will be averaged to determine the final signal-to-noise ratio. Use the following procedure:
   a. Measure the QRS amplitude (mm) for the right arm electrode (V_1). See example below.
   b. Measure the amplitude of the highest artifact wave between the QRS measured and the next QRS waveform. No artifact is equal to 0.
   c. Divide the QRS amplitude by the artifact amplitude to derive the signal to noise ratio:

$$SNR = \frac{QRS \ amplitude}{Artifact \ amplitude}$$

   d. Repeat steps a to c for each electrode, using the QRS complex that occurred at the same time as the QRS complex measured in step a.

APPENDIX C
SKIN COMFORT SCALE

Periodically during this study you will be asked to rate your feelings of skin irritation at the location of your ECG electrode sites. You will be presented with a series of lines like the line below and asked to place a vertical mark through the line that corresponds to how each ECG electrode site feels.

This line represents the way your skin feels. No irritation is like your normal skin and the most skin irritation imaginable is like an unbearable sunburn. To indicate your level of skin irritation place a vertical mark through the line. Marking at the left end indicates you feel no skin irritation, marking at the right end indicates you feel the most irritation imaginable, and marking in the middle indicates you have moderate irritation. Place a mark where your skin irritation is right now.

FOR EXAMPLE:
How do you feel right now?

_____

No   Most Irritation
Irritation   Imaginable

How does the skin under the ECG patch on your **RIGHT SHOULDER** feel right now?

_____

No   Most Irritation
Irritation   Imaginable

How does the skin under the ECG patch on your **LEFT SHOULDER** feel right now?

_____

No   Most Irritation
Irritation   Imaginable

How does the skin under the ECG patch on your **RIGHT ABDOMEN** feel right now?

_____

No   Most Irritation
Irritation   Imaginable

How does the skin under the ECG patch on your **LEFT ABDOMEN** feel right now?

_____

No   Most Irritation
Irritation   Imaginable

How does the skin under the ECG patch in the **MIDDLE OF YOUR CHEST** feel right now?

_____

No   Most Irritation
Irritation   Imaginable

APPENDIX D
SKIN INTEGRITY SCALE

1 = YES 2 = NO	PRE ELECTRODE PLACEMENT					POST ELECTRODE REMOVAL				
	RA	LA	RL	LL	V1	RA	LA	RL	LL	V1
Date/time of assessment										
No abnormalities at electrode site										
Abnormalities at electrode site:										
Redness										
Blisters										
Rash										
Bleeding										
Scraped/abraded skin										
Miscellaneous findings (please describe below)										

APPENDIX E
IMC ECG ELECTRODE STUDY DATA COLLECTION TOOL

Name: _____

Age: ____ years

Sex: ___ (1 = male, 2 = female)

Ethnic origin: ____

Medical Dx: _____

_____

Electrode Assignment:

    RA ___ LA ___ RL ___ LL ___ V_1 ___

Length of Electrode Adherence:

    RA ___ LA ___ RL ___ LL ___ V_1 ___

Ht: _____ inches Wt: __ kg.   BSA:

Skin type: Dry Oily Moist Thin Thick

No lotion/cream application in the 8 hours prior to electrode application:
        NO   YES (if yes, not eligible at this time).

HOURS SINCE APPLICATION

Variables	0	12	24	36	48	60	72
Clock Time							
Electrode A:							
Offset potential							
Signal-to-noise ratio							
Irritation scale							
Skin integrity scale[a]							
Electrode B:							
Offset potential							
Signal-to-noise ratio							
Irritation scale							
Skin integrity scale[a]							
Electrode C:							
Offset potential							
Signal-to-noise ratio							
Irritation scale							
Skin Integrity scale[a]							
Electrode D:							
Offset potential							
Signal-to-noise ratio							
Irritation scale							
Skin integrity scale[a]							
Electrode E:							
Offset potential							
Signal-to-noise ratio							

Variables	0	12	24	36	48	60	72
Irritation scale							
Skin integrity scale[a]							
Miscellaneous							
Temperature > 38.0							
Diaphoretic							

[a]Measurements for these variables occur just prior to electrode application and 10 minutes after electrode removal.

APPENDIX G
SKIN PREPARATION & ELECTRODE PLACEMENT

1. The following five sites will be used for skin preparation and electrode placement. There will be two electrodes at each site, one as the primary (monitoring) electrode and one as the reference electrode (used to check offset potential).
(See attached diagram also)

	Primary	*Reference*
RA	Lateral to right midclavicular line, below clavicle	Medial to primary electrode (touching but not overlapping)
LA	Lateral to left midclavicular line, below clavicle	Medial to primary electrode (touching but not overlapping)
RL	Right abdomen, below 6th rib, lateral to right midclavicular line	Medial to primary electrode (touching but not overlapping)
LL	Left abdomen, below 6th rib, lateral to left midclavicular line	Medial to primary electrode (touching but not overlapping)
V_1	4th intercostal space, right sternal border	Lateral to primary electrode (touching but not overlapping)

2. Electrodes will be applied in the following manner:
   a. Remove backing from electrode, taking care to minimize finger contact with the electrode's adhesive area.
   b. Inspect the electrode's gel pad, verifying that the gel pad is moist. Discard electrode if gel pad is not moist.
   c. Place the gel pad over the prepped area.
   d. Pull the opposite edge of the pad slightly and press down to adhere electrode to skin.
   e. Use finger pressure around the adhesive portion of electrode in a circular motion to promote firm electrode contact. Avoid direct pressure on the gel pad.
3. Connect the appropriate ECG electrode wires to the primary (monitoring) electrode using an alligator spring clip (rather than the snap-on button type).

Effect of Early Ambulation on Patient Comfort
and Bleeding Post Cardiac Catheterization

Principal Investigator:

Mary Welch, RN, MSN

Associate Investigators:

David Bailey, RN   Elizabeth Hilliard, RN, BSN
Patricia Galaviz, RN   Ruthie Pompey, RN
Smita Glosson, RN   Kimberly Webster, RN

SCIENTIFIC JUSTIFICATION

Short-term immobilization and bedrest are necessary to decrease the risk of
postprocedural bleeding after cardiac angiography. Current practice in many
facilities includes bedrest for 6 to 8 hours after removal of the femoral artery
sheath. Prolonged bedrest and restricted movement increase patient discomfort
and extend length of stay.

Bedrest standards vary between institutions, and the optimal time period for
immobilization is unknown. Several investigators recommend ambulation after
3 to 4 hours of bedrest.[1,2,4,5] Barkman and Lunse[1] evaluated patients who am-
bulated either 3 or 6 hours after angiogram and found no delayed bleeding or
palpable hematoma in either study group. Additionally, patients ambulating
after 3 hours of bedrest reported significantly less back pain ($p < 0.05$) compared to patients restricted to 6 hours of bedrest.[1]

The purpose of this study is to examine the effects of early ambulation after
cardiac angiography.

Hypotheses: In postangiography patients:

1. There will be no difference in the incidence of postambulation bleeding
   between the early (3 hour) and routine (6 hour) ambulation groups.
2. There will be a significant decrease in back pain for the early ambulation
   group as compared to the routine ambulation group.

Definition of Terms: The following definitions describe the terms used in
this study:

1. Bleeding: puncture site bleeding after arterial sheath removal; for the purposes of this study, bleeding will be determined using the Groin Assess-

ment Scale (Appendix A) and measurement of maximum hematoma diameter (cm).
2. Back pain: patient's perceived discomfort in the low back area. For the purposes of this study, back pain will be measured with a Visual Analog Scale[6] (VAS, Appendix B).
3. Ambulation: first time walking in room or hallway for a minimum of 2 minutes, in the presence of a nurse, and up ad lib thereafter.
   a. Routine ambulation: walking 6 hours after sheath removal.
   b. Early ambulation: walking 3 hours after sheath removal.

MATERIALS AND METHODS

Study Design. An experimental, comparative design will be used for this study. Consenting subjects will be randomized by computer into either the experimental (early ambulation) or the control group (routine ambulation). The independent variable will be time patients remain on bedrest post cardiac catheterization (6 hours vs. 3 hours). The dependent variables will be incidence of post-sheath removal bleeding and back pain.

Sample Selection. Subjects for this study will be 104 adult ($\geq$ 18 years old) patients scheduled to undergo an elective cardiac catheterization procedure at Moses H. Cone Hospital. Sample size was determined using power analysis (α = 0.05, $1 - \beta$ = 0.80, moderate effect size).[3]

Exclusionary criteria include:

1. Known liver disease
2. Bleeding disorders
3. Systolic blood pressure > 180 mm Hg
4. Diastolic blood pressure > 90 mm Hg
5. Nonambulatory or comatose state
6. Heparin therapy post procedure
7. Severe aortic insufficiency
8. Emergency or nonelective cardiac catheterization
9. Brachial arterial access site
10. Level II or III groin complication or active bleeding at groin site prior to ambulaton
11. Intervention (ie, PTCA, stent) during catheterization
12. Distal extremity complication

Data Collection. All patients who meet the eligibility criteria for the study will have the following procedures carried out:

1. Patients scheduled for elective angiography will be verbally informed about the nature of the study by one of the investigators and written informed consent will be obtained (Appendix C).
2. Demographic data will be collected (Appendix D).

3. Use of the VAS will be explained and demonstrated by one of the investigators. Return demonstration by the patient will be used to verify understanding of VAS completion.

4. Patient will rate perceived back discomfort on VAS.

5. Following current standard protocol, subjects will be instructed about signs and symptoms of groin site bleeding and the need to immediately notify the nurse should groin site bleeding/hematoma occur.

6. Following the angiography, consenting subjects will be screened for presence of any exclusionary criteria. Eligible subjects will be randomly assigned to one of two groups: control or experimental.

7. Both groups will initially be instructed to remain in bed, keeping the affected leg straight and the head of the bed no higher than 30°. The control group will remain on bedrest for 6 hours. The experimental group will remain on bedrest for 3 hours.

8. The standard dressing will be removed per routine postcatheterization orders for the control group; experimental group dressings will be removed immediately prior to ambulation. (See Appendix E.)

9. Following the designated period of bedrest, patients will be assisted, by a nurse, to walk in their room or hallway for a minimum of 2 minutes and then will be up ad lib.

10. Blood pressure, heart rate, groin site stability, groin assessment, pedal pulses, and patient's perceived back pain will be assessed per standard unit routine. In addition to these standard assessments, back pain will be measured at 2, 4, and 7 hours after sheath removal. Groin assessments will occur every 15 to 60 minutes per current postcatheterization protocol.

11. Any cardiopulmonary or bleeding complications that occur will be managed per current Emergency Standing Orders and procedures.

DATA ANALYSIS

Data will be summarized with descriptive statistics. Data will be analyzed with Student's t test (pain, hematoma measurement) and chi square analysis (Groin Assessment Scale). The level of significance for all tests will be $p < 0.05$.

HAZARDS AND PRECAUTIONS, DISCOMFORTS, INCONVENIENCES

The primary hazard associated with this study is the possible risk of groin site hematoma or bleeding with early ambulation. Frequent observation by nurses, as well as careful patient instructions regarding signs and symptoms of bleeding/hematoma, allows for early identification of this complication and reduces the risk of bleeding complications. Patients may be slightly inconvenienced by being asked to rate their pain according to the visual analog scale at 2, 4, and 7 hours post hemostasis achievement. All other discomforts and inconveniences are the same as patients would routinely experience post-cardiac catheterization. Pain medications will be administered as needed according to physician's orders and patient needs.

ETHICAL CONSIDERATIONS AND PROVISIONS/INFORMED CONSENT

Prior to participation in the study, one of the investigators will obtain informed consent. The investigator will explain the study verbally and answer the patient's questions prior to written informed consent being obtained. Confidentiality of the patient will be assured.

REFERENCES

1. Barkman A, Lunse C. The effect of early ambulation on patient comfort and delayed bleeding after cardiac angiogram: A pilot study. Heart & Lung, March/April 1994;112–117.
2. Christenson R, Staab E, Burko M, Foster J. Pressure dressings and post-arteriographic care of the femoral puncture site. Radiology 1976;119:97–99.
3. Cohen L. Statistical power analysis for the behavioral sciences. New York: Academic Press, 1977, pages 311–314.
4. Keeling A, Powers E, Nordt LA, Taylor V, Fisher C. Decreased time-in-bed after cardiac angiography. AACN: Proceedings NTI 1995:104.
5. Klinke W, Kubac G, Talibi T, Lee S. Safety of outpatient cardiac catheterizations. American Journal of Cardiology 1985;56:639–641.
6. Lee K, Kieckhefer G. Measuring human responses using visual analogue scales. Western Journal of Nursing Research 1989;11(1):128–132.

APPENDIX A
GROIN ASSESSMENT SCALE

Level 0
- no bruising or bleeding
- no palpable hematoma

Level I
- bruising/ecchymosis
- minimal bleeding/oozing
- palpable hematoma < 3 cm

Level II
- bleeding not affecting hemodynamic parameters
- pseudoaneurysm
- palpable hematoma > 3 cm

Level III
- bleeding that affects hemodynamic parameters
- retroperitoneal hemorrhage
- palpable hematoma > 3 cm

APPENDIX B
COMFORT SCALE

Periodically during this study you will be asked to rate your feelings of back discomfort or pain. You will be given a series of lines like the line below and asked to place a mark through the line that corresponds to the way you feel right at that moment.

This line represents the way your back feels. At one end "no pain" would be absolutely no discomfort in your back. At the other end of the line, "worst pain," would be the worst pain you could possibly imagine having. Place a vertical mark through the line to show how much, if any, back pain you feel right now.

FOR EXAMPLE: How does your back feel right now?

_____

No pain or discomfort   Worst pain or discomfort

APPENDIX C
CONSENT TO PARTICIPATE AS A RESEARCH SUBJECT IN NURSING RESEARCH

Effect of early ambulation on patient comfort and bleeding post cardiac catheterization.

Principal investigator: Mary Welch, RN, MSN
                              574-7200 or Pager #152

Co-investigators:

David Bailey, RN	Elizabeth Hilliard RN, BSN
Patricia Galaviz, RN	Ruthie Pompey, RN
Smita Glosson, RN	Kimberly Webster, RN

IRB #: 12/95-398

We invite you to take part in a research study for post cardiac catheterization patients. It is important that you read and fully understand the following general principles that apply to all who take part in this study. Taking part in this study is entirely voluntary. Personal benefit may not result from taking part in this study, but knowledge may be gained that will benefit others. Any significant new findings that relate to your treatment will be discussed with you. You may refuse to participate or withdraw from the study at any time without interfering with your regular medical treatment.

The nature of this study, as well as the risks, inconveniences, discomforts, and other important information about this study are described below. You are urged to discuss any questions you have about the study with the staff member who explains it to you.

BACKGROUND INFORMATION AND PURPOSE OF THE STUDY

Following a cardiac catheterization, it is customary to remain in bed for several hours to prevent bleeding from the groin incision area. This period of immobility causes back discomfort for many patients. The length of time for bedrest varies from hospital to hospital, with the optimal time period for immobilization not known. The purpose of this study is to determine if shortening the bedrest period from the current 6-hour period to 3 hours would be more comfortable for cardiac catheterization patients.

PROCEDURES

If you agree to participate, the following will occur as a result of your participation in this research study:

- After returning to your room from the catheterization lab, you will be randomly assigned to be on bedrest for either 3 or 6 hours.
- During your bedrest, you will be asked several times to rate the amount of back discomfort you are feeling.
- Your nurse will help you walk in your room or the hallway after either 3 or 6 hours of bedrest.

All other aspects of your nursing care after the cardiac catheterization will follow standard routines, including frequent checking of your blood pressure, pulse, and incision area, as well as administration of medication as ordered by your doctor for pain and discomfort.

POTENTIAL RISKS

The following risk may result from participation in this trial:

- Potential of increased bleeding at the incision area. Bleeding from the incision area can occur in some patients after catheterization. Any bleeding that occurs at the incision site is usually treated by a brief application of pressure at the site. Previous research on early walking after catheterization, however, did not find any increase in bleeding.

FOR WOMEN OF CHILDBEARING POTENTIAL

There are no potential adverse affects on the mother or unborn child.

POTENTIAL BENEFITS

The primary benefit is that you may have less back discomfort if you are assigned to the 3-hour ambulation (walking) group.

ALTERNATIVES

If you decide not to participate in this research, you will receive the standard nursing care normally given for your condition. Standard nursing care consists of 6 hours of bedrest after cardiac catheterization, followed by walking in your room or hallway. Frequent checking of blood pressure, pulse, and the incision area is done by your nurse before and after walking to identify any complications from the catheterization. Medication for discomfort is administered as needed if prescribed by your physician.

COSTS

There will be no additional costs to you for involvement in this study. In the event of unanticipated physical injury directly resulting from research procedures, financial compensation cannot be provided. Every effort, however, will be made to make available to you the facilities and professional skills of the Moses Cone Health System and its professional staff.

COMPENSATION

No payment or compensation will be made to you because of your participation in this study.

CONFIDENTIALITY

Every effort will be taken to protect the identity of the participants in this study. However, there can be no guarantee that the information cannot be obtained by legal process or court order. No subjects will be identified in any report or publication of this study and its results.

VOLUNTARY PARTICIPATION

Participation in research is voluntary. You have the right to refuse to participate or to withdraw at any point in this study without jeopardizing your medical care. In addition, your participation in this study may be terminated by the Investigator for medical reasons or for noncompliance.

STATEMENT OF CONSENT

I understand that this project has been approved by the committee under the protection of the rights of human subjects at The Moses H. Cone Memorial Hospital. If I believe there is any infringement upon my rights, I may contact the chairman of the committee, **Donald D. Smith, M.D. at (910) 574-8025.**

I understand that in the event of physical injury directly resulting from the research procedures, financial compensation cannot be provided. However, appropriate care will be made available to me through the facilities and professional skills of The Moses H. Cone Memorial Hospital.

I have had this study explained to me and have been given the opportunity to ask questions and discuss my concerns. No guarantees have been made to me regarding outcomes of this study. If I have any further questions about the study or feel I am developing a side effect, I may call the principal investigator, Mary Welch, RN, MSN at 574-7200. I understand that I may withdraw from this study at any time without interfering with my medical care.

My signature below indicates that I agree to participate in this study. I understand that I will receive a copy of this consent form.

_____

Patient Signature   Date

_____

Nurse obtaining consent   Date

_____

Witness signature   Date

APPENDIX D
DEMOGRAPHIC DATA*

Male/Female

Age (years)

Previous angiogram

Chronic back discomfort

ASA

Catheter size (French)

Admission diagnosis

Operating physician

Total units of heparin administered during angiogram

Analgesics administered between 0 and 7 hours post angiogram (time, drug, dose, route)

_____

*Incorporated into Data Collection Form.

APPENDIX E
ROUTINE POST CARDIAC CATHETERIZATION ORDERS

1. Vital signs q15 min ×4, if stable q30min ×4, if stable q2H ×4, if stable q4H till am.
2. Groin and distal extremity assessment with vital signs.
3. Resume previous medication orders except: _____

   _____

   May have _____, q _____ H prn pain.
4. Resume fat modified 4 gm sodium diet. No caffeine.
5. IV fluids: continue pre cath fluid or _____ at _____

   _____
6. Convert IV to saline lock when ambulatory.
7. Flush saline lock q12H.
8. If stable post cath D/C wedge after 4 hours or _____.
9. Activity: bedrest ×6H or _____ post cath then up ad lib.
10. May insert Foley catheter as necessary if patient has difficulty voiding.
11. If present, remove Foley catheter with ambulatory.

APPENDIX F
DATA COLLECTION TOOL

Group: ID #:

[ ] 3 Hour Walk

[ ] 6 Hour Walk

[ ] Consent Signed   Sex ____ (M/F) Operating Physician Name _____

[ ] Baseline Pre-Cath Pain Assessment   Age ____   Diagnosis _____

Arterial Catheter Size _____Fr.   Previous Cardiac Catheterization [ ] Yes [ ] No

Chronic Back Discomfort [ ] Yes [ ] No   Post-Cath Heparin Restart [ ] No [ ] Yes
(If yes, STOP STUDY)

Heparin Bolus during Cath: _____ Units

Post-Cath Sheath Removal Time: _____ (Military Time)

Time Since Sheath Removal	2 Hr.	2.5 Hr.	3 Hr.	4 Hr.	5 Hr.	6 Hr.	7 Hr.
Actual Time (Military)							
Groin Scale: I, II, or III (If > I or active bleed, STOP STUDY)							
Patient Completes Back Comfort Scale (✔ when done)							
Systolic BP < 190 mm/ Diastolic BP < 100 mm (✔)							
Patient walked at assigned time (✔)							
Nurse (Initials)							

ANALGESICS/SEDATIVES/HYPNOTICS GIVEN
(From 4 Hr. Pre-Cath to 7 Hr. Post-Cath)

Time						
Drug						
Dose						
Route						

COMMENTS/Explanation if Study Stopped: _____

Sample Case Report Forms

Chest Pain Assessment Tool
Sugar Case Report Form

Women and Heart Disease—Chest Pain Assessment Tool

Patient Study #: _____   History #: _____

FINAL DIAGNOSIS: ____(pick list)_____   Time presentation to triage: _____
                                            Time ECG done: _____

DESCRIPTION OF SYMPTOMS AT TRIAGE: (Please QUOTE in the EXACT order
of complaint) _____

_____

Description of Symptoms: (Additional questions asked by RN)

P (What PROVOKES this pain)
  ☐ Activity (if so, what was the exact activity _____)
  ☐ Rest
Q (What is the QUALITY of the pain)
  ☐ Pressure   ☐ Ache
  ☐ Sharpness   ☐ Squeezing
  ☐ Dullness   ☐ Heaviness
  ☐ Tightness

R (Does the pain RADIATE to locations other than the chest)
☐ Epigastric area   ☐ Back
☐ Jaw   ☐ R Arm
☐ Neck   ☐ L Arm
☐ R shoulder
☐ L shoulder

S (What is the SEVERITY of the pain on a scale of 1–10) *CIRCLE NUMBER*
    0   1   2   3   4   5   6   7   8   9   10

T (What is the TIMING of the pain)
☐ Time of ONSET of this episode of pain _____?

Other associated symptoms:
☐ Nausea   ☐ SOB
☐ Vomiting   ☐ Syncope
☐ Dizziness   ☐ Weakness
☐ Diaphoresis   ☐ Flushed feeling

Duration of symptoms:
_____From time of onset to time patient states pain free.

AGE:
ETHNICITY: ☐ African American   ☐ Caucasion   ☐ Hispanic   ☐ Other_____

SUGAR CASE REPORT FORM

Patient Study Number: _____
Date of Enrollment: _____

ADDRESSOGRAPH

PATIENT DEMOGRAPHICS
Age:_____   Sex: ☐ Male   ☐ Female
Race: ☐ White   ☐ Black   ☐ Indian   ☐ Hispanic   ☐ Asian   ☐ Other
Referred from: ☐ _____
Surgical Attending: _____
Last grade completed: <6–7–8–9–10–11–12– (circle)
            ☐ 2 Year College   ☐ 4 Year College   ☐ > 4 Year College

MEDICAL HISTORY
Hospital Admission Date: ___/___/___   Hospital Discharge Date:___/___/___
    ☐ Primary Diagnosis: ☐ Elective CABG   ☐ Emergent CABG
    ☐ Non-Insulin Dependent Diabetic (on oral agent)   ☐ IDDM
    ☐ Newly diagnosed diabetic
Events leading to hospitalization: _____
Year diagnosed with diabetes: ___/___/___

LABORATORY DATA (at time of enrollment)
ABC ___/___/___   ChemCS ___/___/___
Other: _____/___

LABORATORY DATA (at time of discharge)
ABC ___/___/___   ChemCS ___/___/___
Other: _____/___

CO-MORBIDITIES
PVD   ☐ Yes   ☐ No   ___/___/___
Renal failure/insufficiency   ☐ Yes   ☐ No   ___/___/___
Retinopathy   ☐ Yes   ☐ No   ___/___/___
Peripheral neuropathies   ☐ Yes   ☐ No   ___/___/___
Gastroenteropathy   ☐ Yes   ☐ No   ___/___/___
Hx Angina   ☐ Yes   ☐ No   ___/___/___
Myocardial Infarction   ☐ Yes   ☐ No   ___/___/___
Prior CABG   ☐ Yes   ☐ No   ___/___/___

COPD	☐ Yes	☐ No	___/___/___
ASHD	☐ Yes	☐ No	___/___/___
HTN	☐ Yes	☐ No	___/___/___
VT/VF	☐ Yes	☐ No	___/___/___
Atrial fibrillation	☐ Yes	☐ No	___/___/___
Stroke	☐ Yes	☐ No	___/___/___
Renal failure/insufficiency	☐ Yes	☐ No	___/___/___
Other:_____	☐ Yes	☐ No	___/___/___

RISK FACTORS

Obesity	☐ Yes	☐ No	___/___/___
Smoking	☐ Yes	☐ No	___/___/___
ETOH/substance abuse	☐ Yes	☐ No	___/___/___
Family history	☐ Yes	☐ No	___/___/___
Age (>65)	☐ Yes	☐ No	___/___/___
Sex (male)	☐ Yes	☐ No	___/___/___
Sedentary lifestyle	☐ Yes	☐ No	___/___/___
History of noncompliance	☐ Yes	☐ No	___/___/___
Other	☐ Yes	☐ No	___/___/___

FOLLOW-UP PLAN

Date 7 day F/U call: ___/___/___

How many readings obtained   ☐ # readings < 200   ☐ # readings > 200

Have you been seen in a clinic/office for assistance with your diabetes since D/C
☐ Yes   ☐ No

Withdrawn from Study?   ☐ Yes   ☐ No   If yes, Date___/___/___

Reason:_____

January 1997

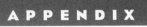

Examples of IRB Forms

Consent forms

> Consent to Participate As a Research Subject in Nursing Research
> Consent for Pain Assessment in Chest Tube Removal with EMLA Cream

IRB Submission forms

> Sample memo for IRB submission
> Blank IRB form for Research Proposal Review
> Duke University Medical Center Institutional Review Board Research Protocol

CONSENT TO PARTICIPATE AS A RESEARCH SUBJECT
IN NURSING RESEARCH

PRINCIPAL INVESTIGATOR: *(Name/Phone #)*

CO-INVESTIGATORS: *(Names/Phone #)*

IRB #:

We invite you to take part in a research study for patients with (*insert clinical condition here*). It is important that you read and fully understand the following general principles that apply to all who take part in this study. Taking part in this study is entirely voluntary. Personal benefit may not result from taking part in this study, but knowledge may be gained that will benefit others. Any significant new findings that relate to your treatment will be discussed with you. You may refuse to participate or withdraw from the study at any time without interfering with your regular medical treatment.

The nature of this study, as well as the risks, inconveniences, discomforts, and other important information about this study are described below. You are urged to discuss any questions you have about the study with the staff member who explains it to you.

BACKGROUND INFORMATION AND PURPOSE OF THE STUDY

(Insert brief explanation of the purpose and rationale of the research study.)

PROCEDURES

If you agree to participate in this research study, the following will occur as a result of your participation.

(Insert an explanation, usually step by step, of all procedures, treatments, drugs, and devices that will be specifically used as part of the research. Avoid technical jargon.)

POTENTIAL RISKS

The following risks and/or discomforts may result from participation in this trial:

(Describe all discomforts and risks to be reasonably expected and what measures the investigator will provide to protect against and to minimize those discomforts and risks.)

FOR WOMEN OF CHILDBEARING POTENTIAL

(Describe any potential adverse effects on the mother or unborn child.)

POTENTIAL BENEFITS

(Describe benefits to subjects that may be reasonably expected.)

ALTERNATIVES

If you decide not to participate in this research, you will receive the standard nursing care normally given for your condition. *(Describe briefly what the standard nursing care includes.)*

COSTS

There will be no additional costs to you for involvement in this study. In the event of unanticipated physical injury directly resulting from research procedures, financial compensation cannot be provided. Every effort, however, will be made to make available to you the facilities and professional skills of the *(insert hospital name)* and its professional staff.

COMPENSATION

No payment or compensation will be made to you because of your participation in this study.

CONFIDENTIALITY

Every effort will be taken to protect the identity of the participants in this study. However, there can be no guarantee that the information cannot be obtained by legal process or court order. No subjects will be identified in any report or publication of this study and its results.

VOLUNTARY PARTICIPATION

Participation in research is voluntary. You have the right to refuse to participate or to withdraw at any point in this study without jeopardizing your medical care. In addition, your participation in this study may be terminated by the Investigator for medical reasons or for noncompliance.

STATEMENT OF CONSENT

I understand that this project has been approved by the committee under the protection of the rights of human subjects at *(insert the name of the hospital or university)*. If I believe there is any infringement upon my rights, I may contact the chairman of the committee, *(insert name and phone number of the appropriate person in bold)*.

I understand that in the event of physical injury directly resulting from the research procedures, financial compensation cannot be provided. However, appropriate care will be made available to me through the facilities and professional skills of *(insert hospital name)*.

I have had this study explained to me and have been given the opportunity to ask questions and discuss my concerns. If I have any further questions about the study or feel I am developing a side effect, I may call the principal investigator, (*insert name and phone number in bold*). I understand that I may withdraw from this study at any time without interfering with my medical care.

My signature below indicates that I agree to participate in this study. I understand that I will receive a copy of this consent form.

_____   _____

PATIENT SIGNATURE   DATE

_____   _____

INVESTIGATOR OBTAINING CONSENT   DATE

_____   _____

WITNESS SIGNATURE   DATE

DUKE UNIVERSITY MEDICAL CENTER

Form
M-03

Duke University Medical Center

MEDICAL RESEARCH CONSENT FORM

Title of Project: Pain Assessment in Chest Tube Removal with EMLA cream

(PAIN-CaRE) Study

Principal Investigator: Pam Boggs, RN
IRB protocol number: 1346-97-9

You are being asked, with the approval of your physician, to take part in a research study involving application of analgesic (pain relieving) cream to your chest tube drainage sites prior to removal of the chest tubes. This study is being conducted by nurses at Duke University Medical Center for the purpose of making the chest tube removal procedure more comfortable for you. Currently, no specific medication is given for the chest tube removal procedure. If you agree to participate in this study, you will be approached on the second day following your surgery by a nurse who will discuss chest tube removal with you and apply a thick white cream around the outside of your chest tube sites. The cream will remain in place for at least one hour and no longer than four hours. The cream will be assigned to you by random selection, similar to flipping a coin, and the cream that you receive may or may not be the analgesic cream. Fifty patients will receive analgesic cream and fifty patients will receive an identical-looking cream without active ingredients, known as a placebo. All patients will be asked questions about their perception of the procedure before and after the chest tubes are removed. You will be given the opportunity to ask and/or clarify any questions you may have both before and after the removal of your chest tubes. The completion of the forms at the time of the procedure should take 30–35 minutes.

You may not benefit personally from taking part in this study, but knowledge may be gained that will benefit others. Taking part in this study is entirely voluntary and you may withdraw from the study at any time. Refusal to participate will not influence your medical or nursing care. This study will not require any extra visits to the hospital. There is no charge or compensation for participating in this study. All information is confidential and material will be kept by the researcher in a locked file. Your responses will be known only to the researcher and will not be revealed to

DUKE UNIVERSITY MEDICAL CENTER

anyone without your consent. You will not be identified in any way when the results of this study are written or reported at meetings or in professional journals.

There is no anticipated risk to you from participation in this study; however, 1–2% of people may develop itching or rash, in which case the cream will be removed. Immediate care is available if necessary, should an individual be injured because of participation in the research project. There is no provision for free medical care or monetary compensation for such injury. Further information may be obtained from the Hospital Risk Management Office (919) 684-3277.

Patient Initials_____

"I have read the above and have been given the opportunity to discuss and to ask questions. I have been informed that I may contact Pam Boggs, RN at (919) 681-3241 to answer any questions I may have during the investigation, and that I may contact the Office of Risk Management at (919) 684-3277 for any questions concerning my rights as a research subject. I agree to participate as a subject with the understanding that I may withdraw at any time without interfering with my regular care."

_____   _____
Patient Signature   Signature of Person Obtaining Consent

_____   _____
Date   Date

TO: Chairman
        Institutional Review Board (IRB)

FROM: Director, Nursing Research and Practice

DATE: January 29, 1997

RE: PROPOSAL REVIEW

The enclosed protocol, "The Effect of Two Different Bathing Techniques on Skin Integrity, Patient Satisfaction, and Cost," is submitted for review by the committee. The proposal has received scientific peer review within the Nursing Department. We would appreciate your consideration of this protocol for expedited review since the study activities meet the IRB's criteria for expedited review. Also, please note that this study is proposing a verbal consenting process only (no written consent documentation) due to the nature of the study. The criteria for exception to the written consenting process (Section 46.117, item c of the Code of Federal Regulations for the Protection of Human Subjects, 45 CFR 46) are applicable to the design and methods of this study, in that there is no risk associated with this study and the use of the alternative bathing technique would not normally require consent outside the research process. All patients eligible for the study will have the study thoroughly explained to them and will be given the opportunity to voluntarily participate in the project.

Attachments:
  Protocol
  IRB forms

COMMITTEE ON THE PROTECTION OF THE RIGHTS
OF HUMAN SUBJECTS—INSTITUTIONAL REVIEW BOARD (IRB)

RESEARCH PROPOSAL REVIEW

Title of Project:

IRB Committee Project Number: _____

Principal Investigator (*include degrees*):

Department:
Mailing Address
Phone:

Type of Proposal: ____New   ____Renewal

Is the proposal being submitted to a granting agency or sponsor?
___No   ___Yes. If yes, name of agency or sponsor: _____

Part I. Considerations to Assure Protection of Human Subjects and Personnel.
Please indicate on the following check list the presence of any of the following situations in your study:

RESEARCH STUDY INCLUDES THE FOLLOWING PROCEDURES / SITUATIONS:	YES	NO
Ionizing radiation; radioactive isotopes		
Experimental devices, instruments, or machines		
Recombinant DNA research		
Fetal tissue		
Surgical pathological tissue		
Drugs under investigation		
Placebo(s)		
Protocol approved at collaborating institution		

SITUATIONS INCLUDED IN RESEARCH STUDY	INVOLVED		AT RISK*	
	YES	NO	YES	NO
Personnel exposure to hazardous substances				
Patients as experimental subjects				
Pregnant subjects				
Non-patient volunteers				
Students and staff as subjects				
Minors (less than 18)				
Non-English speaking subjects				
Mentally incompetent subjects				
Prisoners and parolees as subjects				
Subjects at other institutions				
Videotaping, filming, or voice recording of subjects				

*Human subject risk is regarded as "yes" if the research adds *any* additional risk above and beyond that which would be entailed by conventional and/or routine clinical diagnosis and therapy.

II. Scientific Review (Peer Review) Committee Approval

Date of committee approval: _____ **(Attach signed peer review approval form)**
Peer review approval must be obtained prior to submission of research proposal to IRB.

III. Principal Investigator Agreement

Interval for submission of progress reports to the IRB: _____ per year
(Interval should be appropriate to the degree of risk to subjects, with a minimum frequency of annually.)

The Principal Investigator, whose signature appears below, agrees to a continuing exchange of information or advice with the Committee on the Protection of the Rights of Human Subjects.

The Principal Investigator agrees to communicate with the Committee to obtain its approval before institution of any significant change or additions to the project or before continuing the project beyond the approval date.

The Principal Investigator agrees to inform the Committee and the Hospital Risk Management upon the occurrence of any previously undescribed or serious adverse effects or complications.

Signature _____
Principal Investigator

IV. Summary of Proposal

Please provide a brief summary of the proposed research study. This summary should include the purpose of the study and research methods. A simplified research schema or summary diagram may also be included to clarify study design for the reviewers. The summary should not exceed 1 page in length. **This summary will be read by all IRB Committee members. This summary should be written in language understandable to non-medical members of the IRB Committee.**

SUMMARY OF RESEARCH PROPOSAL

Number of subjects: _____   Age range: _____   Sex: Male   Female

List inclusion/exclusion criteria for subjects:

Duration of study: _____

Copy of informed consent form attached: _____

Copy of detailed research proposal attached: _____

Brief overview summary of research study (**should not exceed 400 words or 1 single-spaced page**):

DUKE UNIVERSITY MEDICAL CENTER INSTITUTIONAL
REVIEW BOARD RESEARCH PROTOCOL

Complete and submit original and 2 copies to the IRB (Room 107, Seeley G. Mudd Bldg., Box 3001) 15 days before meeting

Fax #: _____

P.I.: <u>Pam Boggs, RN</u>   Dept.: <u>Nursing</u>   Phone: 681-4060   PO Box: 3658

Faculty Sponsor: <u>Bradi Granger, RN, MSN</u>   Dept: <u>Nursing</u>   Phone: <u>681-4060</u>   PO Box: <u>3658</u>

Project Title: Pain Assessment in Chest Tube Removal with EMLA Cream (PAIN- CaRE Study)

Previous Registry # (Renewals) _____   Source of Research Funds   <u>None.</u>

Subject Types   [ ] Normal volunteers   [ ] Subjects incapable of giving consent
                  [x] Inpatients   [ ] Prisoners or institutionalized individuals
                  [ ] Outpatients   [ ] Minors
                  [ ] Patient controls   [x] Patient subjects over age 65
                  [ ] Students

Does protocol call for:
Yes   No
_____ x   Subject compensation? Patients $ _____ Volunteers $ _____
_____ x   Investigational devices or drugs? If yes, study phase ____;   letter of indemnification; <u>yes</u>
_____ x   More than minimal physical risk? ____ More than minimal psychological stress?
x   ___   Confidential material (questionnaires, photos, etc.)?
_____ x   Extra costs to the subjects (tests, hospitalization, OPC visits)?
_____ x   The exclusion of pregnant women?
_____ x   Is blood used? Give total amount _____ over time period (days) _____

Are the following used? If yes, obtain appropriate signatures:
Yes   No
_____ x   VA Hospital _____   VA IRB
_____ x   Rankin Ward _____   Clin. Res. Unit Comm.
_____ x   Cancer Related _____   CPRC
_____ x   Hypo/Hyperbaric Unit _____   Safety Comm.
_____ x   Radiation (Ionizing, laser) _____   Radiation Comm.
_____ x   Center for Living _____   Center for Living Res. Comm.
_____ x   Operating Room/Anesthesia Time _____   Minutes required

The following signatures are required before submission to the IRB:

P.I. (and faculty sponsor) _____   Date _____

Dept. IRB Member (Clinical Dept.) _____   Date_____   Date _____
                                                            Received   Signed

Dept. Chairperson _____   Date _____   Date _____
                                                            Received   Signed

DO NOT WRITE BELOW THIS LINE

Assigned IRB Member _____
IRB Action:
[ ] Approved   [ ] Tabled
[ ] Approved with modification [ ] Disapproved
    Approval Termination Date _____   Registry # Assigned _____

    IRB Chairperson _____   Date of Approval _____

**INCLUDE THE ASSIGNED PROTOCOL NUMBER IN ALL
CORRESPONDENCE WITH THE IRB CONCERNING THE PROTOCOL**

Briefly summarize your protocol below (no more than two pages). The summary should include applicable items in the check list under description of the protocol. Additional material may be appended but the brief summary must be provided. Append a consent form. Refer to checklists for content of protocol and consent forms.

PURPOSE: The purpose of this study is to compare the patient's perception of pain during chest tube removal using a new topical anesthetic called EMLA cream (Lidocaine 2.5% and Prilocaine 2.5%) as compared to pain perception in patients receiving standard therapy.

HYPOTHESIS: Patients who receive EMLA cream prior to chest tube removal will perceive less pain than those receiving placebo cream.

BACKGROUND AND SIGNIFICANCE: At Duke, 1505 patients underwent chest tube removal following coronary artery bypass graft surgery in fiscal year 1996. Patients' verbal response as well as informal, subjective observations by members of the health care team during chest tube removal in these patients both indicate a need for improved pain management during this procedure.

Currently, there is no standard for premedication prior to chest tube removal at Duke. Across the country, practice related to premedication for chest tube removal differs from practitioner to practitioner, with some institutions recommending premedication, but none that we identified requiring it. Adult patients have reported in the literature "the most painful part of a cardiothoracic procedure is chest tube removal" (1).

To date, studies using EMLA cream for pain management during line insertion and removal have been done predominantly in the pediatric population (2,3). One study, however, by Valenzuela and colleagues, studied the use of EMLA cream in adults during chest tube removal. This study compared the use of 5 grams EMLA cream with 0.1mg/kg morphine in adults prior to chest tube removal. Patients receiving EMLA cream demonstrated decreased pain behavior as measured by videotape recording of the behavior prior to, during, and after tube removal. This recording was then observed and scored by a blinded reviewer using a 10-cm analogue scale. The McGill Pain Questionnaire was also used to measure patients' reported pain perception, and this tool showed no statistical difference in pain between the two groups. However, due to increased sedation in the morphine group, a number of these patients were unable to complete the McGill questionnaire. This side effect, as well as others including hypotension and respiratory depression, are common occurrences with narcotic administration, and therefore frequently cited as reasons for not premedicating prior to chest tube removal (1).

DESIGN OF STUDY: This is a prospective, randomized trial in coronary artery bypass graft (CABG) patients and CABG/ Valve patients, who require removal of chest tubes following surgery. Patients will be randomized to a blinded treatment strategy of either EMLA Cream® or a white, neutral, placebo cream supplied by the same manufacturer (Astra Pharmaceuticals) and in the same packaging. Randomization will be accomplished by sealed envelope. The planned sample size is 100 patients, 50 in each arm. A formal re-

INCLUDE THE ASSIGNED PROTOCOL NUMBER IN ALL CORRESPONDENCE WITH THE IRB CONCERNING THE PROTOCOL

view of the data by the Data and Safety Monitoring Board (DSMB) will occur after 50 patients have been enrolled.

STUDY POPULATION:
Inclusion Criteria:
- CABG or CABG/Valve patient requiring chest tube removal
- Chest tubes in place ≤ 48 hours
- Less than or equal to 3 total chest tubes
- Patient progressing on clinical pathway
- 18 years or older

Exclusion Criteria:
- Sepsis
- Chest tubes in place > 48 hours
- Off clinical pathway
- Less than 18 years of age
- Transplant patients
- Known allergy to lidocaine or prilocaine

ENDPOINTS:
Primary: Patient perception of pain using subjective and objective measures (see appendices)
Secondary: Cost, time expenditure of the health care team, patient satisfaction

METHODS: The research associate will screen and obtain informed consent on eligible patients. The resident and research associate (RA) will collaborate on a target time for chest tubes to be removed. All demographic information will be collected and recorded by the research associate (Appendix A). The RA will remove the chest tube dressing and apply the treatment cream using sterile technique. The application will be in a circular pattern around the chest tube insertion site, with a margin of at least 1 inch, and at least .25 cm thick. An occlusive dressing will be placed over the chest tubes and cream/treatment area. The application will be left in place for a minimum of one hour. Prior to the chest tube removal, the occlusive dressing will be removed and the treatment cream will be thoroughly removed by wiping with a dry, sterile gauze. Prior to the initiation of the chest tube pull the RA will perform the Time One baseline assessment (see Appendix B). During the procedure the patient will be observed for pain behaviors and changes in physiologic variables for one minute. Immediately after the chest tube is pulled the patient will be asked to rate his/her pain and assess pain location. This assessment period is known as Time Two (see Appendix C). Ten minutes after the procedure the patient's heart rate and blood pressure will be measured and the patient will be asked to rate his/her pain intensity and assess location using the body diagram. This assessment is known as Time Three (see Appendix D). Following all three assessment periods, the patient will be given an opportunity to ask questions or make additional comments.

**INCLUDE THE ASSIGNED PROTOCOL NUMBER IN ALL
CORRESPONDENCE WITH THE IRB CONCERNING THE PROTOCOL**

STATISTICAL ANALYSIS: Inferential and parametric statistics will be used for analysis and will be selected after further statistical consultation.

RISKS: No adverse experiences directly related to administration of study drugs are expected.

COMPENSATION: There is no monetary compensation to the patient.

CONSENT: Informed consent will be obtained on all patients prior to enrollment in the study. Consent may be obtained by the care nurse, charge nurse, or member of the Heart Center enrollment team. The patient will not be asked to participate unless the physician has given approval.

CONFIDENTIALITY: All records will be kept confidential and the patient's name will not be released at anytime. Study patient files will not be released to anyone other than the investigators.

INCLUDE THE ASSIGNED PROTOCOL NUMBER IN ALL CORRESPONDENCE WITH THE IRB CONCERNING THE PROTOCOL

Code of Federal Regulations

NIH Guidelines for Human Research

Department of Health and Human Services
National Institutes of Health Office for Protection from Research Risks

Part 46—Protection of Human Subjects

Revised June 18, 1991

(Effective August 19, 1991)

Sec.

46.205 Additional duties of the Institutional Review Boards in connection with activities involving fetuses, pregnant women, or human in vitro fertilization.

46.206 General limitations.

46.207 Activities directed toward pregnant women as subjects.

46.208 Activities directed toward fetuses *in utero* as subjects.

46.209 Activities directed toward fetuses *ex utero*, including nonviable fetuses, as subjects.

46.210 Activities involving the dead fetus, fetal material, or the placenta.

46.211 Modification or waiver of specific requirements.

Subpart C—Additional DHHS Protections Pertaining to Biomedical and Behavioral Research Involving Prisoners as Subjects

Sec.

46.301 Applicability.

46.302 Purpose.

46.303 Definitions.

46.304 Composition of Institutional Review Boards where prisoners are involved.

46.305 Additional duties of the Institutional Review Boards where prisoners are involved.

46.306 Permitted research involving prisoners.

Subpart D—Additional DHHS Protections for Children Involved as Subjects in Research

Sec.

46.401 To what do these regulations apply?

46.402 Definitions.

46.403 IRB duties.

46.404 Research not involving greater than minimal risk.

46.405 Research involving greater than minimal risk but presenting the prospect of direct benefit to the individual subjects.

46.406 Research involving greater than minimal risk and no prospect of direct benefit to

individual subjects, but likely to yield generalizable knowledge about the subject's disorder or condition.

46.407 Research not otherwise approvable which presents an opportunity to understand, prevent, or alleviate a serious problem affecting the health or welfare of children.

46.408 Requirements for permission by parents or guardians and for assent by children.

46.409 Wards.

Authority: 5 U.S.C. 301; Sec. 474(a), 88 Stat. 352 (42 U.S.C. 2891–3(a)).

Note: As revised, Subpart A of the DHHS regulations incorporates the Common Rule (Federal Policy for the Protection of Human Subjects (56 FR 28003). Subpart D of the HHS regulations has been amended at Section 46.401(b) to reference the revised Subpart A. **The Common Rule (Federal Policy) is also codified at**

7 CFR Part 1c Department of Agriculture

10 CFR Part 745 Department of Energy

14 CFR Part 1230 National Aeronautics and Space Administration

15 CFR Part 27 Department of Commerce

16 CFR Part 1028 Consumer Product Safety Commission

22 CFR Part 225 International Development Cooperation Agency, Agency for International Development

24 CFR Part 60 Department of Housing and Urban Development

28 CFR Part 46 Department of Justice

32 CFR Part 219 Department of Defense

34 CFR Part 97 Department of Education

38 CFR Part 16 Department of Veterans Affairs

40 CFR Part 26 Environmental Protection Agency

45 CFR Part 690 National Science Foundation

49 CFR Part 11 Department of Transportation

PART 46—Protection of Human Subjects

Subpart A—Federal Policy for the Protection of Human Subjects (Basic DHHS Policy for Protection of Human Research Subjects)

Source: 56 FR 28003, June 18, 1991.

§46.101   To what does this policy apply?

(a) Except as provided in paragraph (b) of this section, this policy applies to all research involving human subjects conducted, supported or otherwise subject to regulation by any Federal Department or Agency which takes appropriate administrative action to make the policy applicable to such research. This includes research conducted by Federal civilian employees or military personnel, except that each Department or Agency head may adopt such procedural modifications as may be appropriate from an administrative standpoint. It also includes research conducted, supported, or otherwise subject to regulation by the Federal Government outside the United States.

(1) Research that is conducted or supported by a Federal Department or Agency, whether or not it is regulated as defined in §46.102(e), must comply with all sections of this policy.

(2) Research that is neither conducted nor supported by a Federal Department or Agency but is subject to regulation as defined in §46.102(e) must be reviewed and approved, in compliance with §46.101, §46.102, and §46.107 through §46.117 of this policy, by an Institutional Review Board (IRB) that operates in accordance with the pertinent requirements of this policy.

(b) Unless otherwise required by Department or Agency heads, research activities in which the only involvement of human subjects will be in one or more of the following categories are exempt from this policy:

(1) Research conducted in established or commonly accepted educational settings, involving normal educational practices, such as (i) research on regular and special education instructional strategies, or (ii) research on the effectiveness of or the comparison among instructional techniques, curricula, or classroom management methods.

(2) Research involving the use of educational tests (cognitive, diagnostic, aptitude, achievement), survey procedures, interview procedures or observation of public behavior, unless: (i) information obtained is recorded in such a manner that human subjects can be identified, directly or through identifiers linked to the subjects; and (ii) any disclosure of the human subjects' responses outside the research could reasonably place the subjects at the risk of criminal or civil liability or be damaging to the subjects' financial standing, employability, or reputation.

(3) Research involving the use of educational tests (cognitive, diagnostic, aptitude, achievement), survey procedures, interview procedures, or observation of public behavior that is not exempt under paragraph (b)(2) of this section, if: (i) the human subjects are elected or appointed public officials or candidates for public office; or (ii) Federal statute(s) require(s) without exception that the confidentiality of the personally identifiable information will be maintained throughout the research and thereafter.

(4) Research involving the collection or study of existing data, documents, records, pathological specimens, or diagnostic specimens, if these sources are publicly available or if the information is recorded by the investigator in such a manner that subjects cannot be identified, directly or through identifiers linked to the subjects.

(5) Research and demonstration projects which are conducted by or subject to the approval of Department or Agency heads, and which are designed to study, evaluate, or otherwise examine: (i) Public benefit or service programs; (ii) procedures for obtaining benefits or services under those programs; (iii) possible changes in or alternatives to those programs or procedures; or (iv) possible changes in methods or levels of payment for benefits or services under those programs.

(6) Taste and food quality evaluation and consumer acceptance studies, (i) if wholesome foods without additives are consumed or (ii) if a

food is consumed that contains a food ingredient at or below the level and for a use found to be safe, or agricultural chemical or environmental contaminant at or below the level found to be safe, by the Food and Drug Administration or approved by the Environmental Protection Agency or the Food Safety and Inspection Service of the U.S. Department of Agriculture.

(c) Department or Agency heads retain final judgment as to whether a particular activity is covered by this policy.

(d) Department or Agency heads may require that specific research activities or classes of research activities conducted, supported, or otherwise subject to regulation by the Department or Agency but not otherwise covered by this policy, comply with some or all of the requirements of this policy.

(e) Compliance with this policy requires compliance with pertinent Federal laws or regulations which provide additional protections for human subjects.

(f) This policy does not affect any State or local laws or regulations which may otherwise be applicable and which provide additional protections for human subjects.

(g) This policy does not affect any foreign laws or regulations which may otherwise be applicable and which provide additional protections to human subjects of research.

(h) When research covered by this policy takes place in foreign countries, procedures normally followed in the foreign countries to protect human subjects may differ from those set forth in this policy. [An example is a foreign institution which complies with guidelines consistent with the World Medical Assembly Declaration (Declaration of Helsinki amended 1989) issued either by sovereign states or by an organization whose function for the protection of human research subjects is internationally recognized.] In these circumstances, if a Department or Agency head determines that the procedures prescribed by the institution afford protections that are at least equivalent to those provided in this policy, the Department or Agency head may approve the substitution of the foreign procedures in lieu of the procedural requirements provided in this policy. Except when otherwise required by statute, Executive Order, or the Department or Agency head, notices of these actions as they occur will be published in the **Federal Register** or will be otherwise published as provided in Department or Agency procedures.

(i) Unless otherwise required by law, Department or Agency heads may waive the applicability of some or all of the provisions of this policy to specific research activities or classes of research activities otherwise covered by this policy. Except when otherwise required by statute or Executive Order, the Department or Agency head shall forward advance notices of these actions to the Office for Protection from Research Risks, National Institutes of Health, Department of Health and Human Services (DHHS), and shall also publish them in the **Federal Register** or in such other manner as provided in Department or Agency procedures.[1]

§46.102   Definitions.

(a) *Department or Agency head* means the head of any Federal Department or Agency and any other officer or employee of any Department or Agency to whom authority has been delegated.

(b) *Institution* means any public or private entity or Agency (including Federal, State, and other agencies).

(c) *Legally authorized representative* means an individual or judicial or other body authorized under applicable law to consent on behalf of a prospective subject to the subject's participation in the procedure(s) involved in the research.

---

[1]Institutions with DHHS-approved assurances on file will abide by provisions of Title 45 CFR Part 46 Subparts A–D. Some of the other departments and agencies have incorporated all provisions of Title 45 CFR Part 46 into their policies and procedures as well. However, the exemptions at 45 CFR 46.101(b) do not apply to research involving prisoners, fetuses, pregnant women, or human in vitro fertilization, Subparts B and C. The exemption at 45 CFR 46.101(b)(2), for research involving survey or interview procedures or observation of public behavior, does not apply to research with children, Subpart D, except for research involving observations of public behavior when the investigator(s) do not participate in the activities being observed.

(d) *Research* means a systematic investigation, including research development, testing and evaluation, designed to develop or contribute to generalizable knowledge. Activities which meet this definition constitute research for purposes of this policy, whether or not they are conducted or supported under a program which is considered research for other purposes. For example, some demonstration and service programs may include research activities.

(e) *Research subject to regulation*, and similar terms are intended to encompass those research activities for which a Federal Department or Agency has specific responsibility for regulating as a research activity, (for example, Investigational New Drug requirements administered by the Food and Drug Administration). It does not include research activities which are incidentally regulated by a Federal Department or Agency solely as part of the Department's or Agency's broader responsibility to regulate certain types of activities whether research or non-research in nature (for example, Wage and Hour requirements administered by the Department of Labor).

(f) *Human subject* means a living individual about whom an investigator (whether professional or student) conducting research obtains

(1) data through intervention or interaction with the individual, or

(2) identifiable private information. *Intervention* includes both physical procedures by which data are gathered (for example, venipuncture) and manipulations of the subject or the subject's environment that are performed for research purposes. Interaction includes communication or interpersonal contact between investigator and subject. *Private information* includes information about behavior that occurs in a context in which an individual can reasonably expect that no observation or recording is taking place, and information which has been provided for specific purposes by an individual and which the individual can reasonably expect will not be made public (for example, a medical record). Private information must be individually identifiable (i.e., the identity of the subject is or may readily be ascertained by the investigator or associated with the information) in order for obtaining the information to constitute research involving human subjects.

(g) *IRB* means an Institutional Review Board established in accord with and for the purposes expressed in this policy.

(h) *IRB approval* means the determination of the IRB that the research has been reviewed and may be conducted at an institution within the constraints set forth by the IRB and by other institutional and Federal requirements.

(i) *Minimal risk* means that the probability and magnitude of harm or discomfort anticipated in the research are not greater in and of themselves than those ordinarily encountered in daily life or during the performance of routine physical or psychological examinations or tests.

(j) *Certification* means the official notification by the institution to the supporting Department or Agency, in accordance with the requirements of this policy, that a research project or activity involving human subjects has been reviewed and approved by an IRB in accordance with an approved assurance.

§46.103 Assuring compliance with this policy—research conducted or supported by any Federal Department or Agency.

(a) Each institution engaged in research which is covered by this policy and which is conducted or supported by a Federal Department or Agency shall provide written assurance satisfactory to the Department or Agency head that it will comply with the requirements set forth in this policy. In lieu of requiring submission of an assurance, individual Department or Agency heads shall accept the existence of a current assurance, appropriate for the research in question, on file with the Office for Protection from Research Risks, National Institutes Health, DHHS, and approved for Federalwide use by that office. When the existence of an DHHS-approved assurance is accepted in lieu of requiring submission of an assurance, reports (except certification) required by this policy to be made to Department and Agency heads shall also be made to the Office for Protection from Research Risks, National Institutes of Health, DHHS.

(b) Departments and agencies will conduct or support research covered by this policy only if the institution has an assurance approved as provided in this section, and only if the institution has certified to the Department or Agency head that the research has been reviewed and approved by an IRB provided for in the assurance, and will be subject to continuing review by the IRB. Assurances applicable to federally supported or conducted research shall at a minimum include:

(1) A statement of principles governing the institution in the discharge of its responsibilities for protecting the rights and welfare of human subjects of research conducted at or sponsored by the institution, regardless of whether the research is subject to Federal regulation. This may include an appropriate existing code, declaration, or statement of ethical principles, or a statement formulated by the institution itself. This requirement does not preempt provisions of this policy applicable to Department- or Agency-supported or regulated research and need not be applicable to any research exempted or waived under §46.101 (b) or (i).

(2) Designation of one or more IRBs established in accordance with the requirements of this policy, and for which provisions are made for meeting space and sufficient staff to support the IRB's review and recordkeeping duties.

(3) A list of IRB members identified by name; earned degrees; representative capacity; indications of experience such as board certifications, licenses, etc., sufficient to describe each member's chief anticipated contributions to IRB deliberations; and any employment or other relationship between each member and the institution; for example: full-time employee, part-time employee, member of governing panel or board, stockholder, paid or unpaid consultant. Changes in IRB membership shall be reported to the Department or Agency head, unless in accord with §46.103(a) of this policy, the existence of a DHHS-approved assurance is accepted. In this case, change in IRB membership shall be reported to the Office for Protection from Research Risks, National Institutes of Health, DHHS.

(4) Written procedures which the IRB will follow (i) for conducting its initial and continuing review of research and for reporting its findings and actions to the investigator and the institution; (ii) for determining which projects require review more often than annually and which projects need verification from sources other than the investigators that no material changes have occurred since previous IRB review; and (iii) for ensuring prompt reporting to the IRB of proposed changes in a research activity, and for ensuring that such changes in approved research, during the period for which IRB approval has already been given, may not be initiated without IRB review and approval except when necessary to eliminate apparent immediate hazards to the subject.

(5) Written procedures for ensuring prompt reporting to the IRB, appropriate institutional officials, and the Department or Agency head of (i) any unanticipated problems involving risks to subjects or others or any serious or continuing noncompliance with this policy or the requirements or determinations of the IRB; and (ii) any suspension or termination of IRB approval.

(c) The assurance shall be executed by an individual authorized to act for the institution and to assume on behalf of the institution the obligations imposed by this policy and shall be filed in such form and manner as the Department or Agency head prescribes.

(d) The Department or Agency head will evaluate all assurances submitted in accordance with this policy through such officers and employees of the Department or Agency and such experts or consultants engaged for this purpose as the Department or Agency head determines to be appropriate. The Department or Agency head's evaluation will take into consideration the adequacy of the proposed IRB in light of the anticipated scope of the institution's research activities and the types of subject populations likely to be involved, the appropriateness of the proposed initial and continuing review procedures in light of the probable risks, and the size and complexity of the institution.

(e) On the basis of this evaluation, the Department or Agency head may approve or disapprove the assurance, or enter into negotiations to develop an approvable one. The Department or Agency head may limit the period during which any particular approved assurance or class of approved assurances shall remain effective or otherwise condition or restrict approval.

(f) Certification is required when the research is supported by a Federal Department or Agency and not otherwise exempted or waived under §46.101 (b) or (i). An institution with an approved assurance shall certify that each application or proposal for research covered by the assurance and by §46.103 of this policy has been reviewed and approved by the IRB. Such certification must be submitted with the application or proposal or by such later date as may be prescribed by the Department or Agency to which the application or proposal is submitted. Under no condition shall research covered by §46.103 of the policy be supported prior to receipt of the certification that the research has been reviewed and approved by the IRB. Institutions without an approved assurance covering the research shall certify within 30 days after receipt of a request for such a certification from the Department or Agency, that the application or proposal has been approved by the IRB. If the certification is not submitted within these time limits, the application or proposal may be returned to the institution.
(Approved by the Office of Management and Budget under Control Number 9999–0020.)

§§46.104—46.106 [Reserved]

§46.107   IRB membership

(a) Each IRB shall have at least five members, with varying backgrounds to promote complete and adequate review of research activities commonly conducted by the institution. The IRB shall be sufficiently qualified through the experience and expertise of its members, and the diversity of the members, including consideration of race, gender, and cultural backgrounds and sensitivity to such issues as community attitudes, to promote respect for its advice and counsel in safeguarding the rights and welfare of human subjects. In addition to possessing the professional competence necessary to review specific research activities, the IRB shall be able to ascertain the acceptability of proposed research in terms of institutional commitments and regulations, applicable law, and the standards of professional conduct and prac-

tice. The IRB shall therefore include persons knowledgeable in these areas. If an IRB regularly reviews research that involves a vulnerable category of subjects, such as children, prisoners, pregnant women, or handicapped or mentally disabled persons, consideration shall be given to the inclusion of one or more individuals who are knowledgeable about and experienced in working with these subjects.

(b) Every nondiscriminatory effort will be made to ensure that no IRB consists entirely of men or entirely of women, including the institution's consideration of qualified persons of both sexes, so long as no selection is made to the IRB on the basis of gender. No IRB may consist entirely of members of one profession.

(c) Each IRB shall include at least one member whose primary concerns are in scientific areas and at least one member whose primary concerns are in nonscientific areas.

(d) Each IRB shall include at least one member who is not otherwise affiliated with the institution and who is not part of the immediate family of a person who is affiliated with the institution.

(e) No IRB may have a member participate in the IRB's initial or continuing review of any project in which the member has a conflicting interest, except to provide information requested by the IRB.

(f) An IRB may, in its discretion, invite individuals with competence in special areas to assist in the review of issues which require expertise beyond or in addition to that available on the IRB. These individuals may not vote with the IRB.

§46.108   IRB functions and operations.

In order to fulfill the requirements of this policy each IRB shall:

(a) Follow written procedures in the same detail as described in §46.103(b)(4) and to the extent required by §46.103(b)(5).

(b) Except when an expedited review procedure is used (see §46.110), review proposed research at convened meetings at which a majority of the members of the IRB are present, including at least one member whose primary concerns are in nonscientific areas. In order for the research to be approved, it shall receive the approval of a majority of those members present at the meeting.

§46.109   IRB review of research.

(a) An IRB shall review and have authority to approve, require modifications in (to secure approval), or disapprove all research activities covered by this policy.

(b) An IRB shall require that information given to subjects as part of informed consent is in accordance with §46.116. The IRB may require that information, in addition to that specifically mentioned in §46.116, be given to the subjects when in the IRB's judgment the information would meaningfully add to the protection of the rights and welfare of subjects.

(c) An IRB shall require documentation of informed consent or may waive documentation in accordance with §46.117.

(d) An IRB shall notify investigators and the institution in writing of its decision to approve or disapprove the proposed research activity, or of modifications required to secure IRB approval of the research activity. If the IRB decides to disapprove a research activity, it shall include in its written notification a statement of the reasons for its decision and give the investigator an opportunity to respond in person or in writing.

(e) An IRB shall conduct continuing review of research covered by this policy at intervals appropriate to the degree of risk, but not less than once per year, and shall have authority to observe or have a third party observe the consent process and the research.
(Approved by the Office of Management and Budget under Control Number 9999–0020.)

§46.110   Expedited review procedures for certain kinds of research involving no more than minimal risk, and for minor changes in approved research.

(a) The Secretary, HHS, has established, and published as a Notice in the **Federal Register**, a list of categories of research that may be reviewed by the IRB through an expedited review procedure. The list will be amended, as appropriate, after consultation with other departments and agencies, through periodic republication by the Secretary, HHS, in the **Federal Register.** A copy of the list is available from the Office for Protection from Research Risks, National Institutes of Health, DHHS, Bethesda, Maryland 20892.

(b) An IRB may use the expedited review procedure to review either or both of the following:

(1) some or all of the research appearing on the list and found by the reviewer(s) to involve no more than minimal risk,

(2) minor changes in previously approved research during the period (of one year or less) for which approval is authorized.

Under an expedited review procedure, the review may be carried out by the IRB chairperson or by one or more experienced reviewers designated by the chairperson from among members of the IRB. In reviewing the research, the reviewers may exercise all of the authorities of the IRB except that the reviewers may not disapprove the research. A research activity may be disapproved only after review in accordance with the non-expedited procedure set forth in §46.108(b).

(c) Each IRB which uses an expedited review procedure shall adopt a method for keeping all members advised of research proposals which have been approved under the procedure.

(d) The Department or Agency head may restrict, suspend, terminate, or choose not to authorize an institution's or IRB's use of the expedited review procedure.

§46.111   Criteria for IRB approval of research.

(a) In order to approve research covered by this policy the IRB shall determine that all of the following requirements are satisfied:

(1) Risks to subjects are minimized: (i) by using procedures which are consistent with sound research design and which do not unnecessarily expose subjects to risk, and (ii) whenever appropriate, by using procedures already being performed on the subjects for diagnostic or treatment purposes.

(2) Risks to subjects are reasonable in relation to anticipated benefits, if any, to subjects, and the importance of the knowledge that may

reasonably be expected to result. In evaluating risks and benefits, the IRB should consider only those risks and benefits that may result from the research (as distinguished from risks and benefits of therapies subjects would receive even if not participating in the research). The IRB should not consider possible long-range effects of applying knowledge gained in the research (for example, the possible effects of the research on public policy) as among those research risks that fall within the purview of its responsibility.

(3) Selection of subjects is equitable. In making this assessment the IRB should take into account the purposes of the research and the setting in which the research will be conducted and should be particularly cognizant of the special problems of research involving vulnerable populations, such as children, prisoners, pregnant women, mentally disabled persons, or economically or educationally disadvantaged persons.

(4) Informed consent will be sought from each prospective subject or the subject's legally authorized representative, in accordance with, and to the extent required by §46.116.

(5) Informed consent will be appropriately documented, in accordance with, and to the extent required by §46.117.

(6) When appropriate, the research plan makes adequate provision for monitoring the data collected to ensure the safety of subjects.

(7) When appropriate, there are adequate provisions to protect the privacy of subjects and to maintain the confidentiality of data.

(b) When some of all of the subjects are likely to be vulnerable to coercion or undue influence, such as children, prisoners, pregnant women, mentally disabled persons, or economically or educationally disadvantaged persons, additional safeguards have been included in the study to protect the rights and welfare of these subjects.

§46.112   Review by institution.

Research covered by this policy that has been approved by an IRB may be subject to further appropriate review and approval or disapproval by officials of the institution. However, those officials may not approve the research if it has not been approved by an IRB.

§46.113   Suspension or termination of IRB approval of research.

An IRB shall have authority to suspend or terminate approval of research that is not being conducted in accordance with the IRB's requirements or that has been associated with unexpected serious harm to subjects. Any suspension or termination of approval shall include a statement of the reasons for the IRB's action and shall be reported promptly to the investigator, appropriate institutional officials, and the Department or Agency head.
(Approved by the Office of Management and Budget under Control Number 9999–0020.)

§46.114   Cooperative research.

Cooperative research projects are those projects covered by this policy which involve more than one institution. In the conduct of cooperative research projects, each institution is responsible for safeguarding the rights and welfare of human subjects an for complying with this policy. With the approval of the Department or Agency head, an institution participating in a cooperative project may enter into a joint review arrangement, rely upon the review of another qualified IRB, or make similar arrangements for avoiding duplication of effort.

§46.115   IRB records.

(a) An institution, or when appropriate an IRB, shall prepare and maintain adequate documentation of IRB activities, including the following:

(1) Copies of all research proposals reviewed, scientific evaluations, if any, that accompany the proposals, approved sample consent documents, progress reports submitted by investigators, and reports of injuries to subjects.

(2) Minutes of IRB meetings which shall be in sufficient detail to show attendance at the meetings; actions taken by the IRB; the vote on these actions including the number of members voting for, against, and abstaining; the basis for requiring changes in or disapproving research; and a written summary of the discussion of controverted issues and their resolution.

(3) Records of continuing review activities.

(4) Copies of all correspondence between the IRB and the investigators.

(5) A list of IRB members in the same detail as described in §46.103(b)(3).

(6) Written procedures for the IRB in the same detail as described in §46.103(b)(4) and §46.103(b)(5).

(7) Statements of significant new findings provided to subjects, as required by §46.116(b)(5).

(b) The records required by this policy shall be retained for at least 3 years, and records relating to research which is conducted shall be retained for at least 3 years after completion of the research. All records shall be accessible for inspection and copying by authorized representatives of the Department or Agency at reasonable times and in a reasonable manner.

(Approved by the Office of Management and Budget under Control Number 9999–0020.)

§46.116 General requirements for informed consent.

Except as provided elsewhere in this policy, no investigator may involve a human being as a subject in research covered by this policy unless the investigator has obtained the legally effective informed consent of the subject or the subject's legally authorized representative. An investigator shall seek such consent only under circumstances that provide the prospective subject or the representative sufficient opportunity to consider whether or not to participate and that minimize the possibility of coercion or undue influence. The information that is given to the subject or the representative shall be in language understandable to the subject or the representative. No informed consent, whether oral or written, may include any exculpatory language through which the subject or the representative is made to waive or appear to waive any of the subject's legal rights, or releases or appears to release the investigator, the sponsor, the institution or its agents from liability for negligence.

(a) Basic elements of informed consent. Except as provided in paragraph (c) or (d) of this section, in seeking informed consent the following information shall be provided to each subject:

(1) a statement that the study involves research, an explanation of the purposes of the research and the expected duration of the subject's participation, a description of the procedures to be followed, and identification of any procedures which are experimental;

(2) a description of any reasonably foreseeable risks or discomforts to the subject;

(3) a description of any benefits to the subject or to others which may reasonably be expected from the research;

(4) a disclosure of appropriate alternative procedures or courses of treatment, if any, that might be advantageous to the subject;

(5) a statement describing the extent, if any, to which confidentiality of records identifying the subject will be maintained;

(6) for research involving more than minimal risk, an explanation as to whether any compensation and an explanation as to whether any medical treatments are available if injury occurs and, if so, what they consist of, or where further information may be obtained;

(7) an explanation of whom to contact for answers to pertinent questions about the research and research subjects' rights, and whom to contact in the event of a research-related injury to the subject; and

(8) a statement that participation is voluntary, refusal to participate will involve no penalty or loss of benefits to which the subject is otherwise entitled, and the subject may discontinue participation at any time without penalty or loss of benefits to which the subject is otherwise entitled.

(b) additional elements of informed consent. When appropriate, one or more of the following elements of information shall also be provided to each subject:

(1) a statement that the particular treatment or procedure may involve risks to the subject (or to the embryo or fetus, if the subject is or may become pregnant) which are currently unforeseeable;

(2) anticipated circumstances under which the subject's participation may be terminated by the investigator without regard to the subject's consent;

(3) any additional costs to the subject that may result from participation in the research;

(4) the consequences of a subject's decision to withdraw from the research and procedures

for orderly termination of participation by the subject;

(5) A statement that significant new findings developed during the course of the research which may relate to the subject's willingness to continue participation will be provided to the subject; and

(6) the approximate number of subjects involved in the study.

(c) An IRB may approve a consent procedure which does not include, or which alters, some or all of the elements of informed consent set forth above, or waive the requirement to obtain informed consent provided the IRB finds and documents that:

(1) the research or demonstration project is to be conducted by or subject to the approval of state or local government officials and is designed to study, evaluate, or otherwise examine: (i) public benefit or service programs; (ii) procedures for obtaining benefits or services under those programs; (iii) possible changes in or alternatives to those programs or procedures; or (iv) possible changes in methods or levels of payment for benefits or services under those programs; and

(2) the research could not practicably be carried out without the waiver or alteration.

(d) An IRB may approve a consent procedure which does not include, or which alters, some or all of the elements of informed consent set forth in this section, or waive the requirements to obtain informed consent provided the IRB finds and documents that:

(1) the research involves no more than minimal risk to the subjects;

(2) the waiver or alteration will not adversely affect the rights and welfare of the subjects;

(3) the research could not practicably be carried out without the waiver or alteration; and

(4) whenever appropriate, the subjects will be provided with additional pertinent information after participation.

(e) The informed consent requirements in this policy are not intended to preempt any applicable Federal, State, or local laws which require additional information to be disclosed in order for informed consent to be legally effective.

(f) Nothing in this policy is intended to limit the authority of a physician to provide emergency medical care, to the extent the physician is permitted to do so under applicable Federal, State, or local law.

(Approved by the Office of Management and Budget under Control Number 9999–0020.)

§46.117 Documentation of informed consent.

(a) Except as provided in paragraph (c) of this section, informed consent shall be documented by the use of a written consent form approved by the IRB and signed by the subject or the subject's legally authorized representative. A copy shall be given to the person signing the form.

(b) Except as provided in paragraph (c) of this section, the consent form may be either of the following:

(1) A written consent document that embodies the elements of informed consent required by §46.116. This form may be read to the subject or the subject's legally authorized representative, but in any event, the investigator shall give either the subject or the representative adequate opportunity to read it before it is signed; or

(2) A short form written consent document stating that the elements of informed consent required by §46.116 have been presented orally to the subject or the subject's legally authorized representative. When this method is used, there shall be a witness to the oral presentation. Also, the IRB shall approve a written summary of what is to be said to the subject or the representative. Only the short form itself is to be signed by the subject or the representative. However, the witness shall sign both the short form and a copy of the summary, and the person actually obtaining consent shall sign a copy of the summary. A copy of the summary shall be given to the subject or the representative, in addition to a copy of the short form.

(c) An IRB may waive the requirement for the investigator to obtain a signed consent form for some or all subjects if it finds either:

(1) That the only record linking the subject and the research would be the consent docu-

ment and the principal risk would be potential harm resulting from a breach of confidentiality. Each subject will be asked whether the subject wants documentation linking the subject with the research, and the subject's wishes will govern; or

(2) That the research presents no more than minimal risk of harm to subjects and involves no procedures for which written consent is normally required outside of the research context.

In cases in which the documentation requirement is waived, the IRB may require the investigator to provide subjects with a written statement regarding the research.

(Approved by the Office of Management and Budget under Control Number 9999–0020.)

§46.118 Applications and proposals lacking definite plans for involvement of human subjects.

Certain types of applications for grants, cooperative agreements, or contracts are submitted to departments or agencies with the knowledge that subjects may be involved within the period of support, but definite plans would not normally be set forth in the application or proposal. These include activities such as institutional type grants when selection of specific projects is the institution's responsibility; research training grants in which the activities involving subjects remain to be selected; and projects in which human subjects' involvement will depend upon completion of instruments, prior animal studies, or purification of compounds. These applications need not be reviewed by an IRB before an award may be made. However, except for research exempted or waived under §46.101 (b) or (i), no human subjects may be involved in any project supported by these awards until the project has been reviewed and approved by the IRB, as provided in this policy, and certification submitted, by the institution, to the Department or Agency.

§46.119 Research undertaken without the intention of involving human subjects.

In the event research is undertaken without the intention of involving human subjects, but it is later proposed to involve human subjects in the research, the research shall first be reviewed and approved by an IRB, as provided in this policy, a certification submitted, by the institution, to the Department or Agency, and final approval given to the proposed change by the Department or Agency.

§46.120 Evaluation and disposition of applications and proposals for research to be conducted or supported by a Federal Department or Agency.

(a) The Department or Agency head will evaluate all applications and proposals involving human subjects submitted to the Department or Agency through such officers and employees of the Department or Agency and such experts and consultants as the Department or Agency head determines to be appropriate. This evaluation will take into consideration the risks to the subjects, the adequacy of protection against these risks, the potential benefits of the research to the subjects and others, and the importance of the knowledge gained or to be gained.

(b) On the basis of this evaluation, the Department or Agency head may approve or disapprove the application or proposal, or enter into negotiations to develop an approvable one.

§46.121 [Reserved]

§46.122 Use of Federal funds.

Federal funds administered by a Department or Agency may not be expended for research involving human subjects unless the requirements of this policy have been satisfied.

§46.123 Early termination of research support: Evaluation of applications and proposals.

(a) The Department or Agency head may require that Department or Agency support for any project be terminated or suspended in the manner prescribed in applicable program requirements, when the Department or Agency head finds an institution has materially failed to comply with the terms of this policy.

(b) In making decisions about supporting or approving applications or proposals covered by this policy the Department or Agency head may take into account, in addition to all other eligibility requirements and program criteria, factors such as whether the applicant has been subject to a termination or suspension under paragraph (a) of this section and whether the applicant or the person or persons who would direct or has/have directed the scientific and technical aspects of an activity has/have, in the judgment of the Department or Agency head, materially failed to discharge responsibility for the protection of the rights and welfare of human subjects (whether or not the research was subject to Federal regulation).

§46.124 Conditions.

With respect to any research project or any class of research projects the Department or Agency head may impose additional conditions prior to or at the time of approval when in the judgment of the Department or Agency head additional conditions are necessary for the protection of human subjects.

Subpart B—Additional DHHS Protections Pertaining to Research, Development, and Related Activities Involving Fetuses, Pregnant Women, and Human In Vitro Fertilization

Source: 40 FR 33528, Aug. 8, 1975, 43 FR 1758, January 11, 1978; 43 FR 51559, November 3, 1978.

§46.201 Applicability.

(a) The regulations in this subpart are applicable to all Department of Health and Human Services grants and contracts supporting research, development, and related activities involving: (1) the fetus, (2) pregnant women, and (3) human *in vitro* fertilization.

(b) Nothing in this subpart shall be construed as indicating that compliance with the procedures set forth herein will in any way render inapplicable pertinent State or local laws bearing upon activities covered by this subpart.

(c) The requirements of this subpart are in addition to those imposed under the other subparts of this part.

§46.202 Purpose.

It is the purpose of this subpart to provide additional safeguards in reviewing activities to which this subpart is applicable to assure that they conform to appropriate ethical standards and relate to important societal needs.

§46.203 Definitions.

As used in this subpart:

(a) "Secretary" means the Secretary of Health and Human Services and any other officer or employee of the Department of Health and Human Services (DHHS) to whom authority has been delegated.

(b) "Pregnancy" encompasses the period of time from confirmation of implantation (through any of the presumptive signs of pregnancy, such as missed menses, or by a medically acceptable pregnancy test), until expulsion or extraction of the fetus.

(c) "Fetus" means the product of conception from the time of implantation (as evidenced by any of the presumptive signs of pregnancy, such as missed menses, or a medically acceptable pregnancy test), until a determination is made, following expulsion or extraction of the fetus, that it is viable.

(d) "Viable" as it pertains to the fetus means being able, after either spontaneous or induced delivery, to survive (given the benefit of available medical therapy) to the point of independently maintaining heart beat and respiration. The Secretary may from time to time, taking into account medical advances, publish in the **Federal Register** guidelines to assist in determining whether a fetus is viable for purposes of this subpart. If a fetus is viable after delivery, it is a premature infant.

(e) "Nonviable fetus" means a fetus *ex utero* which, although living, is not viable.

(f) "Dead fetus" means a fetus *ex utero* which exhibits neither heartbeat, spontaneous respiratory activity, spontaneous movement of voluntary muscles, nor pulsation of the umbilical cord (if still attached).

(g) "*In vitro* fertilization" means any fertilization of human ova which occurs outside the body of a female, either through admixture of donor human sperm and ova or by any other means.

§46.204 Ethical Advisory Boards.

(a) One or more Ethical Advisory Boards shall be established by the Secretary. Members of these Board(s) shall be so selected that the Board(s) will be competent to deal with medical, legal, social, ethical, and related issues and may include, for example, research scientists, physicians, psychologists, sociologists, educators, lawyers, and ethicists, as well as representatives of the general public. No Board member may be a regular, full-time employee of the Department of Health and Human Services.

(b) At the request of the Secretary, the Ethical Advisory Board shall render advice consistent with the policies and requirements of this part as to ethical issues, involving activities covered by this subpart, raised by individual applications or proposals. In addition, upon request by the Secretary, the Board shall render advice as to classes of applications or proposals and general policies, guidelines, and procedures.

(c) A Board may establish, with the approval of the Secretary, classes of applications or proposals which: (1) must be submitted to the Board, or (2) need not be submitted to the Board. Where the Board so establishes a class of applications or proposals which must be submitted, no application or proposal within the class may be funded by the Department or any component thereof until the application or proposal has been reviewed by the Board and the Board has rendered advice as to its acceptability from an ethical standpoint.

§46.205   Additional duties of the Institutional Review Boards in connection with activities involving fetuses, pregnant women, or human in vitro fertilization.

(a) In addition to the responsibilities prescribed for Institutional Review Boards under Subpart A of this part, the applicant's or offeror's Board shall, with respect to activities covered by this subpart, carry out the following additional duties:

(1) determine that all aspects of the activity meet the requirements of this subpart;

(2) determine that adequate consideration has been given to the manner in which potential subjects will be selected, and adequate provision has been made by the applicant or offeror for monitoring the actual informed consent process (e.g., through such mechanisms, when appropriate, as participation by the Institutional Review Board or subject advocates in: (i) overseeing the actual process by which individual consents required by this subpart are secured either by approving induction of each individual into the activity or verifying, perhaps through sampling, that approved procedures for induction of individuals into the activity are being followed, and (ii) monitoring the progress of the activity and intervening as necessary through such steps as visits to the activity site and continuing evaluation to determine if any unanticipated risks have arisen);

(3) carry out such other responsibilities as may be assigned by the Secretary.

(b) No award may be issued until the applicant or offeror has certified to the Secretary that the Institutional Review Board has made the determinations required under paragraph (a) of this section and the Secretary has approved these determinations, as provided in §46.120 of Subpart A of this part.

(c) Applicants or offerors seeking support for activities covered by this subpart must provide for the designation of an Institutional Review Board, subject to approval by the Secretary, where no such Board has been established under Subpart A of this part.

§46.206   General limitations.

(a) No activity to which this subpart is applicable may be undertaken unless:

(1) appropriate studies on animals and nonpregnant individuals have been completed;

(2) except where the purpose of the activity is to meet the health needs of the mother or the particular fetus, the risk to the fetus is minimal and, in all cases, is the least possible risk for achieving the objectives of the activity;

(3) individuals engaged in the activity will have no part in: (i) any decisions as to the timing, method, and procedures used to terminate the pregnancy, and (ii) determining the viability of the fetus at the termination of the pregnancy; and

(4) no procedural changes which may cause greater than minimal risk to the fetus or the pregnant woman will be introduced into the

procedure for terminating the pregnancy solely in the interest of the activity.

(b) No inducements, monetary or otherwise, may be offered to terminate pregnancy for purposes of the activity.

Source: 40 FR 33528, Aug. 8, 1975, as amended at 40 FR 51638, Nov. 6, 1975.

§46.207 Activities directed toward pregnant women as subjects.

(a) No pregnant woman may be involved as a subject in an activity covered by this subpart unless: (1) the purpose of the activity is to meet the health needs of the mother and the fetus will be placed at risk only to the minimum extent necessary to meet such needs, or (2) the risk to the fetus is minimal.

(b) An activity permitted under paragraph (a) of this section may be conducted only if the mother and father are legally competent and have given their informed consent after having been fully informed regarding possible impact on the fetus, except that the father's informed consent need not be secured if: (1) the purpose of the activity is to meet the health needs of the mother; (2) his identity or whereabouts cannot reasonably be ascertained; (3) he is not reasonably available; or (4) the pregnancy resulted from rape.

§46.208 Activities directed toward fetuses *in utero* as subjects.

(a) No fetus *in utero* may be involved as a subject in any activity covered by this subpart unless: (1) the purpose of the activity is to meet the health needs of the particular fetus and the fetus will be placed at risk only to the minimum extent necessary to meet such needs, or (2) the risk to the fetus imposed by the research is minimal and the purpose of the activity is the development of important biomedical knowledge which cannot be obtained by other means.

(b) An activity permitted under paragraph (a) of this section may be conducted only if the mother and father are legally competent and have given their informed consent, except that the father's consent need not be secured if: (1) his identity or whereabouts cannot reasonably be ascertained, (2) he is not reasonably available, or (3) the pregnancy resulted from rape.

§46.209 Activities directed toward fetuses *ex utero*, including nonviable fetuses, as subjects.

(a) Until it has been ascertained whether or not a fetus *ex utero* is viable, a fetus *ex utero* may not be involved as a subject in an activity covered by this subpart unless:

(1) there will be no added risk to the fetus resulting from the activity, and the purpose of the activity is the development of important biomedical knowledge which cannot be obtained by other means, or

(2) the purpose of the activity is to enhance the possibility of survival of the particular fetus to the point of viability.

(b) No nonviable fetus may be involved as a subject in an activity covered by this subpart unless:

(1) vital functions of the fetus will not be artificially maintained,

(2) experimental activities which of themselves would terminate the heartbeat or respiration of the fetus will not be employed, and

(3) the purpose of the activity is the development of important biomedical knowledge which cannot be obtained by other means.

(c) In the event the fetus *ex utero* is found to be viable, it may be included as a subject in the activity only to the extent permitted by and in accordance with the requirements of other subparts of this part.

(d) An activity permitted under paragraph (a) or (b) of this section may be conducted only if the mother and father are legally competent and have given their informed consent, except that the father's informed consent need not be secured if: (1) his identity or whereabouts cannot reasonably be ascertained, (2) he is not reasonably available, or (3) the pregnancy resulted from rape.

§46.210 Activities involving the dead fetus, fetal material, or the placenta.

Activities involving the dead fetus, mascerated fetal material, or cells, tissue, or organs excised from a dead fetus shall be conducted only in accordance with any applicable State or local laws regarding such activities.

§46.211 Modification or waiver of specific requirements.

Upon the request of an applicant or offeror (with the approval of its Institutional Review Board), the Secretary may modify or waive specific requirements of this subpart, with the approval of the Ethical Advisory Board after such opportunity for public comment as the Ethical Advisory Board considers appropriate in the particular instance. In making such decisions, the Secretary will consider whether the risks to the subject are so outweighed by the sum of the benefit to the subject and the importance of the knowledge to be gained as to warrant such modification or waiver and that such benefits cannot be gained except through a modification or waiver. Any such modifications or waivers will be published as notices in the **Federal Register.**

Subpart C—Additional DHHS Protections Pertaining to Biomedical and Behavioral Research Involving Prisoners as Subjects

Source: 43 FR 53655, Nov. 16, 1978.

§46.301 Applicability.

(a) The regulations in this subpart are applicable to all biomedical and behavioral research conducted or supported by the Department of Health and Human Services involving prisoners as subjects.

(b) Nothing in this subpart shall be construed as indicating that compliance with the procedures set forth herein will authorize research involving prisoners as subjects, to the extent such research is limited or barred by applicable State or local law.

(c) The requirements of this subpart are in addition to those imposed under the other subparts of this part.

§46.302 Purpose.

Inasmuch as prisoners may be under constraints because of their incarceration which could affect their ability to make a truly voluntary and uncoerced decision whether or not to participate as subjects in research, it is the purpose of this subpart to provide additional safeguards for the protection of prisoners involved in activities to which this subpart is applicable.

§46.303 Definitions.

As used in this subpart:

(a) "Secretary" means the Secretary of Health and Human Services and any other officer or employee of the Department of Health and Human Services to whom authority has been delegated.

(b) "DHHS" means the Department of Health and Human Services.

(c) "Prisoner" means any individual involuntarily confined or detained in a penal institution. The term is intended to encompass individuals sentenced to such an institution under a criminal or civil statute, individuals detained in other facilities by virtue of statutes or commitment procedures which provide alternatives to criminal prosecution or incarceration in a penal institution, and individuals detained pending arraignment, trial, or sentencing.

(d) "Minimal risk" is the probability and magnitude of physical or psychological harm that is normally encountered in the daily lives, or in the routine medical, dental, or psychological examination of healthy persons.

§46.304 Composition of Institutional Review Boards where prisoners are involved.

In addition to satisfying the requirements in §46.107 of this part, an Institutional Review Board, carrying out responsibilities under this part with respect to research covered by this subpart, shall also meet the following specific requirements:

(a) A majority of the Board (exclusive of prisoner members) shall have no association with the prison(s) involved, apart from their membership on the Board.

(b) At least one member of the Board shall be a prisoner, or a prisoner representative with appropriate background and experience to serve in that capacity, except that where a particular research project is reviewed by more than one

Board only one Board need satisfy this requirement.

§46.305 Additional duties of the Institutional Review Boards where prisoners are involved.

(a) In addition to all other responsibilities prescribed for Institutional Review Boards under this part, the Board shall review research covered by this subpart and approve such research only if it finds that:

(1) the research under review represents one of the categories of research permissible under §46.306(a)(2);

(2) any possible advantages accruing to the prisoner through his or her participation in the research, when compared to the general living conditions, medical care, quality of food, amenities and opportunity for earnings in the prison, are not of such a magnitude that his or her ability to weigh the risks of the research against the value of such advantages in the limited choice environment of the prison is impaired;

(3) the risks involved in the research are commensurate with risks that would be accepted by nonprisoner volunteers;

(4) procedures for the selection of subjects within the prison are fair to all prisoners and immune from arbitrary intervention by prison authorities or prisoners. Unless the principal investigator provides to the Board justification in writing for following some other procedures, control subjects must be selected randomly from the group of available prisoners who meet the characteristics needed for that particular research project;

(5) the information is presented in language which is understandable to the subject population;

(6) adequate assurance exists that parole boards will not take into account a prisoner's participation in the research in making decisions regarding parole, and each prisoner is clearly informed in advance that participation in the research will have no effect on his or parole; and

(7) where the Board finds there may be a need for follow-up examination or care of participants after the end of their participation, adequate provision has been made for such examination or care, taking into account the varying lengths of individual prisoners' sentences, and for informing participants of this fact.

(b) The Board shall carry out such other duties as may be assigned by the Secretary.

(c) The institution shall certify to the Secretary, in such form and manner as the Secretary may require, that the duties of the Board under this section have been fulfilled.

§46.306 Permitted research involving prisoners.

(a) Biomedical or behavioral research conducted or supported by DHHS may involve prisoners as subjects only if:

(1) the institution responsible for the conduct of the research has certified to the Secretary that the Institutional Review Board has approved the research under §46.305 of this subpart; and

(2) in the judgment of the Secretary the proposed research involves solely the following:

(A) study of the possible causes, effects, and processes of incarceration, and of criminal behavior, provided that the study presents no more than minimal risk and no more than inconvenience to the subjects;

(B) study of prisons as institutional structures or of prisoners as incarcerated persons, provided that the study presents no more than minimal risk and no more than inconvenience to the subjects;

(C) research on conditions particularly affecting prisoners as a class (for example, vaccine trials and other research on hepatitis which is much more prevalent in prisons than elsewhere; and research on social and psychological problems such as alcoholism, drug addiction, and sexual assaults) provided that the study may proceed only after the Secretary has consulted with appropriate experts including experts in penology, medicine, and ethics, and published notice, in the **Federal Register,** of his intent to approve such research; or

(D) research on practices, both innovative and accepted, which have the intent and reasonable probability of improving the health or well-being of the subject. In cases in which those studies require the assignment of prisoners in a manner consistent with protocols approved by the IRB to control groups which may not benefit from the research, the study may proceed only after the Secretary has consulted with appropriate experts, including experts in penology, medicine, and ethics, and published notice, in the **Federal Register,** of the intent to approve such research.

(b) Except as provided in paragraph (a) of this section, biomedical or behavioral research conducted or supported by DHHS shall not involve prisoners as subjects.

Subpart D—Additional DHHS Protections for Children Involved as Subjects in Research.

Source: 48 FR 9818, March 8, 1983; 56 FR 28032, June 18, 1991.

§46.401   To what do these regulations apply?

(a) This subpart applies to all research involving children as subjects, conducted or supported by the Department of Health and Human Services.

(1) This includes research conducted by Department employees, except that each head of an Operating Division of the Department may adopt such nonsubstantive, procedural modifications as may be appropriate from an administrative standpoint.

(2) It also includes research conducted or supported by the Department of Health and Human Services outside the United States, but in appropriate circumstances, the Secretary may, under paragraph (i) of §46.101 of Subpart A, waive the applicability of some or all of the requirements of these regulations for research of this type.

(b) Exemptions at §46.101(b)(1) and (b)(3) through (b)(6) are applicable to this subpart. The exemption at §46.101(b)(2) regarding educational tests is also applicable to this subpart. However, the exemption at §46.101(b)(2) for research involving survey or interview procedures or observations of public behavior does

not apply to research covered by this subpart, except for research involving observation of public behavior when the investigator(s) do not participate in the activities being observed.

(c) The exceptions, additions, and provisions for waiver as they appear in paragraphs (c) through (i) of §46.101 of Subpart A are applicable to this subpart.

§46.402   Definitions.

The definitions in §46.102 of Subpart A shall be applicable to this subpart as well. In addition, as used in this subpart:

(a) "Children" are persons who have not attained the legal age for consent to treatments or procedures involved in the research, under the applicable law of the jurisdiction in which the research will be conducted.

(b) "Assent" means a child's affirmative agreement to participate in research. Mere failure to object should not, absent affirmative agreement, be construed as assent.

(c) "Permission" means the agreement of parent(s) or guardian to the participation of their child or ward in research.

(d) "Parent" means a child's biological or adoptive parent.

(e) "Guardian" means an individual who is authorized under applicable State or local law to consent on behalf of a child to general medical care.

§46.403   IRB duties.

In addition to other responsibilities assigned to IRBs under this part, each IRB shall review research covered by this subpart and approve only research which satisfies the conditions of all applicable sections of this subpart.

§46.404   Research not involving greater than minimal risk.

DHHS will conduct or fund research in which the IRB finds that no greater than minimal risk to children is presented, only if the IRB finds that adequate provisions are made for soliciting the assent of the children and the permission of their parents or guardians, as set forth in §46.408.

§46.405 Research involving greater than minimal risk but presenting the prospect of direct benefit to the individual subjects.

DHHS will conduct or fund research in which the IRB finds that more than minimal risk to children is presented by an intervention or procedure that holds out the prospect of direct benefit for the individual subject, or by a monitoring procedure that is likely to contribute to the subject's well-being, only if the IRB finds that:

(a) the risk is justified by the anticipated benefit to the subjects;

(b) the relation of the anticipated benefit to the risk is at least as favorable to the subjects as that presented by available alternative approaches; and

(c) adequate provisions are made for soliciting the assent of the children and permission of their parents or guardians, as set forth in §46.408.

§46.406 Research involving greater than minimal risk and no prospect of direct benefit to individual subjects, but likely to yield generalizable knowledge about the subject's disorder or condition.

DHHS will conduct or fund research in which the IRB finds that more than minimal risk to children is presented by an intervention or procedure that does not hold out the prospect of direct benefit for the individual subject, or by a monitoring procedure which is not likely to contribute to the well-being of the subject, only if the IRB finds that:

(a) the risk represents a minor increase over minimal risk;

(b) the intervention or procedure presents experiences to subjects that are reasonably commensurate with those inherent in their actual or expected medical, dental, psychological, social, or educational situations;

(c) the intervention or procedure is likely to yield generalizable knowledge about the subjects' disorder or condition which is of vital importance for the understanding or amelioration of the subjects' disorder or condition; and

(d) adequate provisions are made for soliciting assent of the children and permission of their parents or guardians, as set forth in §46.408.

§46.407 Research not otherwise approvable which presents an opportunity to understand, prevent, or alleviate a serious problem affecting the health or welfare of children.

DHHS will conduct or fund research that the IRB does not believe meets the requirements of §46.404, §46.405, or §46.406 only if:

(a) the IRB finds that the research presents a reasonable opportunity to further the understanding, prevention, or alleviation of a serious problem affecting the health or welfare of children; and

(b) the Secretary, after consultation with a panel of experts in pertinent disciplines (for example: science, medicine, education, ethics, law) and following opportunity for public review and comment, has determined either:

(1) that the research in fact satisfies the conditions of §46.404, §46.405, or §46.406, as applicable, or (2) the following:

(i) the research presents a reasonable opportunity to further the understanding, prevention, or alleviation of a serious problem affecting the health or welfare of children;

(ii) the research will be conducted in accordance with sound ethical principles;

(iii) adequate provisions are made for soliciting the assent of children and the permission of their parents or guardians, as set forth in §46.408.

§46.408 Requirements for permission by parents or guardians and for assent by children.

(a) In addition to the determinations required under other applicable sections of this subpart, the IRB shall determine that adequate provisions are made for soliciting the assent of the children, when in the judgment of the IRB the children are capable of providing assent. In determining whether children are capable of assenting, the IRB shall take into account the ages, maturity, and psychological state of the children involved. This judgment may be made for all children to be involved in research under a particular protocol, or for each child, as the IRB deems appropriate. If the IRB determines that the capability of some or all of the children is so limited that they cannot reasonably be consulted or that the intervention or procedure involved in the research holds out a prospect of direct benefit that is important to the health or well-being of the children and is available only in the context of the research, the assent of the children is not a necessary condition for proceeding with the research. Even where the IRB determines that the subjects are capable of assenting, the IRB may still waive the assent requirement under circumstances in which consent may be waived in accord with §46.116 of Subpart A.

(b) In addition to the determinations required under other applicable sections of this subpart, the IRB shall determine, in accordance with and to the extent that consent is required by §46.116 of Subpart A, that adequate provisions are made for soliciting the permission of each child's parents or guardian. Where parental permission is to be obtained, the IRB may find that the permission of one parent is sufficient for research to be conducted under §46.404 or §46.405. Where research is covered by §46.406 and §46.407 and permission is to be obtained from parents, both parents must give their permission unless one parent is deceased, unknown, incompetent, or not reasonably available, or when only one parent has legal responsibility for the care and custody of the child.

(c) In addition to the provisions for waiver contained in §46.116 of Subpart A, if the IRB determines that a research protocol is designed for conditions or for a subject population for which parental or guardian permission is not a reasonable requirement to protect the subjects (for example, neglected or abused children), it may waive the consent requirements in Subpart A of this part and paragraph (b) of this section, provided an appropriate mechanism for protecting the children who will participate as subjects in the research is substituted, and provided further that the waiver is not inconsistent with Federal, State, or local law. The choice of an appropriate mechanism would depend upon the nature and purpose of the activities described in the protocol, the risk and anticipated benefit to the research subjects, and their age, maturity, status, and condition.

(d) Permission by parents or guardians shall be documented in accordance with and to the extent required by §46.117 of Subpart A.

(e) When the IRB determines that assent is required, it shall also determine whether and how assent must be documented.

§46.409 Wards.

(a) Children who are wards of the State or any other agency, institution, or entity can be included in research approved under §46.406 or §46.407 only if such research is:

(1) related to their status as wards; or

(2) conducted in schools, camps, hospitals, institutions, or similar settings in which the majority of children involved as subjects are not wards.

(b) If the research is approved under paragraph (a) of this section, the IRB shall require appointment of an advocate for each child who is a ward, in addition to any other individual acting on behalf of the child as guardian or in loco parentis. One individual may serve as advocate for more than one child. The advocate shall be an individual who has the background and experience to act in, and agrees to act in, the best interests of the child for the duration of the child's participation in the research and who is not associated in any way (except in the role as advocate or member of the IRB) with the research, the investigator(s), or the guardian organization.

RESEARCH ACTIVITIES WHICH MAY BE REVIEWED THROUGH EXPEDITED REVIEW PROCEDURES

Research activities involving no more than minimal risk *and* in which the only involvement of human subjects will be in one or more of the following categories (carried out through standard methods) may be reviewed by the Institutional Review Board through expedited review procedure authorized in §46.110 of 45 CFR Part 46.

(1) Collection of: hair and nail clippings, in a nondisfiguring manner; deciduous teeth; and permanent teeth if patient care indicates a need for extraction.

(2) Collection of excreta and external secretions including sweat, uncannulated saliva, placenta removed at delivery, and amniotic fluid at the time of rupture of the membrane prior to or during labor.

(3) Recording of data from subjects 18 years of age or older using noninvasive procedures routinely employed in clinical practice. This includes the use of physical sensors that are applied either to the surface of the body or at a distance and do not involve input of matter or significant amounts of energy into the subject or an invasion of the subject's privacy. It also includes such procedures as weighing, testing, sensory acuity, electrocardiography, electroencephalography, thermography, detection of naturally occurring radioactivity, diagnostic echography, and electroretinography. It does not include exposure to electromagnetic radiation outside the visible range (for example, x-rays, microwaves).

(4) Collection of blood samples by venipuncture, in amounts not exceeding 450 milliliters in an eight-week period and no more often than two times per week, from subjects 18 years of age or older and who are in good health and not pregnant.

(5) Collection of both supra- and subgingival dental plaque and calculus, provided the procedure is not more invasive than routine prophylactic scaling of the teeth and the process is accomplished in accordance with accepted prophylactic techniques.

(6) Voice recordings made for research purposes such as investigations of speech defects.

(7) Moderate exercise by healthy volunteers.

(8) The study of existing data, documents, records, pathological specimens, or diagnostic specimens.

(9) Research on individual or group behavior or characteristics of individuals, such as studies of perception, cognition, game theory, or test development, where the investigator does not manipulate subjects' behavior and the research will not involve stress to subjects.

(10) Research on drugs or devices for which an investigational new drug exemption or an investigational device exemption is not required.

Source: 46 FR 8392; January 26, 1981.

PUBLIC LAW 103–43—JUNE 10, 1993

National Institutes of Health Revitalization Act Of 1993

TITLE I—GENERAL PROVISIONS REGARDING TITLE IV
OF PUBLIC HEALTH SERVICE ACT

Subtitle A—Research Freedom

PART II—Research On Transplantation Of Fetal Tissue

SEC. 111. Establishment Of Authorities.

Part G of title IV of the Public Health Service Act (42 U.S.C. 289 et seq.) is amended by inserting after section 498 the following section:

"RESEARCH ON TRANSPLANTATION OF FETAL TISSUE

"SEC. 498A. (a) ESTABLISHMENT OF PROGRAM.—

"(1) IN GENERAL.—The Secretary may conduct or support research on the transplantation of human fetal tissue for therapeutic purposes.

"(2) SOURCE OF TISSUE.—Human fetal tissue may be used in research carried out under paragraph (1) regardless of whether the tissue is obtained pursuant to a spontaneous or induced abortion or pursuant to a stillbirth.

"(b) INFORMED CONSENT OF DONOR.—

"(1) IN GENERAL.—In research carried out under subsection (a), human fetal tissue may be used only if the woman providing the tissue makes a statement, made in writing and signed by the woman, declaring that—

"(A) the woman donates the fetal tissue for use in research described in subsection (a);

"(B) the donation is made without any restriction regarding the identity of individuals who may be the recipients of transplantations of the tissue; and

"(C) the woman has not been informed of the identity of any such individuals.

"(2) ADDITIONAL STATEMENT.—In research carried out under subsection (a), human fetal tissue may be used only if the attending physician with respect to obtaining the tissue from the woman involved makes a statement, made in writing and signed by the physician, declaring that—

"(A) in the case of tissue obtained pursuant to an induced abortion—

"(i) the consent of the woman for the abortion was obtained prior to requesting or obtaining consent for a donation of the tissue for use in such research;

"(ii) no alteration of the timing, method, or procedures used to terminate the pregnancy was made solely for the purposes of obtaining the tissue; and

"(iii) the abortion was performed in accordance with applicable State law;

"(B) the tissue has been donated by the woman in accordance with paragraph (1); and

"(C) full disclosure has been provided to the woman with regard to—

"(i) such physician's interest, if any, in the research to be conducted with the tissue; and

"(ii) any known medical risks to the woman or risks to her privacy that might be associated with the donation of the tissue and that are in addition to risks of such type that are associated with the woman's medical care.

"(c) INFORMED CONSENT OF RESEARCHER AND DONEE.—In research carried out under subsection (a), human fetal tissue may be used only if the individual with the principal responsibility for conducting the research involved makes a statement, made in writing and signed by the individual, declaring that the individual—

"(1) is aware that—

"(A) the tissue is human fetal tissue;

"(B) the tissue may have been obtained pursuant to a spontaneous or induced abortion or pursuant to a stillbirth; and

"(C) the tissue was donated for research purposes;

"(2) has provided such information to other individuals with responsibilities regarding the research;

"(3) will require, prior to obtaining the consent of an individual to be a recipient of a transplantation of the tissue, written acknowledgment of receipt of such information by such recipient; and

"(4) has had no part in any decisions as to the timing, method, or procedures used to terminate the pregnancy made solely for the purposes of the research.

"(d) AVAILABILITY OF STATEMENTS FOR AUDIT.—

"(1) IN GENERAL.—In research carried out under subsection (a), human fetal tissue may be used only if the head of the agency or other entity conducting the research involved certifies to the Secretary that the statements required under subsections (b)(2) and (c) will be available for audit by the Secretary.

"(2) CONFIDENTIALITY OF AUDIT.—Any audit conducted by the Secretary pursuant to paragraph (1) shall be conducted in a confidential manner to protect the privacy rights of the individuals and entities involved in such research, including such individuals and entities involved in the donation, transfer, receipt, or transplantation of human fetal tissue. With respect to any material or information obtained pursuant to such audit, the Secretary shall—

"(A) use such material or information only for the purposes of verifying compliance with the requirements of this section;

"(B) not disclose or publish such material or information, except where required by Federal law, in which case such material or information shall be coded in a manner such that the identities of such individuals and entities are protected; and

"(C) not maintain such material or information after completion of such audit, except where necessary for the purposes of such audit.

"(e) APPLICABILITY OF STATE AND LOCAL LAW.—

"(1) RESEARCH CONDUCTED BY RECIPIENTS OF ASSISTANCE.—The Secretary may not provide support for research under subsection (a) unless the applicant for the financial assistance involved agrees to conduct the research in accordance with applicable State law.

"(2) RESEARCH CONDUCTED BY SECRETARY.—The Secretary may conduct research under subsection (a) only in accordance with applicable State and local law.

"(f) REPORT.—The Secretary shall annually submit to the Committee on Energy and Commerce of the House of Representatives, and to the Committee on Labor and Human Resources of the Senate, a report describing the activities carried out under this section during the preceding fiscal year, including a description of whether and to what extent research under subsection (a) has been conducted in accordance with this section.

"(g) DEFINITION.—For purposes of this section, the term 'human fetal tissue' means tissue or cells obtained from a dead human embryo or fetus after a spontaneous or induced abortion, or after a stillbirth.".

SEC. 112. Purchase Of Human Fetal Tissue; Solicitation Or Acceptance Of Tissue As Directed Donation For Use In Transplantation.

Part G of title IV of the Public Health Service Act, as amended by section 111 of this Act, is amended by inserting after section 498A the following section:

"PROHIBITIONS REGARDING HUMAN FETAL TISSUE

"Sec. 498B. (a) Purchase of Tissue.—It shall be unlawful for any person to knowingly acquire, receive, or otherwise transfer any human fetal tissue for valuable consideration if the transfer affects interstate commerce.

"(b) Solicitation or Acceptance of Tissue as Directed Donation for Use in Transplantation.—It shall be unlawful for any person to solicit or knowingly acquire, receive, or accept a donation of human fetal tissue for the purpose of transplantation of such tissue into another person if the donation affects interstate commerce, the tissue will be or is obtained pursuant to an induced abortion, and—

"(1) the donation will be or is made pursuant to a promise to the donating individual that the donated tissue will be transplanted into a recipient specified by such individual;

"(2) the donated tissue will be transplanted into a relative of the donating individual; or

"(3) the person who solicits or knowingly acquires, receives, or accepts the donation has provided valuable consideration for the costs associated with such abortion.

"(c) Criminal Penalties for Violations.—

"(1) In general.—Any person who violates subsection (a) or (b) shall be fined in accordance with title 18, United States Code, subject to paragraph (2), or imprisoned for not more than 10 years, or both.

"(2) Penalties applicable to persons receiving consideration.—With respect to the imposition of a fine under paragraph (1), if the person involved violates subsection (a) or (b)(3), a fine shall be imposed in an amount not less than twice the amount of the valuable consideration received.

"(d) Definitions.—For purposes of this section:

"(1) The term 'human fetal tissue' has the meaning given such term in section 498A(f).

"(2) The term 'interstate commerce' has the meaning given such term in section 201(b) of the Federal Food, Drug, and Cosmetic Act.

"(3) The term 'valuable consideration' does not include reasonable payments associated with the transportation, implantation, processing, preservation, quality control, or storage of human fetal tissue.".

SEC. 113. Nullification Of Moratorium.

(a) In General.—Except as provided in subsection (c), no official of the executive branch may impose a policy that the Department of Health and Human Services is prohibited from conducting or supporting any research on the transplantation of human fetal tissue for therapeutic purposes. Such research shall be carried out in accordance with section 498A of the Public Health Service Act (as added by section 111 of this Act), without regard to any such policy that may have been in effect prior to the date of the enactment of this Act.

(b) Prohibition Against Withholding of Funds in Cases of Technical and Scientific Merit.—

(1) In general.—Subject to subsection (b)(2) of section 492A of the Public Health Service Act (as added by section 101 of this Act), in the case of any proposal for research on the transplantation of human fetal tissue for therapeutic purposes, the Secretary of Health and Human Services may not withhold funds for the research if—

(A) the research has been approved for purposes of subsection (a) of such section 492A;

(B) the research will be carried out in accordance with section 498A of such Act (as added by section 111 of this Act); and

(C) there are reasonable assurances that the research will not utilize any human fetal tissue that has been obtained in violation of section 498B(a) of such Act (as added by section 112 of this Act).

(2) STANDING APPROVAL REGARDING ETHICAL STATUS.—In the case of any proposal for research on the transplantation of human fetal tissue for therapeutic purposes, the issuance in December 1988 of the Report of the Human Fetal Tissue Transplantation Research Panel shall be deemed to be a report—

(A) issued by an ethics advisory board pursuant to section 492A(b)(5)(B)(ii) of the Public Health Service Act (as added by section 101 of this Act); and

(B) finding, on a basis that is neither arbitrary nor capricious, that the nature of the research is such that it is not unethical to conduct or support the research.

(c) AUTHORITY FOR WITHHOLDING FUNDS FROM RESEARCH.—In the case of any research on the transplantation of human fetal tissue for therapeutic purposes, the Secretary of Health and Human Services may withhold funds for the research if any of the conditions specified in any of subparagraphs (A) through (C) of subsection (b)(1) are not met with respect to the research.

(d) DEFINITION.—For purposes of this section, the term "human fetal tissue" has the meaning given such term in section 498A(f) of the Public Health Service Act (as added by section 111 of this Act).

Answers for Exercises

Following are the answers to the Exercises found throughout the text. While some questions have universal answers, others ask you to evaluate procedures in your own institution or discuss your own experiences.

EXERCISE 2–1
(page 31)

1. a,b,c,& d
2. answer depends on the situation in your own facility
3. answer depends on your finding in you own facility

EXERCISE 2–2
(page 32)

All answers should be based on the situation at your own institution.

EXERCISE 3–1
(page 49)

Cost terms:

1. Direct: a, b, c, e, f, g, h, j, k, l, o, p
2. Indirect: d, i, m, n
3. Fixed: d, m, n

4. Semi-fixed: a, b, h, i
5. Variable: c, e, f, g, j, k, l, o
6. Semi-variable: f
7. Marginal: (none)
8. Incremental: p
9. Induced: p

EXERCISE 3–2
(page 51)

	Measurable Costs	Associated Cost Drivers
1.	• Continuous cardiac output machine • Standard cardiac output equipment • Nursing time required for each method	• Treatment-related factors • Provider-related factors • Geographic/economic factors
2.	• In-line sampling tubing • Standard tubing • Nursing time required for each method	• Treatment-related factors • Provider-related factors • Geographic/economic factors
3.	• In-line suction catheter and circuit • Standard suction catheter • Nursing time required for each method	• Patient-related factors • Treatment-related factors • Provider-related factors • Geographic/economic factors
4.	• Triflow equipment • Vibrator or other equipment used for chest physio-therapy (CPT) • PT fee or nursing time required for each method	• Patient-related factors • Treatment-related factors • Provider-related factors • Geographic/economic factors
5.	• Equipment for administration of bolus and continuous feeds • Nursing time required for each method	• Patient-related factors • Treatment-related factors • Provider-related factors • Geographic/economic factors
6.	• Total cost of drug required in each method • Nursing time required to obtain and administer drug in each method	• Patient-related factors • Treatment-related factors • Provider-related factors • Geographic/economic factors

EXERCISE 3–3
(page 54)

Answers should be based on your own research question.

EXERCISE 3–4
(page 57)

Answers should be based on your own research question.

EXERCISE 4–1
(page 67)

Answers should be based on your own research team members.

EXERCISE 4–2
(page 72)

Answers should be based on your own study time line.

EXERCISE 5–1
(page 82)

Answers should be based on your own research question.

EXERCISE 5–2
(page 83)

Answers given within the exercise.

EXERCISE 5–3
(page 84)

Answers should be based on your own research question.

EXERCISE 6–1
(page 102)

The example can be broken down as follows:

Problem/background: In the United States, the difficulty of early diagnosis of myocardial infraction has led to 1.6 million unnecessary hospital days and $600 million in hospital costs annually. In an attempt to expedite patient diagnosis and treatment, and reduce unnecessary hospital charges, many institutions are experimenting with the use of early serum-enzyme markers.

Research Question: This study will compare sensitivity, specificity, and time to completed result, using one promising marker, Troponin-T, and the standard serum marker, CK-MB.

Methods: Two hundred and fifty consecutive adult patients presenting to the emergency department in a large teaching hospital with complaints of chest pain will be asked to participate. Troponin levels will be drawn by the care nurse every 4 hours for 8 hours, and results will be compared with concomitantly drawn samples of the standard marker, CK-MB, in each of the patients. Functional study results and cardiac catheterization results will also be collected.

Analysis: Descriptive and inferential statistics will be used to analyze the relationship between Tropinin-T and positive coronary artery disease.

EXERCISE 6–2
(page 103)

Answer should be based on your own problem statement.

EXERCISE 6–3
(page 105)

Answers should be based on your own research question.

EXERCISE 6–4A
(page 109)

1. What: Internal cardioverter-defibrillator (ICD) recipient's perceived quality of life (QOL)
   How: Descriptive, comparative design
2. What: CABG patients response to bedbath
   How: Within subjects, repeated-measures design
3. Answers should be based on your design

EXERCISE 6–4B
(page 110)

Answers should be based on your own study design and variables.

EXERCISE 6–5
(page 112)

1. Who: Patients with chest pain and no ECG changes
   Where: Emergency department
2. Who: 198 consecutive patients with gun shot wounds
   Where: ICU
3. Who: Patients in acute asthmatic crisis
   Where: Pediatric ICU
4. Who: Patients who died following CPR from January 97-98
   Where: In any area of the hospital (this is feasible in a chart review)
5. Answers should be based on your design

EXERCISE 6–6
(page 114)

Case A
What: Demographic data form, QLI:CV and a consent form
When: Following discharge from ICD implant (should say how long following discharge)
How: Survey packets were mailed; reminders were sent out (How the patients were accrued should be stated)
Who: TO whom: 182 adult ICU patients who received an ICD.
By whom: the investigators

Case B
What: Demographic, clinical, and outcome data was collected in 42 ICUs
When: From May 1988 to Feb. 1990
How: Using the APACHE III prognostic system and questionnaires completed on each study unit. ICUs were selected using stratified, random sampling criteria related to region, bed size, and teaching status.
Who: APACHE III collected ICU data, we aren't told who completed the questionnaires. By whom: the investigators administered the questionnaires

EXERCISE 6–7
(page 118)

Answers should be based on your own data collection processes.

EXERCISE 7–1
(page 142)

Complete checklist based on your own project status.

EXERCISE 9–1
(page 162)

Complete based on your own nursing specialty area.

EXERCISE 9–2
(page 164)

Answers should be based on your own research findings.

Index

THE Xs AND WHYs OF ALGEBRA
Key Ideas and Common Misconceptions
Anne Collins and Linda Dacey

Stenhouse Publishers
www.stenhouse.com

Library of Congress Cataloging-in-Publication Data
Collins, Anne, 1950-
  The Xs and whys of algebra : key ideas and common misconceptions / Anne Collins and Linda Dacey.
    p. cm.
  Includes bibliographical references.
  ISBN 978-1-57110-857-9 (pbk. : alk. paper)—ISBN 978-1-57110-927-9 (e-book)
  1. Algebra—Study and teaching (Middle school)
I. Dacey, Linda Schulman, 1949– II. Title.
  QA159.C64 2011
  512.0071'2—dc23

                                        2011016558

Cover, interior design, and typesetting by MPS Limited, a Macmillan Company

Manufactured in the United States of America
17 16 15 14 13 12   9 8 7 6 5 4 3 2

Stenhouse Publishers
Portland, Maine

CONTENTS

Introduction

Algebra is so integral to many of today's careers that the class is often referred to as a gatekeeper course. It is also the cornerstone on which all higher mathematics is built. The long-term advantages to successful learners are so great that Robert Moses, the founder of the Algebra Project and a noted civil rights leader, has identified the learning of algebra as a civil right. Though algebraic reasoning is introduced in the earlier grades, most students usually enter into a more formal study of algebra in grade eight.

Too often, educators pay inadequate attention to the conceptual development of algebraic ideas as they focus almost exclusively on procedural knowledge. In fact, many teachers believe that algebra is simply the manipulation of variables and symbols, and that mastery of that manipulation is the goal for a successful algebra program. Further, there is a vast discrepancy among teachers about how algebra should be taught, how it relates to arithmetic, and how it connects to real-world experiences. It is no wonder, then, that teachers are often unable to identify algebra's key ideas or address students' common misconceptions.

By the end of grade eight, all students should have a strong foundation for algebra and should be able to reason about and make sense of algebra. This reasoning and sense making is essential to students' future success in mathematics. This flipchart will focus on the following key ideas:

- using variables meaningfully
- using multiple representations for expressions
- connecting algebra with number
- connecting algebra with geometry
- manipulating symbols with understanding

The thirty modules in this flipchart are designed to engage all students in mathematical learning that develops conceptual understanding, addresses common misconceptions, and builds key ideas essential to future learning. The modules are research based and can be used to support response to intervention (RTI), a philosophy that utilizes quality interventions matched to student needs. They offer suggestions and resources for teachers seeking material for students identified as most likely to benefit from tier 1 or 2 supports as well as enrichment activities and challenges for all students.

Following the recommendations of the National Council of Teachers of Mathematics (2010) and the National Governors Association along with the Council of Chief State School Officers (2010), we have organized the modules at this level into three sections: Expressions, Equations, and Functions. Each module begins with the identification of its **Mathematical Focus** and the **Potential Challenges and Misconceptions** associated with those ideas. **In the Classroom** then suggests instructional strategies and specific activities to implement with your students. **Meeting Individual Needs** offers ideas for adjusting the activities to reach a broader range of learners. All modules are supported by one or more reproducibles (located in the appendix), and **References/Further Reading** provides resources for enriching your knowledge of the topic and gathering more ideas.

We encourage you to keep this resource on your desk or next to your plan book so that you will have these ideas at your fingertips throughout the year.

REFERENCES/FURTHER READING

Collins, Anne, and Linda Dacey. 2010. *Zeroing in on Number and Operations: Key Ideas and Common Misconceptions, Grades 7–8.* Portland, ME: Stenhouse.

National Council of Teachers of Mathematics (NCTM). 2000. *Principles and Standards for School Mathematics.* Reston, VA: NCTM.

———. 2006. *Curriculum Focal Points for Prekindergarten Through Grade 8 Mathematics: A Quest for Coherence.* Reston, VA: NCTM.

National Council of Teachers of Mathematics (NCTM), National Governors Association (NGA) and Council of Chief State School Officers (CCSSO). 2010. *Reaching Higher: The Common Core State Standards Validation Committee: A Report from the National Governors Association Center for Best Practices and the Council of Chief State School Officers.* Washington, DC: NGA Center and CCSSO.

National Mathematics Advisory Panel. 2008. *Foundations for Success: The Final Report of the National Mathematics Advisory Panel.* Washington, DC: U.S. Department of Education.

EXPRESSIONS

Walking the Cartesian Coordinate Plane

Mathematical Focus
- Identify points in all four quadrants.
- Identify x- and y- intercepts.

Potential Challenges and Misconceptions

Many students confuse the sequence of the coordinates in an ordered pair, interpreting the first coordinate as the y-value and the second as the x-value. Some students mistakenly believe they must mark the x-value on the x-axis before plotting the y-value on the y-axis. These students erroneously see two points instead of one ordered pair. For example, they would mark (3, 0) and (0, 4) for the ordered pair (3, 4). Students who have multiple opportunities to physically plot points have a good chance of overcoming these misconceptions.

In the Classroom

One teacher moves all the student desks to the perimeter of the room and draws a large Cartesian coordinate plane on the classroom floor, using liquid shoe polish—a washable material custodians prefer—to mark the axes and label the intervals. If the floor is tiled, it is convenient to use the seams on the floor for the intervals. If the floor is carpeted, you might use masking tape to mark the coordinate plane.

This teacher instructs one volunteer to stand on the origin on the floor grid, a second volunteer to go to the board, and a third volunteer to go to the overhead. The teacher dictates an ordered pair. The student at the origin on the floor must graph the ordered pair by moving to the appropriate point on the grid; the student at the board records the ordered pair and indicates in which quadrant it will be located. The ordered pairs and the quadrants in which they are located remain on the board to allow all students to examine the growing list to identify any patterns they notice about the signs of the coordinates and their corresponding quadrants. The third student plots the point on a grid which is projected for all students to examine. Students at their seats also plot the point and label the

quadrant in which the point lies either on individual whiteboards or in their notebooks. After ensuring all students have correctly labeled the quadrant and correctly plotted the point, the teacher has students rotate through the roles. Each student has a turn to "walk the Cartesian coordinate plane."

This teacher makes sure to include ordered pairs that fall in each of the four quadrants as well as points that lie on the x- and y-axes. She also reviews the meanings of the terms that the students will use when playing the *Match It* game (see the *Match It Cards* reproducible on pages A1 and A2 in the appendix). The class reviews the terms *quadrant I*, *quadrant II*, *quadrant III*, *quadrant IV*, *x-intercept*, *y-intercept*, *origin*, *abscissa*, *ordinate*, *x-axis*, and *y-axis*. Then students pair up to play *Match It*, a game similar to concentration. Cards are dealt facedown in an array and students take turns trying to match a term with its mathematical representation. If a player makes a match, he or she takes another turn. If the player doesn't make a match, the other player takes a turn. The game ends when all the cards have been matched.

Meeting Individual Needs

Some students may benefit from taping a template that shows the direction in which the positive and negative integers move to their desks. For instance, assuming the values for x and y are positive:

$+x$ goes $\longrightarrow$ $+y$ goes $\uparrow$ $-x$ goes $\longleftarrow$ $-y$ goes $\downarrow$

Other students benefit from playing *Paper Battleship*. They see the relevance of using ordered pairs when set in either a game format or a real-world context. Directions are available at http://en.wikipedia.org/wiki/Battleship_game.

REFERENCE/FURTHER READING
Bay, Jennifer, and Deanna Wasman. 2000. "Sharing Teaching Ideas: Making the Coordinate Grid Come to Life with Human Graphing." *Mathematics Teacher* 93 (7): 553–554.

Simplifying Expressions

Mathematical Focus

- Simplify expressions with variables.
- Model operations with integers.

Potential Challenges and Misconceptions

Many students struggle to understand the difference between operators and positive and negative signs. For instance, $+4b$ or $+(+4b)$ means *add a positive* $4b$, while $+(-4b)$ means *add a negative* $4b$. Also, $+(-4b)$ means *add a negative* $4b$, while $-(+4b)$ means *subtract a positive* $4b$. Notice the operator is the first sign and the integer sign is the second sign. The greatest challenge for students is to interpret which operation to perform if there is only one sign given, such as $2b - 3b$. Students must recognize that the operation is subtraction and the lack of a second sign indicates a positive integer. So the difference in this case is $-1b$ or just $-b$.

In the Classroom

One teacher introduces algebra tiles (see the *Algebra Tiles Template* reproducible on page A3 in the appendix) to engage students in developing an understanding of simplifying expressions. The class agrees to call the rectangular tile b. They agree that the square tiles are b^2 since the length and width are both b units long. She asks her students what the sum of 5 plus its opposite, -5, would equal. All agree it is 0. Next she queries her students to tell her what the sum of b plus its opposite, $-b$ equals. Again all students answer 0. She introduces the term *zero pairs* and reminds the students that any term plus its opposite is zero.

The teacher distributes copies of the *Chip Board* reproducible on page A4 to the students and challenges them to model each of the following expressions using the tiles (from page A3 in the appendix) on their chip boards: $+3$, -2, $b + 4$, $b - 8$. She also has them record a pictorial model of each expression in their notebooks. She follows this with simple addition computations, emphasizing the need to simplify. For instance, when demonstrating $b + 5 + 2b + (-6)$, students should simplify their mat to show $3b + (-1)$, as shown in the following figures. Students identify zero pairs and remove them from their mats.

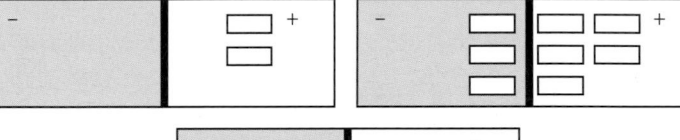

Modeling subtraction is helpful, as is thinking about the subtraction symbol as "do the opposite of." This teacher provides her students with the expression $2b - 5b$ and has a volunteer show how that would look using algebra tiles (see figures below).

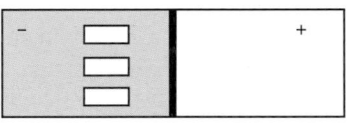

Next, the class begins a round-robin activity, which is described on the *Equivalent Expressions Round-Robin* reproducible on page A5 in the appendix, to reinforce students' understanding of simplifying expressions.

Meeting Individual Needs

Provide students with many experiences to use the chip boards until they show proficiency. As students become more proficient, you may increase the number of terms on the chip board or challenge the students to work in pairs creating and simplifying their own expressions.

REFERENCE/FURTHER READING

Leitze, Annette Ricks, and Nancy A. Kitt. 2000. "Algebra for All: Using Homemade Algebra Tiles to Develop Algebra and Prealgebra Concepts." *Mathematics Teacher* 93 (6): 462–466.

Generalizing Patterns

Mathematical Focus

- Model the distributive property.
- Model an expression with algebra tiles.
- Convert an expression in factored form into expanded form.

Potential Challenges and Misconceptions

Many students struggle with understanding how to simplify expressions that include variables and operation signs. Some ignore the variable altogether; for example, they assume the sum of $3x + 4$ is 7. Many students do not believe an operator can be contained within an equivalent answer, so they think that $r + s = rs$ or that $3s + 5 = 8s$. Other students neglect to understand the notation or importance of parentheses. If they are given the following rectangle, with a length of 7 and a width of $w + 4$, they indicate the area as $7 \times w + 4$ or $w + 4 \times 7$.

In the Classroom

Research indicates that student learning occurs in three phases, from the concrete to the pictorial to the abstract. Students move through the stages at different rates. One teacher requires her students to model, draw a picture in their notebooks, then write an expression in expanded form for each factored expression she provides. She uses the chip board in the *Chip Board* reproducible on page A4 in the appendix to engage students in modeling the distributive property. She begins by instructing her students to use algebra tiles (see page A3 in the appendix) to model $2(a + 1)$. She calls upon a student to go to the overhead to model and explain what he did. He says he placed the quantity of $(a + 1)$ twice to get a product of $2a + 2$, as shown in the following figure.

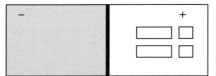

The students record the expanded expression $2a + 2$. They discuss whether the expression is equivalent or if they could represent it as $4a$. This engenders a conversation about whether the students can combine the a tile with a unit tile. Students agree it is not possible.

The teacher provides a second expression: $3(a - 2)$. She calls upon a student to share her solution at the overhead. The student explains that she multiplied both the a and the -2 by 3 by using the distributive property to arrive at a product of $3a - 6$, as shown in the following figure.

The class moves on to distributing a negative factor in the expression $-2(b + 1)$. As the teacher walks around, she listens for *accountable talk* (which includes using correct mathematical vocabulary and restating what someone else has said).

The teacher brings the class together to share the students' strategies and assigns the *Working with Expressions* reproducible on page A6 in the appendix.

Meeting Individual Needs

The amount of time students need to rely on the manipulatives varies. Allow students unrestricted use of the manipulatives until they decide they are ready to work pictorially or abstractly. Some students benefit from drawing a picture of the algebra tiles to ensure they have correctly simplified the symbolic expressions.

REFERENCE/FURTHER READING

Chappell, Michaele F., and Marilyn E. Strutchens. 2001. "Creating Connections: Promoting Algebraic Thinking with Concrete Models." *Mathematics Teaching in the Middle School* 7 (1): 20–25.

Mathematical Focus

- Create an expression to generalize a geometric pattern.
- Identify equivalent expressions.
- Connect expressions to visual representations.

Potential Challenges and Misconceptions

Teachers often use visual representations of patterns as a way to concretize algebraic relationships. Unfortunately, rather than building strong figural reasoning, they often direct students to make a table to find the pattern. This oversimplification of the task means that students merely count to complete a table and then ignore the visual model. Generalizations then result from iterative thinking (*I just need to add five each time*), guessing and checking, or the application of rote procedures, rather than an understanding of the structural relationships within the model. Wallace concludes that as a result, "Students who can provide a formula to solve a problem are usually unable to explain why it works" (2007, 511).

In the Classroom

Teachers can show geometric patterns on interactive whiteboards or projectors, as available. One teacher presents the following pattern to his students:

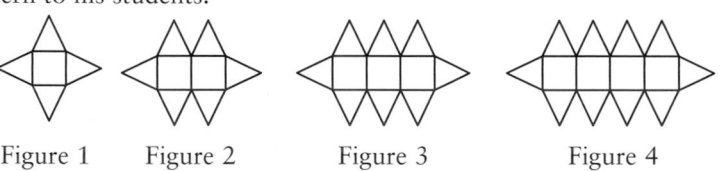

Figure 1   Figure 2   Figure 3   Figure 4

He then distributes a written list of tasks for the students to consider in groups:

1. Describe Figure 5.
2. Draw a sketch of Figure 10.
3. If there were 20 squares, how many triangles would there be? How do you know?
4. If there were 20 squares, how many total pieces (triangles and squares) would there be? What if there were n squares? How do you know?

The teacher walks from table to table as the students work. He notes whether students sketch freely or appear hesitant. He notices who makes a table and who does not. He is particularly interested in the explanations students give to one another. He then brings the groups back together for a discussion of their findings.

Students identify two expressions for the total number of pieces for a figure with n squares: $3n + 2$ and $2n + n + 2$. The teacher records these and the students decide that the expressions are equivalent. Then the teacher asks the students where they can *see* these expressions in the figures. Students who made tables to form a generalization refer to seeing a difference of three in the total. Reid explains, "It keeps going up by three each time."

Squares	1	2	3	4	5	10	20
Triangles	4	6	8	10	12	22	42
Total pieces	5	8	11	14	17	32	62

The teacher again asks about the figures. Julie explains, "Each time there is a row of squares, there are two rows of triangles. The numbers are the same. So our group came up with n plus $2n$ to show the one row of squares and the two rows of triangles. Then we added 2 for the two triangles at the ends."

Jacob added, "Our group just saw the three rows as the same, so we wrote *3n plus 2*." To help them practice this thinking, he has students to complete the *See the Pattern* reproducible on page A7 in the appendix.

Meeting Individual Needs

Some students will almost always prefer to make a table and rely on numerical methods, while others gravitate toward the visual images. Allow your students to begin with their preferred technique, but then encourage them to make connections. For example, ask a student who finds a generalization using a table to then look for those features in the figures.

REFERENCE/FURTHER READING

Wallace, Ann H. 2007. "Anticipating Student Responses to Improve Problem Solving." *Mathematics Teaching in the Middle School* 12 (9): 504–511.

Equivalence of Expressions

Mathematical Focus

- Determine equivalence among representations.
- Simplify expressions to determine equivalence.

Potential Challenges and Misconceptions

Changing the symbolic form of an expression or equation, while maintaining equivalence, is considered a transformational algebraic activity (Driscoll 2010, 13). It is crucial that students become proficient in recognizing and collecting like terms, factoring, expanding, substituting, simplifying, and solving expressions and equations. These skills help students become proficient at taking an expression and either expanding it or simplifying it into an equivalent expression. Many students struggle with simplifying the general form of $(n + 1)^2 - n^2$ by expanding it to $n^2 + 2n + 1 - n^2$ and finding it is equivalent to $2n + 1$, with n being any integer. Yet if they were presented with an arithmetic expression such as $(5 + 1)^2 - 5^2$, most would easily recognize it as $36 - 25$, which is equivalent to 11.

In the Classroom

One teacher provides every student with multiple opportunities to work with expressions. She begins one lesson with a *range question* designed to let her gauge the students' prior knowledge. She posts the following task on the projection device:

List everything you can about the expression $8 - 2(a + 3) + 2$.

She records their observations and notices that many students suggest they have to subtract before distributing. She tailors her lesson to address that misconception.

She continues the lesson by presenting the following expression: $4 + 3(n + 5)$. She instructs them to simplify it on their individual whiteboards and when finished to hold their whiteboards up for her to see. She examines the whiteboards for common misconceptions such as adding $4 + 3$ before distributing the 3 over the quantity of $n + 5$. After discussing the solution, she groups the students into threes and plays *Equivalent Expressions Round-Robin* (see page A5 in the appendix for directions). This allows her to intervene as soon

as she perceives a student is struggling. She conducts the following activities on other days.

- *Do You Have a _____?*: The game *Do You Have a _____?* is similar to go fish. Students play in groups of two or three. One student deals four cards to each participant. The player to the dealer's left begins the game by asking one of the other players, for example, "Do you have a $3n - 15$?" If the second player has an equivalent expression, he or she reads, for example, "I have $3(n - 5)$." If the first player receives the card requested and makes a match, he or she takes another turn. If the second player does not have a matching expression, he or she states, "No match; draw an expression." The first player draws a card and his or her turn ends. Play alternates among the players until they've made all the matches. The *Do You Have a _____?* reproducible on pages A8–A10 in the appendix contains a set of sample expression cards to use for this game.
- *I Have _____; Who Has _____?*: In this game, each student receives one or two cards with a question and a statement. The statement tells the rest of the class what expression the student has, and the question asks the rests of the students if they have an equivalent expression. The game begins with one student asking, "Who has _____?" Whichever student has a match responds, "I have _____." The *I Have _____; Who Has _____?* reproducible on pages A11–A13 in the appendix has sample cards to use for this game.

Meeting Individual Needs

When students demonstrate proficiency, the teacher challenges them to pose a problem that each expression on the game cards might represent. She instructs those students who need more time to master the concept to model each expression with algebra tiles. She also encourages them to sketch each expression if they need a visual representation.

REFERENCE/FURTHER READING

Driscoll, Mark. 2010. "Learning and Teaching Algebra in Secondary School Classrooms." In *Teaching and Learning Mathematics: Translating Research for Secondary School Teachers*, ed. Frank Lester, 13–20. Reston, VA: National Council of Teachers of Mathematics.

A14

Mathematical Focus

- Create tables and graphs to represent real-world situations.
- Translate between natural language and algebraic expressions.

Potential Challenges and Misconceptions

Diana Steele states, "Algebraic thinking includes the ability to analyze and recognize patterns, to represent the quantitative relationships between the patterns, and to generalize these quantitative relationships" (2005, 142). Beginning in the elementary grades, teachers often introduce *Guess My Rule* games to motivate such thinking. Students suggest values for *x* and the game leader discloses the corresponding values for *y*. This process continues until students can guess the rule, that is, identify the expression that generalizes the relationship between the *x*- and *y*-values. Playing such games familiarizes students with the notion of inputs and outputs and with creating generalizations to connect them. Unfortunately, teachers pay far less attention to helping students connect tables of input and output values to contextual situations, leading students to form incomplete concepts.

When students translate natural language to an algebraic statement, they often translate in the order that the information is given. For example, they are likely to misrepresent a relationship such as *there are three times as many crayons as markers* as $3c = m$. This misconception is known as a syntactic error and accounts for many of the difficulties students experience in the solution of word problems. Though identified many years ago, the misconception persists.

In the Classroom

Connecting situations to tables and graphs first, instead of moving immediately to finding expressions that generalize the relationships, can help students recognize errors in their thinking. Describe a situational relationship to students such as *There are four times as many children as adults at the picnic*. Ask: *Are there more children or adults at the picnic? What is one possible answer for how many adults and children there could be at the picnic? If there are six adults, how many children are there?* Ask for additional possibilities and record these responses in a table with the *x*-column labeled Adults and the *y*-column labeled Children. Challenge students to work in groups to write an expression that will allow them to identify the *output* (number of children) if they know the *input* (number of adults). Do not be surprised if some of the students reverse the relationship and state that four times the number of children tells the number of adults. Encourage them to check their ideas by seeing if they work for the ordered pairs in the table. Finally, point to a particular ordered pair in the table and ask, *What does this pair tell us about this situation?*

Talk explicitly with the students about this common error and help them develop ways to check their thinking.

1. Find one ordered pair that works.
2. Pay attention to which variable is greater.
3. Think about how to balance the relationship when you write your expression.
4. Check your idea with your ordered pair.

Continue to explore examples (both linear and nonlinear), sometimes asking the students to make a table, sometimes asking them to make a graph. After several examples, ask, *How can you predict whether the graph will be a straight line or not?* Students can practice these ideas by completing the *It's a Relationship* reproducible on page A14 in the appendix.

Meeting Individual Needs

Working in pairs or small groups can be helpful to students because they can talk about their thinking. You may want to have students record a procedure similar to the four-step process listed in the previous section and keep the list in view.

For students ready for a greater challenge, have them identify the differences between the values in the *y*-column of the tables when the *x*-values are listed from least to greatest and the intervals between them are equal. What do they notice when the relationships are linear? What about when they are nonlinear? Why do they think this is so?

REFERENCES/FURTHER READING

Clement, John. 1982. "Algebra Word Problem Solutions: Thought Processes Underlying a Common Misconception." *Journal for Research in Mathematics Education* 13 (1): 16–30.

Steele, Diana. 2005. "Using Writing to Access Students' Schemata Knowledge for Algebraic Thinking." *School Science and Mathematics* 105 (3): 142–154.

Mathematical Focus
- Identify and select appropriate problem-solving strategies.
- Identify and generalize mathematical patterns in given situations.

Potential Challenges and Misconceptions

There is a pervasive misconception that one has to have a good memory to be successful in mathematics. Contrary to that belief, Booth and Koedinger (2008) found that conceptual understanding is key to solving algebraic problems. It is essential to *not* encourage students to rely on cute sayings or tricks to work through procedures. Strategies are tools or representations that can be applied to any problem situation, thereby eliminating the need for memory and tricks.

In the Classroom

One teacher poses problems such as the following:

> Altogether, how many rectangles are there in this figure?

"And," she adds, "what if the figure has n rectangles?"

Some of the students call out, "There is only one; the rest are squares." This response initiates a short conversation about the attributes of squares and rectangles.

After giving students some time to think about the problem, the teacher asks them to tell her how many rectangles they found. She lists the numbers. She then asks groups to report out the strategies they used.

Jeremy's group made an organized list for identifying all the rectangles. (See following figure.)

1	2	3	4	5	6	7	8	9	10

1-2, 2-3, 3-4, 4-5, 5-6, 6-7, 7-8, 8-9, 9-10   9

1-2-3, 2-3-4, 3-4-5, 4-5-6, 5-6-7, 6-7-8, 7-8-9, 8-9-10   8

1-2-3-4, 2-3-4-5, 3-4-5-6, 4-5-6-7, 5-6-7-8, 6-7-8-9, 7-8-9-10   7

And so on for 6 + 5 + 4 + 3 + 2 + 1

Henry's group solved a simpler problem, drew a picture, and found a pattern, as shown in the following figure:

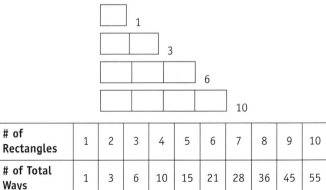

# of Rectangles	1	2	3	4	5	6	7	8	9	10	n
# of Total Ways	1	3	6	10	15	21	28	36	45	55	

The class then discusses the strategies and solutions, identifying similarities and differences in how the students were thinking about the problem.

To give students additional practice with similar problems, hand out copies of the *Express It* reproducible on page A15 in the appendix.

Meeting Individual Needs

When one teacher assigns a problem, she asks her students to think individually about which problem-solving strategy would be appropriate to use. After a minute of individual think time, she instructs her students to share their strategies with their partners. After a brief discussion, the students report their strategies and the teacher records them on the board. This allows all students to access the problem by choosing one of the reported strategies if they could not decide on one by themselves.

REFERENCE/FURTHER READING

Booth, Julie, and Kenneth R. Koedinger. 2008. "Key Misconceptions in Algebraic Problem Solving." In *Proceedings of the 30th Annual Conference of the Cognitive Science Society*, ed. B. C. Love, K. McRae, and V. M. Sloutsky, 571–576. Austin, TX: Cognitive Science Society.

Posing Problems

Mathematical Focus
- Analyze representations.
- Make connections among representations.
- Write story problems.

Potential Challenges and Misconceptions

Rarely are students asked to actually pose problems; rather, they are given word problems that always provide the question to be answered. "When students begin posing their own original mathematical questions and see these questions become the focus of discussion, their perception of the subject is profoundly altered. When they get to spend time working on these questions, their ownership of the experience produces excitement and motivation" (Abrams 2003, 1). Posing problems builds on curiosity, a rare commodity in too many mathematics classes. Knowing what question to ask is a key component in the inquiry and problem-solving process.

In the Classroom

It is important for teachers to model problem posing before assigning such a task to students. When students hear questions such as *I wonder what would happen if . . .* and *What if . . .* as part of regular conversations, they often begin to raise questions themselves. One teacher begins her discussion of problem posing by presenting her students with the following values: *n*, 3, and 5. She challenges her students to use all the values in a problem situation.

Rylie's group writes the following problem:

Write an expression for the following situation. Charlie has five more than three times the number of video games his cousin Walter has.

Amanda's group poses this problem:

Deesha sold three less than five times the number of chocolate chip cookies Marty sold at the school fair. Write an expression for this situation.

Next, the teacher presents a table, as shown in the following figure.

Input	2	4	6	8	n
Output	40	50	60	70	$5n + 30$

She instructs her students to write a story problem for which the table would fit. Students share their problems during a class discussion. Before assigning the situations in the *So What's the Problem?* reproducible on page A16 in the appendix, the teacher instructs her students to pose a story problem for the following stack of triangles.

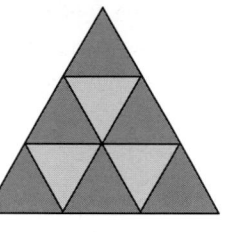

She is pleased with the assorted questions, which include the following:

- How many triangles would be in row 7?
- If there were *n* rows, how many triangles would row *n* have?
- What is the surface area of the triangle?
- How might you find the volume of the triangle?
- What patterns do you notice?

Meeting Individual Needs

To help students who struggle with posing problems, instruct them to examine a familiar problem and change the numerical values. Any time the values change, a new problem is posed. A second strategy is to examine a familiar problem but ask a different question. For example, if the original question is *How long did it take?* students can change the problem by asking, *What was the rate of change?* or even *How far did they go?* Still another strategy is to change the representation that is given. For example, if an original problem gives a table and asks for a graph, students can provide a graph and ask for the data to be represented in a table or give an equation and ask for a graph or a table.

REFERENCES/FURTHER READING
Abrams, Joshua. 2003. "Problem Posing." *Teacher Handbook*. Education Development Center. http://www2.edc.org/makingmath/mathproj.asp#rsskil.
Collier, C. Patrick. 2000. *Menu Collection: Problems Adapted from "Mathematics Teaching in the Middle School,"* 73–74. Reston, VA: National Council of Teachers of Mathematics.

Equal Sign as a Balance

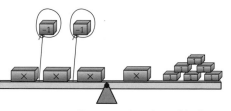

Mathematical Focus

- Develop a relational understanding of the equal sign.
- Apply algebraic thinking to find values of weights on a balance scale.

Potential Challenges and Misconceptions

Young students often develop the misconception that the equal sign is operational, that is, it tells them to carry out a procedure and indicates where to record the result of that operation. For many students this inaccurate view of the equal sign persists through the middle grades. In fact, Knuth et al. (2006) concluded that students' understanding of the equal sign as relational (identifying that two expressions have the same value) does not increase significantly from grade six to grade eight. Most important, these researchers found that those students who did have a relational understanding of the equal sign were more successful in solving algebraic equations.

In the Classroom

Pan balances are often recommended to support the understanding of equality. You can activate prior knowledge of the pan balance model by offering problems such as the following one and telling students that weights of the same shape have the same mass. Such problems provide students with the opportunity to develop important concepts of algebraic thinking such as substitution and "doing the same thing to each side" to maintain balance.

Given:

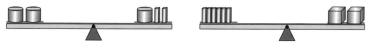

How many cylinders does it take to balance four cubes? (six cylinders)

In order to illustrate a variety of algebraic expressions on the balance, you must include ways to represent negative values. Reeves and Webb (2004) suggest using raised balloons to indicate negative integers. The idea can be applied to variables as well. The pan balance in the following figure would then indicate that $3x - 2 = x + 6$.

You may want to illustrate the idea of balloons representing the opposite of gravity or weight by showing a clip from the movie *Up*, a film about a seventy-eight-year-old man who tied thousands and thousands of balloons to his house to fly to South America. To help students gain confidence with this model, present several examples and ask questions to probe understanding. For example, given the balance shown above, you could ask:

- If two more -1 balloons were placed on the left pan, would that side become heavier or lighter?
- If both -1 balloons were removed from the left pan, what could we do to the right pan to keep the scale balanced?
- If we removed the x from the right pan, what could we do to the left pan to keep the scale balanced?
- What equation could we write to represent what is shown on the scale?

Following such questions, have students find the value of x.

The *In Balance* reproducible on page A17 in the appendix provides additional problems for students to explore.

Meeting Individual Needs

For students who would benefit from additional practice, the National Library of Virtual Manipulatives has two Java applets that allow students to manipulate blocks on pan balances to solve linear equations. They can be found at http://nlvm.usu.edu/en/nav/category_g_3_t_2.html. The site also uses the image of a balloon to illustrate a negative number or variable.

REFERENCES/FURTHER READING

Knuth, Eric J., Ana C. Stephens, Nicole M. McNeil, and Martha W. Alibali. 2006. "Does Understanding the Equal Sign Matter? Evidence from Solving Equations." *Journal for Research in Mathematics Education* 37 (4): 297–312.

Reeves, Charles A., and Darcy Webb. 2004. "Balloons on the Rise: A Problem-Solving Introduction to Integers." *Mathematics Teaching in the Middle School* 9 (9): 476–482.

Mathematical Focus

- Solve equations.
- Use inverse operations to solve equations.
- Work backward to solve equations.

Potential Challenges and Misconceptions

Some misconceptions that students share result from not remembering the rules for solving equations. If students engaged in developing an understanding of what is happening in equations and of the "undoing" that occurs when solving equations, there would be fewer students making the following errors: if $\frac{x}{3} = 6$, then $x = 2$; if $x + 4 = 9$, then $x = 4 + 9 = 13$; and if $x - (-8) = 0$, then $x = 8$.

In the Classroom

It is important that students understand and can apply the algebraic properties when finding equivalent expressions or solving equations. One teacher insists that her students list each property as they work through a solution until they demonstrate understanding. She begins her class by posing a series of *range questions*—questions that allow her to assess the range of understanding her students bring to the discussion. She projects equations on the overhead one at a time and instructs her students to identify the property on their individual whiteboards. The students write the property and hold the whiteboards up for the teacher to see. She determines whether they know the additive identity and inverse, multiplicative identity and inverse, distributive property, and commutative and associative properties for addition and multiplication.

She continues by asking her students to model the equation $3a + 4 = 2a + 6$ on the *Equation Mat* (found on page A18 in the appendix) using their algebra tiles. The figure on the far left below shows how they modeled the equation.

She instructs them to solve the equation, sketching a picture of each equation and each step in their notebooks and indicating which property is used in each step. Students then share their strategies.

Ben: I used the equality property and subtracted two a's from each side of the equation to maintain the balance. (See middle figure below.)

   Then I subtracted four units from each side, again to maintain the balance. I got a equals two for my solution. (See figure on the far right below.)

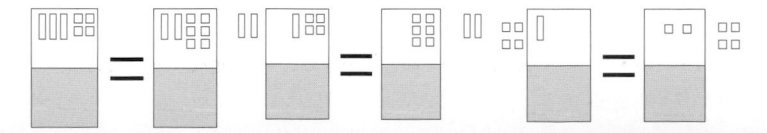

I checked to be sure I was correct and substituted 2 for a and got $3(2) + 4 = 2(2) + 6$, or $6 + 4 = 4 + 6$.

Lauren: I used zero pairs to solve the equation. First I added $-2a$ to both sides. (See figure on the far left below.)

   This is the additive inverse. I removed the zero pairs. Next I added -4 to both sides. (See middle figure below.)

   This is the additive inverse. I removed the zero pairs and got my solution, $a = 2$. (See figure on the far right below.)

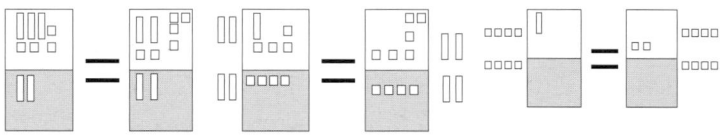

Additive inverse   Additive inverse

After students display proficiency with modeling, the teacher engages them in a game of *Equation Bingo*. (A game board template is provided in the *Equation Bingo* reproducible on page A19 in the appendix; sample equations and answers are included on page A20 in the appendix.) To play the game, students place integers from -12 to 12 randomly on the bingo boards. The teacher reads an equation or displays it on the overhead. Students place a disc or other marker on the correct answer. Play continues until a student has five in a row, column, or diagonal.

Meeting Individual Needs

Encouraging students to model equations for as long as they need a concrete model is appropriate. Ensure that students who are ready to solve equations symbolically know why each step works and that they can identify the algebraic properties to support the symbolic manipulation. For students who need more of a challenge, instruct them to write story problems that match the equations.

REFERENCES/FURTHER READING

Driscoll, Mark. 2010. "Learning and Teaching Algebra in Secondary School Classrooms." In *Teaching and Learning Mathematics: Translating Research for Secondary School Teachers*, ed. Frank Lester, 13–20. Reston, VA: National Council of Teachers of Mathematics.

Foster, David. 2007. "Making Meaning in Algebra: Examining Students' Understandings and Misconceptions." In *Assessing Mathematical Proficiency*, ed. Alan H. Schoenfeld, 163–178. Berkeley, CA: Mathematical Sciences Research Institute.

Mathematical Focus
- Graph equations on the Cartesian coordinate plane.
- Use a graphing calculator to check paper-and-pencil work.

Potential Challenges and Misconceptions

Algebraic (symbolic) representations and graphical representations illuminate each other. Graphing should be taught in conjunction with equations, tables, and charts so that students develop representational fluency. This includes translation tasks, such as matching graphs to equations (Leinhardt, Zaslavsky, and Stein 1990). Students who are expected to solve or graph data void of contexts demonstrate greater challenges and misconceptions than students who solve contextual problems.

In the Classroom

One teacher continues to use the floor-size model of the Cartesian coordinate plane (introduced in the first module) as her students work on setting up, solving, and graphing linear equations. She assigns the following problem:

> Mari earns $7.50 an hour baby-sitting plus a total bonus of $5.00 if there is more than one child. If she baby-sits twin girls for 3 hours, how much money will she earn? What if she baby-sits for 5 hours? What if she baby-sits for 7 hours?

The teacher instructs the students to use the *Multiple Representations* reproducible on page A21 in the appendix to show all their work. After an allotted period of time, the teacher calls on various groups to report their findings by forming a human line on the floor-size grid. Each member of a group stands on an ordered pair the group identified in its table, which represents the relationship between the number of hours worked and the amount of money earned. By inspecting where the students stand, she and the rest of the class can determine if the graph is correct. Because they are investigating linear equations, they know that if the students form a straight line, the ordered pairs are correct. Another group shares its work using the projector. The class discusses each representation.

This teacher also introduces the graphing calculator and explains how it can support their work. She walks them through the procedures for entering equations and using the trace button. She also demonstrates how the students can adjust the window settings and use the table settings. She then challenges them to duplicate their paper-and-pencil tables and graphs on their graphing calculators. Volunteers go to the overhead to share their graphing calculator settings, graphs, and tables.

Following are additional activities designed to develop proficiency in working with graphs, tables, and equations.

- *Gallery Walk*: Write an equation, a graph, and a table at the top of three sheets of easel paper and hang them around the room. Have students work in groups of three to write equations, create tables, and draw graphs for each posted representation. For instance, on the easel sheet with an equation, students must post a table and a graph for that equation. On the sheet with the graph, students must post an equation and a table, and so on. After the gallery walk, you can assign the *AKA: Also Known As* reproducible on page A22 in the appendix, which provides a table, a graph, and an equation for students to translate.
- *Where Am I?*: Give students graph paper. Each student individually identifies a place on the graph that holds a buried treasure and an equation that will lead to the treasure. Students then work in pairs and give clues to their partners that will help them locate the buried treasure. Clues should include the equation of the line, the slope, and the y-intercept. For example, suppose a student's treasure is located at $(3, 6)$. The student might offer this clue: "The treasure is located on a path represented by the equation $y = 2x$." The treasure seeker may guess, "The treasure is buried at $(1, 2)$." The student might respond, "No, but you are on the correct path."

Meeting Individual Needs

Many students will need more time working with the translation between tables and equations. Using a table to determine an explicit relationship is often challenging. It is helpful for students who struggle to write the ratio of the output to the input for many ordered pairs to identify the slope of the line. Other students find it more helpful to graph the data from the table to find the slope and y-intercept.

REFERENCES/FURTHER READING
Leinhardt, Gaea, Orit Zaslavsky, and Mary K. Stein. 1990. "Functions, Graphs, and Graphing: Tasks, Learning, and Teaching." *Review of Educational Research* 60 (1): 1–64.

Noyce, Pendred. 2010. *Lost in Lexicon: An Adventure in Words and Numbers*. Boston: Tumblehome.

Solving Linear Equations

Mathematical Focus

- Explore linear situations.
- Represent linear equations in equations, tables, and graphs.

Potential Challenges and Misconceptions

Students who learn algebra contextually have fewer misconceptions than those who learn procedures and skills in isolation (Booth and Koedinger 2008). An extremely effective way of helping students develop algebraic skills is to engage them in interesting problems or tasks. It's more beneficial to require students to generate data, record the data in a table, and create a graphical representation of the data than to artificially separate work with the three representations. Many students struggle to understand the meaning of the x- and y-intercepts. If, however, they begin their work with a contextual situation, students are much more likely to understand.

In the Classroom

"Make a list of everything you know about linear equations," one teacher instructs as she begins a lesson on equations. She uses this *range question* to shed light on the span of understanding her students bring to class. She lists their responses on the conjecture board. Each statement remains on the conjecture board until the class finds a counterexample or can negate the comment.

This teacher continues her lesson by showing her students a stack of foam drinking cups and engaging them in an exploration of the relationship between the number of cups and the height of the stack. Following are the directions for this activity.

1. Provide each group of students with seven foam cups, a copy of the *Stacking Cups* reproducible from page A23 in the appendix, and a ruler.
2. Instruct students to measure and record the height of one cup.
3. Have students add one cup at a time, nesting one cup into another, measuring and recording the height of the stack each time they add a cup.
4. Ask students to predict and record their prediction of the height of a stack of ten cups, fifteen cups, and n cups.
5. Instruct students to graph their data.
6. Have students write an equation for the relationship of the number of foam cups and the height of the stack.
7. After the students complete their tables, graphs, and equations, instruct them to check their work using a graphing calculator. Tell them to input their predicted height for ten and fifteen cups using the trace function on the calculator.

The teacher raises several questions as the students are working, including these:

- Is the height of the cups the independent or dependent variable?
- Why doesn't the graph begin at (0, 0)?
- What part of your equation relates to the height of the first cup?
- Do you expect your graph to be linear or nonlinear? How do you know?

Building on the previous exploration, the teacher introduces the next problem:

Carly, Jamal, and Joaquin hope to raise money in the annual Walk Your Pet for Healthy Pets Awareness event. Each walker has listed the amount of money he or she will ask sponsors to donate in the following chart.

Walk Your Pet Service

	Rate
Carly	$20 per day
Jamal	$10.00 plus $2.50 per hour
Joaquin	$5 plus $3.50 per hour

Which walker will earn the most money? Justify your answer.

It is extremely informative to discover how your students are thinking about the problem; instruct them to make a prediction about which plan will raise the most money. Direct the students to record their predictions in their notebooks before they solve the problem. The *Pet Health Awareness Walk* reproducible on page A24 in the appendix is a student recording sheet for this activity. This teacher encourages her students to check their tables, graphs, and equations using their graphing calculators.

Meeting Individual Needs

Some students may work better in a pair than a small group; assign accordingly. For students who need an additional challenge, ask them to predict how many cups it will take to make a stack as tall as you. Challenge them to pose other problems that might be represented by the graph they made from the cup-stacking data.

REFERENCE/FURTHER READING

Booth, Julie, and Kenneth Koedinger. 2008. "Key Misconceptions in Algebraic Problem Solving." In *Proceedings of the 30th Annual Cognitive Science Society*, ed. B. C. Love, K. McRae, and V. M. Sloutsky, 571–576. Austin, TX: Cognitive Science Society.

Mathematical Focus

- Write standard forms of a linear equation.
- Identify equivalent forms of equations.

Potential Challenges and Misconceptions

All too often the work students do with linear equations is represented by the slope-intercept form of an equation. The result is that when many students are asked what they know about linear equations, they reply, "I know *y* equals *mx* plus *b*." Although this is one form of a linear equation, it is necessary for students to recognize and be able to transfer among equivalent representations depending on the data given or the problem being solved. Students should have multiple experiences with representing situations with the standard form of a linear equation ($ax + by = c$) before working with the slope-intercept form of the equation. The standard form lends itself to making a table and visualizing what is happening with the data, an experience that benefits all students.

In the Classroom

More often than not, the information given in a problematic situation requires students to work with the standard form of a linear equation if they are to represent it realistically. For example, the following two problems lend themselves to being represented in the standard form of a linear equation. That is, it makes sense to write the parts as addends that equal a sum. Here's the first problem:

> Suppose you decide to make and sell beaded bracelets. You plan to spend $72 on two different types of beads. Glass beads cost $3.50 each while ceramic beads cost only $1.75 each. How many of each type of bead might you purchase?

As you walk around the class listening to the students' conversations, you may want to ask various questions. *Engaging questions* might include *How might you organize your data to represent all possible combinations of beads? How do you know you have identified all the possible combinations? What patterns did you notice in your table?*

You might also ask *clarifying questions*, such as *What happens to the number of glass beads as the number of ceramic beads increases? How might you represent the data from your equation, 3.50g plus 1.75c equals 72, in a graph? How can you be sure your graph accurately represents the data in your table? Why are you trying to rewrite your equation?* and *Why is it a linear equation?*

The second problem is a type that many students enjoy solving. It involves finding the number of specific animals present, given only the number of legs and heads of different classes of animals.

> Rancher Bill counts 48 heads and 134 legs among the ducks and cows on his ranch. How many cows and how many ducks does he have?

In one class, Ella shares her way of thinking about the problem to her group: "I divided the number of heads, 48, by 2 because there are two types of animals. That gives me 24 animals, but it assumes all the animals have the same number of legs. But, that gives me 96 cow legs plus 48 duck legs for a total of 144 legs. I am close to the 134 legs, but I think I have too many cows, so I am going to try 20 cows and 28 ducks. That gives me 80 cow legs and 56 duck legs for 136 total legs. I am only off 2 legs, so I am going to try 19 cows for 76 cow legs and 29 ducks for 58 duck legs and a total of 134 legs and 48 heads."

During the reporting portion of the lesson, the teacher asks Ella to share her thinking after students share their organized lists and tables. She wants to validate both the tables and lists with the accompanying reasoning and sense making. This teacher also challenges her students to write a system of equations to represent the number of animals and the number of legs.

To reinforce the understanding of equivalence, and help students translate between two forms of a linear equation, pass out the equations from the *Equivalence Cards* reproducible (see pages A25–A26 in the appendix) randomly to your students. Instruct the students to move about the classroom to find the peer with a card that is equivalent to the one they received. After all matches are made, students share the equivalent pairs of equations with the class.

Meeting Individual Needs

A lack of organizational skills can make these problems particularly challenging for some students. When solving the second problem, it might be helpful for these students to work with a template written on graph paper that has columns labeled Cows, Hens, Heads, and Total Legs. This would enable them to track the total number of legs with the number of heads.

REFERENCE/FURTHER READING

Shultz, Harris S. 1999. "The Postage-Stamp Problem, Number Theory, and the Programmable Calculator." *Mathematics Teacher* 92 (1): 20–22.

Mathematical Focus

- Represent slope as steepness of a line.
- Represent slope as rate of change.

Potential Challenges and Misconceptions

A widespread misconception among students is that slope is simply the rise over the run. This belief is based on the way in which we have traditionally taught slope. Helping students develop the conceptual understanding that slope is a ratio is an important component of building this key idea in algebra. The challenge students face is to develop flexibility in their thinking about slope. Slope may be represented as rate of change, the steepness of a line, or to indicate directions. No matter which interpretation students encounter, it is crucial that they recognize slope as a ratio or a relationship between two variables. To help students develop a full understanding of the concept of slope, provide them with contextual situations that include steepness of the line and rate of change.

In the Classroom

Any time we can engage our students in a realistic application of mathematics, we should. One teacher takes her students to different staircases in her building and challenges them to find their slopes. She directs the students to measure the height and depth of one step. She instructs them to determine the ratio of the height to the depth. Next she suggests they find two points on the handrail. Armed with meter sticks and measuring tapes, small groups measure the vertical and horizontal difference between the two points they chose, as illustrated in the following figure.

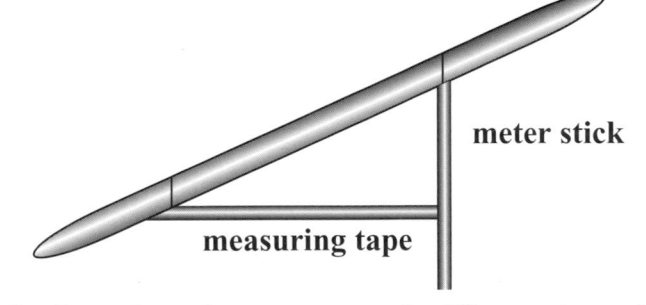

meter stick

measuring tape

She directs the students to represent the differences in a ratio of the vertical to the horizontal and to compare this ratio to the ratio of the height and the depth of the stairs. If there is time, she has her students repeat their data collection on multiple staircases within the school. When they return to the classroom, they discuss the two ratios and why they are the same.

One teacher requires her students to solve problems about mixtures, such as paint, hot chocolate, or juice, using multiple repre-

relates to another. The ratio of red paint powder to water determines how reddish a paint mixture will be. Here's one problem she assigns:

> If you wanted to make the reddest red paint possible, which of the following ratios of red powder to water would you choose: one part paint to four parts water, two parts paint to five parts water, three parts paint to seven parts water, or four parts paint to eleven parts water? Which mixture is the reddest?

Unless directed otherwise, most students would simply convert the mixtures to decimals—0.25, 0.40, 0.43, and 0.36—and order them. In this class, students must include multiple representations to justify their solutions. (See the *Multiple Representations* organizer on page A21 in the appendix.) The graphical representation provides students with an opportunity to visualize how each ratio relates to the others. (See figure.)

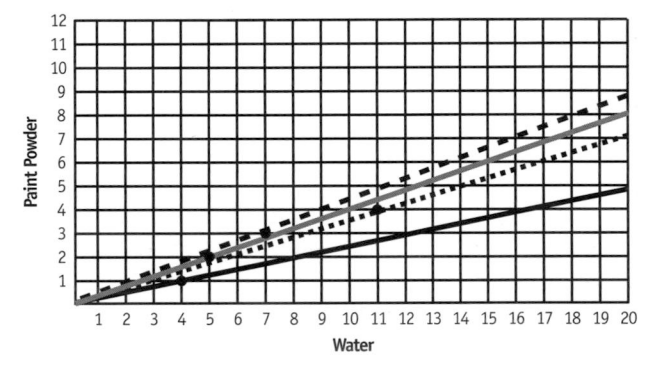

Notice that the ray closest to the *y*-axis is the reddest and the ray closest to the *x*-axis is the most watery. Graphing ratios reinforces the concept that ratios represent slopes and the steeper the ray, the greater the value.

This teacher finds that her students display a better understanding of slope after completing these types of activities. More contextual problems are provided in the *Slippery Slopes* reproducible on page A27 in the appendix.

Meeting Individual Needs

Students who struggle with the concept of slope may find it easier to think about slope as rise over run. If students do use this approach, it is important that they pay close attention to the direction in which the line is going to help them determine whether the slope is positive or negative.

REFERENCE/FURTHER READING

Cheng, Ivan. 2010. "Fractions: A New Slant on Slope." *Mathematics Teaching in the Middle School 16 (1): 34–41.*

Mathematical Focus

- Use slope to find rate of change.
- Use the steepness of a line to find rate of change.

Potential Challenges and Misconceptions

Students demonstrate many misconceptions about slope, including the following:

- A fraction always represents a wider slope (a slope that is less steep) than an integer.
- The change in x goes in the numerator because it comes before y in the alphabet.
- The height of a line (or point) on a graph, rather than the slope, represents which object's speed is greater at a particular time.
- A vertical slope is optimal because it is the steepest slope possible.

Teachers must address each of these erroneous ideas in ways that help students make sense of slope.

In the Classroom

Following are some interactive experiments designed to help students apply the concept of slope:

- Conduct an experiment to determine what happens to the distance a car travels with various slopes. Give each group a 4-by-6-inch strip of cardstock, which will be used as a ramp. Have students fold up the long sides of the strips by a half inch on each side to create curbs, then rest the ramps against one math textbook lying on a table. Next students roll a toy car down the ramp and measure and record the distance the car travels beyond the end of the ramp before coming to a stop in a table. Next they stack two math textbooks, rest the ramp against the top book, and roll the toy car down this slightly steeper ramp. Students continue the experiment until the ramp is vertical (resting against the height of the stack of textbooks) and the car crashes against the table. The class discusses the relationship between the height of the ramp and the distance the toy car travels. Students can record their work on the *Investigating Ramps and Travel Distance* reproducible on page A28 in the appendix. (Note: You might want to teach this activity collaboratively with the science teacher, since many middle schools have a science unit called "Ramps and Motion.")
- If possible, take your class to the gymnasium to examine the controls on a treadmill. If that is not possible, explain what controls are on a treadmill and how they work.

Point out the option to change the incline of the treadmill and explain that the incline, given as a percent, raises the treadmill platform to increase the effort expended to walk or run. Change the incline from 0 to 7 to demonstrate how the treadmill responds, or demonstrate the way it works using a simulation. For example, place a ruler flat on a table to represent 0 percent and raise one end to a height of 1.2 inches above the table to represent a 10 percent rise (0.10×12 inches). After investigating the treadmill, assign the following problem.

- Get Fit Sports sells a treadmill that allows the user to choose the incline at which he or she wants to jog or walk. If the treadmill is 60 inches long, and you set the incline to 5%, how high will the treadmill rise?

As the students work on the solution, listen for conversation that includes a link between the percent of rise and the slope. Encourage students to also talk about the rate of change between the treadmill at rest and how far above the floor it rests after applying the slope or incline.

- Students need to appreciate the difference between positive and negative slope and to identify slopes from graphs. Assign some problems represented on graphs, such as those in the *Aquarium Problems* reproducible on page A29 in the appendix. Challenge the students to answer the questions based on the graphs.

Meeting Individual Needs

Instruct students who need more of a challenge to write the equation of a line for the data they collected during the toy car activity. Encourage students to represent data from a graph in a table and data from a table in a graph, and ask them to examine the tables for either *explicit* patterns (involving the relation between the input and the output) or *recursive* patterns (involving the difference between one output value and the next output value).

REFERENCES/FURTHER READING

Joram, Elana, and Vicki Oleson. 2007. "How Fast Do Trees Grow? Using Tables and Graphs to Explore Slope." *Mathematics Teaching in the Middle School* 13 (5): 260–265.

Wagener, Lauren L. 2009. "A Worthwhile Task to Teach Slope." *Teaching Mathematics in the Middle School* 15 (3): 168–174.

Interpreting Graphs

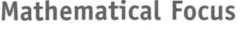

Mathematical Focus
- Connect descriptions of situations to their graphic representations.
- Create contextual situations to match graphs.
- Interpret slope and y-intercepts within graphic representations of change.

Potential Challenges and Misconceptions

Interpreting graphs is a key mathematical ability that is often applied in other subject areas and in real-world situations. Yet too often classroom instruction is limited to having students plot points from information presented in a table or an equation. Such activities do not provide students with opportunities to interpret relationships among variables presented graphically or to connect real-world situations to given graphs. Such limited perspectives often lead to misconceptions.

Unfortunately, when students are asked to create a graph to represent a real-world scenario, they often make an iconic interpretation, that is, they draw an actual picture of the real event. For example, consider the following scenario: *Jenna is going on an exercise walk. She walks at a constant rate from her house to the town hall and back.* Students often make a graph that shows the to-and-from motion (see the figure on the left below) rather than one that shows the distance walked increases as the walk continues, regardless of the direction (see the figure on the right below).

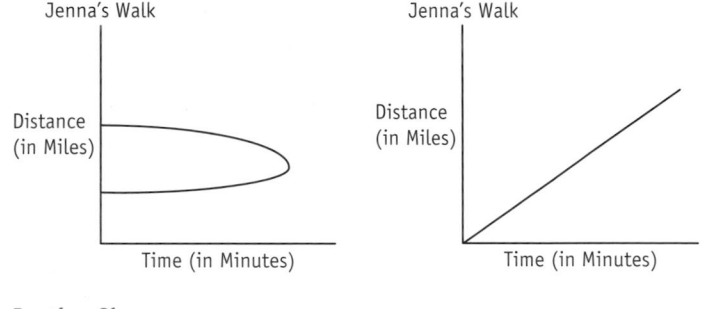

In the Classroom

One teacher begins by presenting the following two graphs about the number of pretzels in two children's bowls over time. He tells the students to each turn to a partner and talk about what they know from analyzing the graphs.

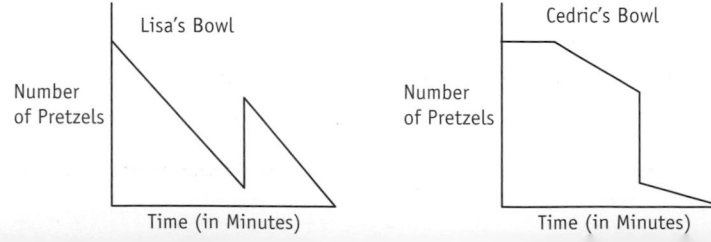

Once the students have had time to become familiar with the graphs, he asks a variety of questions:

- How did the number of pretzels each child had at the beginning compare? (They started with the same number of pretzels.)
- Cedric's graph begins with a line segment that is parallel to the x-axis. What does that tell you? (He didn't start eating right away.)
- When eating, who ate more quickly, Lisa or Cedric? How do you know? (Lisa ate more quickly because the steepness of her descending line segments are greater.)
- What about the graphs might support the idea that Cedric wasn't hungry? (The number of pretzels in Lisa's bowl went up while the number in Cedric's bowl decreased by that same amount. He may have given his pretzels to Lisa because he wasn't hungry.)

After the students discuss their ideas, the teacher presents another graph, shown below. This time he asks the students to work in their groups to create labels for the graph and an accompanying story that the graph could represent. After a class discussion of their ideas, the teacher distributes copies of the *Tell a Story* reproducible on page A30 in the appendix.

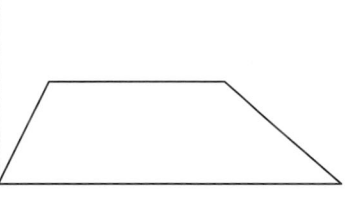

Meeting Individual Needs

Some learners have a strong preference for numerical, rather than visual, representations. Encourage such students to estimate some numbers along the x-axis and y-axis. These numbers can anchor students' thinking, providing them with access to the task.

English language learners may be challenged by the storytelling. You may want them to work with supportive partners, consider the task ahead of time, or dictate their stories to an aide or into a recording device.

REFERENCES/FURTHER READING

Stylianou, Despina A., Beverly Smith, and James J. Kaput. 2005. "Math in Motion: Using CBRs [Calculator-Based Rangers] to Enact Functions." *Journal of Computers in Mathematics and Science Teaching* 24 (3): 299–324.

Wiest, Lynda R. 2009. "Take Time for Action: How Students Interpret Graphs." *Mathematics Teaching in the Middle School* 15 (4): 188–190.

Systems of Linear Equations

Mathematical Focus

- Compare representations of a situation with multiple rates.
- Determine the breaking point between two equations.
- Interpret the meaning of multiple graphs on one set of axes.

Potential Challenges and Misconceptions

Traditional textbooks present methods for solving systems of linear equations as discrete topics, introducing first one method, then another, then the third, while rarely making connections among the three. This approach causes difficulties for many students who are unable to see the connections or the value in deciding when to choose which procedure.

When given data in a list or table, many students tend to draw a bar graph unless otherwise instructed. By grade eight students are expected to understand when it is appropriate to use a bar graph and when it is more fitting to use a line graph.

Many students have experience with plotting points and translating data from tables to graphs but lack experience in interpreting data presented in graphical form. As a result, they face difficulties when it is time to interpret the meaning of multiple lines on one set of axes.

In the Classroom

Relating algebraic concepts to real situations makes the mathematics meaningful to most students. Considering the popularity of walking to raise money for various charitable causes, it makes sense for students to study the results of various donation plans. One teacher poses the following problem:

> Luke, Sam, and Neil are running to raise money for team uniforms. Luke decides that he is going to charge $15 plus $2 for each mile he runs. Sam is going to ask for $25 from each donor. Neil plans on asking for $10 plus $3 for each mile he runs. Which student will raise the most money if they all run the same distance? Justify your answer.

She instructs her students to solve the problem using tables, graphs, and equations. As she decides which group will be first to report its work, she selects the one group who uses a bar graph instead of a line graph to represent the data. (See figure.)

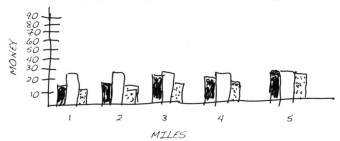

Parker speaks for this group, explaining, "We saw in our table and graph that up to 5 miles, Sam makes the most money even if he does not run a single mile. After 5 miles, Neil makes the most money. We used a bar graph to show that all three make the same amount of money at 5 miles."

Next, Ibby describes what his group did: "We agree with Parker's group, but we used a line graph and found the go-ahead point at twenty-six dollars. All three were even at 5 miles, raising twenty-five dollars." (See figure below.)

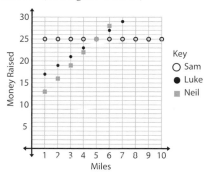

The class discusses when it is appropriate to use a bar graph. Kenny states, "You only use a bar graph with categorical data, like when you want to know how many kids prefer cookie dough ice cream compared with chocolate, or stuff like that."

Jessa says, "Bar graphs tell a frequency."

After this discussion the students work with more problems, which can be found in the *Systems, Strategies, and Solutions* reproducible on page A31 in the appendix.

Meeting Individual Needs

Many students benefit from working with graphing calculators to compare and contrast data in tables, graphs, and equations before generating those representations themselves. Using the trace function on the calculator helps students identify the intersection of all donation plans, allows them to enter a specific mile number and get its corresponding dollar amount, or helps them find a y-value for any given x-value. They also benefit from using the split-screen function on the calculator to compare the data in a table with that of the graph in one window. Most students benefit from experimenting with the window settings as they grapple with the concept of domain and range.

REFERENCE/FURTHER READING

Zaslavsky, Orit, Hagit Sela, and Uri Leron. 2002. "Being Sloppy About Slope: The Effect of Changing the Scale." *Educational Studies in Mathematics* 49 (1): 119–140.

Mathematical Focus

- Represent inequalities on a number line.
- Solve problems involving inequalities.

Potential Challenges and Misconceptions

Studies have shown that students have difficulties with inequalities in the following three areas: (1) regarding inequalities as equations (Vaiyavutjamai and Clements 2006), (2) relating and using different solution techniques (Tsamir and Almog 2001), and (3) interpreting solutions (Tsamir and Bazzini 2004). Much of students' confusion about inequalities can be attributed to vocabulary used to describe inequalities—phrases like *less than*, *greater than*, *at least*, *at most*, and *no more than*.

In the Classroom

One activity designed to prevent misconceptions from developing and help students understand how inequalities might look involves manipulating a classroom-size open number line. First make and hang a long, laminated open number line in the front of the room. Adhere magnetic tape to this open number line as well as on the backs of laminated nonshaded and shaded circles, integers, line segments, and arrows, all of which will be used to represent inequalities.

Then pose a situation such as *Anyone who collects twenty or more signatures on his or her student council nomination form is eligible to run for president of the student council.* Ask all students to represent the situation individually on the *Number Lines* reproducible on page A32 in the appendix. Then have a volunteer go to the class number line and attach the appropriate arrow, integers, and circle, as shown in the first figure below. Notice that the first solution, which was shared by many students, uses an open circle at 20 indicating the exclusion of twenty signatures. A closed circle is necessary to signify that twenty or more signatures are needed. Instruct a second volunteer to write the symbolic representation on the board. Ask the students if anyone did it differently or if anyone got a different answer. In one class, a third volunteer shared her correct number line and inequality, as shown in the second figure.

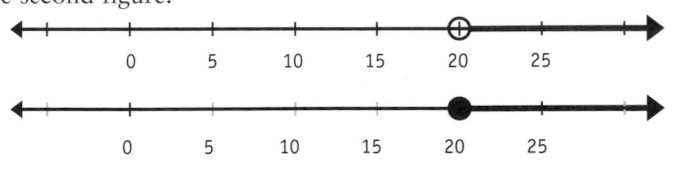

The class discussed the two solutions, focusing on the mathematical meaning behind the two representations and the difference between an open and a closed circle.

Continue posing additional problems such as this:

> Steve is on the middle school wrestling team. To be in class one, he can weigh at most 103 pounds, and to be in class two, he can weigh more than 103 pounds but no more than 130 pounds. Steve is hoping to wrestle in class two. How much is he allowed to weigh?

Following are questions you might want to ask your students:

- What are the parameters for Steve's weight?
- What is the most he can weigh?
- What is the least he can weigh?
- How might you represent this situation on a number line?

After an allotted period of time, direct a volunteer to show the solution on the magnetic number line. Before discussing the solution, ask the class if anyone got anything different. In one class the students showed decidedly different representations on the number line (see the following figure). The class discussed the differences in representations. Of particular interest to many students was the fact that the second representation included both a shaded and a nonshaded circle. Jessie exclaimed, "Wow! I didn't think we could use both an open circle and a filled circle on the same number line."

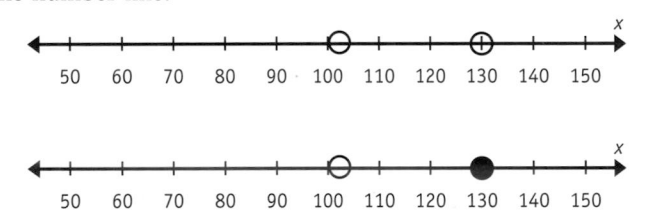

Meeting Individual Needs

English language learners may struggle more than usual because of the language that is used in the problems they must represent. For these students, it is helpful to spend time clarifying the phrases *at least*, *at most*, *no more than*, *less than*, *greater than*, and *equal to or less than*. Students often find it helpful to work in small groups with the teacher or aide and model the terms on the class-size number line before solving inequality problems.

REFERENCES/FURTHER READING

Tsamir, Pessia, and Nava Almog. 2001. "Students' Strategies and Difficulties: The Case of Algebraic Inequalities." *International Journal of Mathematical Education in Science and Technology* 32 (4): 513–524.

Tsamir, Pessia, and Luciana Bazzini. 2004. "Consistencies and Inconsistencies in Students' Solutions to Algebraic 'Single-Value' Inequalities." *International Journal of Mathematical Education in Science and Technology* 35 (6): 793–812.

Vaiyavutjamai, Pongchawee, and M. A. Clements. 2006. "Effects of Classroom Instruction on Student Performance on, and Understanding of, Linear Equations and Linear Inequalities." *Mathematical Thinking and Learning* 8 (2): 113–147.

Mathematical Focus
- Represent systems of inequalities on the Cartesian coordinate plane.
- Solve problems using inequalities.

Potential Challenges and Misconceptions
"Students who think a variable must represent only one value find it extremely difficult to grasp that it has the ability to cover an (un)limited range of numbers. This becomes a major barrier to students' interpretation of the possible solutions to an inequality" (Blanco and Garrote 2007, 227). It is often difficult for students to represent, understand, and use the specific mathematical language of inequalities and to illustrate them on a graph.

In the Classroom
Inequality problems that involve a relationship between two variables require graphing on the Cartesian coordinate plane. One teacher starts with a problem that has a familiar context.

> Claire mixed a batch of hot chocolate with a ratio of two parts chocolate to three parts milk. Her friends said it was too sweet. Claire then mixed a second batch with a ratio of three parts chocolate and five parts milk. Her friends told her it was not chocolatey enough. What are some chocolate-to-milk ratios she can use to make a better-tasting batch of hot chocolate?

As the teacher walks around listening to students discuss the problem, she hears Devon state, "A number line won't work, so let's use a graph."

She pauses to ask Devon a *clarifying question*. "What criteria do you need to draw a graph?"

She also hears Jamal ask, "If we draw a ray, we can't use open circles; what do you think shows the values come close to but don't equal a number?" She listens to Charlie ask, "Do you think we color in the space between the rays or leave it blank?"

After an allotted period of time, Charlie's group shares its work (see figure).

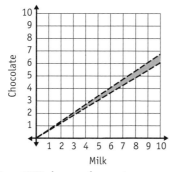

Charlie explains, "We knew the ratio was greater than three-fifths but less than two-thirds, so we decided to shade in the space between the two ratios. The only thing we could think of was to use dashed lines to show the amounts come close to but don't equal those ratios." The class discusses the suggested representation before examining the next problem.

> Ross and Max are planting a garden of pumpkins and watermelons. They have room for no more than 60 plants. They plan on planting more pumpkins than watermelons. How many of each plant might they plant?

Many students find this problem more challenging than the previous one since they have to solve the system of inequalities before graphing it. One teacher engages his students in a facilitated solution process to ensure that all students understand this important concept. He first instructs the students to read the entire problem and discuss it until he is satisfied that the students know what the problem is asking. He then instructs the students to write a symbolic representation for the data in the problem. After a very short period of time, he asks a volunteer to write the inequalities on the board. He asks if anyone did it differently. He asks a volunteer to write the solution on the board. She writes p ≤ 60 − w *and* p > w. The class discusses it, agreeing that it is correct. Next, groups graph the solution on easel-size paper. When they've finished, students hang their graphs on the board. The teacher challenges the class to examine all the graphs and decide which is the most accurate and why. After much discussion, the class agrees that the graph in the following figure is correct.

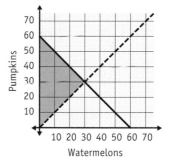

Meeting Individual Needs
To ensure that all students understand the symbols used on both the number line and the Cartesian coordinate plane, assign pairs of students to complete the *Matching Inequalities* reproducible on page A33 in the appendix. After cutting out the cards and mixing them up, each pair of students must match the cards with written inequalities to the cards with symbolic and graphical representations. Students should take turns sharing their matches, defending their selections as necessary.

REFERENCE/FURTHER READING
Blanco, Lorenzo J., and Manuel Garrote. 2007. "Difficulties in Learning Inequalities in Students of the First Year of Pre-University Education in Spain." *Eurasia Journal of Mathematics, Science and Technology Education* 3 (3): 221–229.

A34

Mathematical Focus

- Pose problems that include number line inequalities.
- Pose problems that include Cartesian coordinate plane inequalities.

Potential Challenges and Misconceptions

When teachers give students mathematical expressions, equations, graphs, or tables, they often instruct the class to compute, simplify, solve, or graph information presented without any context. Rarely do they ask students to pose questions about the data or representations. This lack of experience dampens students' curiosity and makes it challenging for them to identify appropriate questions or problems to research. "When students begin posing their own original mathematical questions and see these questions become the focus of discussion, their perception of the subject is profoundly altered. When they get to spend time working on these questions, their ownership of the experience produces excitement and motivation" (Cuoco, Manes, and Dash 2003). This is especially true when inequalities are involved.

In the Classroom

One teacher begins a lesson on problem posing by stating, "I need you to help me make sense of this open number line. What situations might the original question represent?"

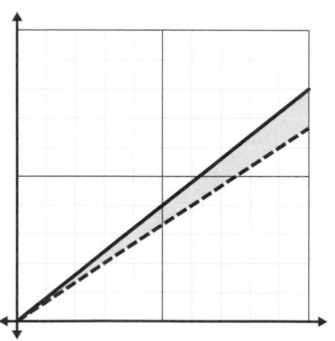

Students work in small groups to identify appropriate contexts. Isabel's group offers this idea:

> If we have fifty girls in our eighth-grade class and our total enrollment is more than 75 but no more than 100 students, how many boys might be in the class?

The teacher shows another representation to her students, which indicates a relationship between two variables. She challenges them to pose problems that might be represented by the following graph.

Max's group suggests a problem similar to ones the class has studied before:

> What mixtures of hot chocolate to milk will be richer than two parts hot chocolate to three parts milk but no richer than the mixture of four parts hot chocolate to five parts milk?

Sabrina's group reports next:

> Levi is challenging Brandi and Brett to a walking race. He claims he walks at a rate that is faster than Brandi's and less than Brett's. If Brandi walks two meters in three seconds and Brett no faster than four meters in five seconds, at what rate might Levi walk?

The most challenging problem-posing situations are prompted by the following two representations.

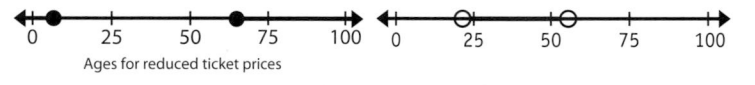

Ages for reduced ticket prices

Students need assistance with identifying potential situations for these compound inequalities. The teacher suggests the students brainstorm about times when exceptions are made for people of different ages. After an allotted period of time, students share the following circumstances: at the movies you pay less if you are under twelve or over sixty-five; on a bus you pay less fare if you are under six or over sixty-five; at an amusement park children pay less than adults and senior citizens. After the brainstorming exercise, the students pose a variety of different problems. For the figure on the left, one group suggests a question about movie ticket prices:

> The Show Me Cinema charges $10.50 to see a movie. They have reduced rates for senior citizens and children. At what ages does the Show Me Cinema discount their rates?

The group writes the inequality as $y \geq 65$ or $y \leq 6$.
For the figure on the right, another group proposes this problem:

> Jill's favorite cookies contain 7 grams of fat. Jill usually eats more than three small cookies and usually fewer than eight small cookies. How many grams of fat might Jill consume?

The group represents the inequality as $21 < f < 56$.
The *Problem-Posing Representations* reproducible on page A34 in the appendix provides inequalities in various forms for students to write story problems about.

Meeting Individual Needs

Putting inequalities into contextual situations is most beneficial for students who struggle with using algorithms for the sake of algorithms. We have found that when our students represent situations that they confront in their own lives, they are better able to make sense of the algebraic representations and reason through them. Some students need help in identifying when those situations occur. Most benefit from brainstorming ideas.

REFERENCE/FURTHER READING

Cuoco, Al, Michelle Manes, and Terry Dash. 2003. *Making Mathematics.* Newton, MA: Educational Development Center. www2.edu.org/makingmath/handbook/Teacher/ProblemPosing.asp.

Absolute Value as Distance

Mathematical Focus

- Represent absolute value equations on a number line.
- Solve absolute value equations.

Potential Challenges and Misconceptions

The concept of absolute value is extremely challenging. Students become confused when they are told that the solution of an absolute value equation must be positive. They develop several common misconceptions, including the following: (1) the solution of an absolute problem can never be negative; (2) any solutions to an absolute problem must be made positive; (3) there is only one solution to an absolute value problem; and (4) when there are two solutions to an absolute value problem, they are always a number and its opposite.

In the Classroom

One teacher begins by asking a student volunteer to go to the floor-size number line and stand at 0. She asks another student volunteer to go to the board to record the first student's actions and directs the students at their desks to draw a set of number lines, model each example, and record the mathematical notation. She directs the student "traveler" to move 5 units to the west (left) and the student at the board to record this motion. The student at the board records $0 + (-5) = -5$. The teacher asks a seated student *how far* from 0 the student is now standing. The student replies, "Five units from 0." The teacher uses this example as a stepping-stone to introduce the notation for absolute value. She explains that the absolute value indicates the difference or distance from zero. She shows the students that they should represent the distance as $|0 - (-5)| = 5$ and should read the equation as *the absolute value of zero minus negative five is equal to five*. They discuss the concept that the $| \ |$ symbol indicates that after the action of $|0 - (-5)|$ is completed, the difference is $+5$ since distance cannot be negative. If the first traveler moved five units to the right they would represent that as $|0 - 5| = 5$ and would be read as *the absolute value of zero minus five is equal to five*.

Next she invites two different students, one to the number line and one to the board, to model and record the next process. The traveler stands on 0 and moves to the right 6 units. The student at the board records $|0 - 6| = 6$. The teacher reads the notation as "the absolute value of zero minus six equals six." The traveler then stands on 0 and moves to the left 6 units. The student at the board records $|0 - (-6)| = 6$. This teacher continues with different students assuming the roles of the traveler and recorder until all students have an opportunity to perform both roles.

The teacher quickly moves on to working with situations with variables since they cause more difficulty than simply working with integers. Again a student traveler models the problem while a second one records the notation. She challenges her students to determine where the traveler might have begun a number line journey if the distance of his starting location is 2 units from the position of 5 on the number line. The recorder notates $2 = |x - 5|$. The traveler stands at 2, then walks 5 units east (right) and identifies a possible beginning location at 7. The traveler returns to 2 and walks 5 units west and erroneously identifies a possible beginning location at -3. The teacher asks the class if anyone did it differently. Many students raise their hands and Brody demonstrates and explains, "First, I start at 5 and move to the east 2 units, ending at 7. Then I return to 5 and move west 2 units, ending at 3."

The teacher asks the students what caused them the most confusion. Colin answers, "I think the hardest part of doing these is realizing that the answer to the absolute value part of the equation tells the *distance* that we travel, and we have to remember to travel both east and west on the number line to find both possible starting points."

The teacher distributes copies of the reproducible *Distance Is Always Positive* (see page A35 in the appendix) to give students additional opportunities to model and solve absolute value problems.

Meeting Individual Needs

Interpreting absolute value problems can be very difficult, much more so than the mechanics of completing the computations. Many students struggle with trying to make sense of absolute value and have a better chance of understanding when the problems consistently refer to units of measurement such as distance, volume, and capacity. We suggest that you restrict "naked" computation until after students demonstrate a conceptual understanding of absolute value through problem solving. It is crucial to emphasize the fact that if students check their solutions by substituting their answers in the original equations, they can determine if the answers are correct.

REFERENCE/FURTHER READING

Wei, S. 2005. "Solving Absolute Value Equations Algebraically and Geometrically." *Mathematics Teacher* 99 (1): 72–74.

Absolute Value Inequalities

Mathematical Focus

- Represent absolute value inequalities symbolically and graphically.
- Solve problems that include absolute value inequalities.

Potential Challenges and Misconceptions

When we combine two difficult concepts such as absolute value and inequalities, we have a perfect storm for misconceptions and challenges. Some of the challenges students face include correctly identifying the meaning when variables are located on the right side of the inequality; that inequalities cannot be read left to right and right to left in the same way; that compound inequalities can be written as one statement or as two statements joined by a keyword; and that the keyword may not be included in the wording of the problem. When conducting lessons on absolute value inequalities, some teachers tell students to use shortcuts such as *solve the positive case, then reverse the inequality sign and the sign of the constant on the side opposite the variable when solving the negative case.* These shortcuts inevitably cause difficulty for students who have not developed a deep understanding of the concept.

In the Classroom

Just as with simple absolute value equations, it is necessary to teach absolute value inequalities and compound absolute value inequalities by engaging students in modeling the problems using the number line.

One teacher begins her work with absolute value inequalities by building on the work she did with absolute value equalities. (See "Absolute Value as Distance.") She invites a student to model an absolute value inequality on the floor-size number line and a second student to record the absolute value inequality and solution on the board. Students at their desks do the same problem using individual number lines. She poses the following situation: *If I traveled less than 2 units from the position of 6 on the number line, where might my starting point have been?* The recorder writes the equation $|x - 6| < 2$ and draws a number line to represent the answer. The traveler moves to 6 on the number line and explains, "I have to move to the right (east) 2 units to 8."

The teacher asks a seated student what the solution is. Lauren replies, "The answer is any value between six and eight, but it does not include eight." The traveler returns to 6 and moves 2 units west (left) to 4. She explains that the points of 4 and 8 are the lower and upper bounds and that any value in between could be where she started. As the symbolic representation of the solution begins notice the absolute value notation becomes parentheses.

The recorder has written the following for the first inequality:

$$(x - 6) < 2$$
$$x - 6 < 2$$
$$x < 8$$

She announces that she does not know what to do next. The teacher asks what the opposite of less than two is. After an allotted period of time, David replies, "The opposite of less than two is greater than two." The recorder writes $(x - 6) > 2$.

The teacher asks whether they can just reverse the inequality sign. Dante says, "I think since what is in the absolute value can be positive or negative, we have to make the 2 negative." The teacher records the correct symbolic representation on the board, explaining, "Notice I multiplied the quantity of $(x - 6)$ by -1 and reversed the inequality sign."

$$-(x - 6) < 2$$
$$(x - 6) > -2$$
$$x > 4$$

The teacher asks the recorder to show the two solutions on one number line. (See figure.)

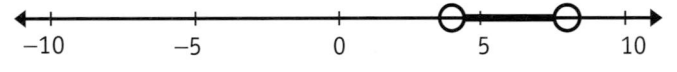

The teacher poses another situation: *How might you represent all numbers whose distance from 3 is greater than or equal to 4?* A student volunteer goes to the number line while another goes to the board. The traveler stands on 3 and moves to the right 4 units, stopping at 7. The recorder notes $|x - 3| \geq 4$. He simplifies it to $x - 3 \geq 4$. He continues by writing $x \geq 7$. The traveler returns to the 3 on the number line and walks 4 units to the left, stopping at -1. The recorder writes $-|x - 3| \geq 4$ followed by $-(x - 3) \geq 4$ and $x - 3 \leq -4$. Finally he records $x \leq 4 + 3$, solves it as $x \leq -1$, and draws the number line. (See figure.)

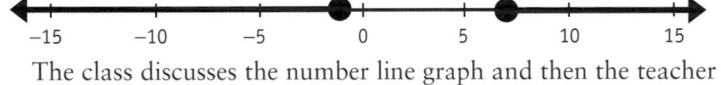

The class discusses the number line graph and then the teacher hands out copies of the *What Is My Range?* reproducible on page A36 in the appendix to provide additional practice.

Meeting Individual Needs

Since absolute value with inequalities poses a compounded set of challenges for students, it is important to ensure that students who have struggled with inequalities have multiple opportunities to reinforce that concept before adding the absolute value component. This scaffolding will give all students the opportunity to succeed with modeling and solving absolute value with inequalities.

REFERENCE/FURTHER READING

Ponce, Gregorio A. 2008. "Using, Seeing, Feeling, and Doing Absolute Value for Deeper Understanding." *Mathematics Teaching in the Middle School* 14 (4): 234–240.

Am I a Function?

A37

Mathematical Focus

- Recognize and identify the characteristics of functions.
- Work with linear functions.

Potential Challenges and Misconceptions

Traditionally, when teachers introduce the concept of function, they emphasize the representation of function rather than the *functional relationships* that comprise the function. Students often find it very challenging to relate the symbolic, tabular, and graphic representations to functions when they lack opportunities to think about the functional relationships in contextual situations. As a result, many students also struggle to explain why the "vertical line test" works to determine whether a graph represents a function. It is common for students to mistakenly believe that the graph of a function cannot stop at a given point; that horizontal lines are not functions; and that familiar graphs are functions—for instance, a circle is a function because it looks familiar. Although the Common Core State Standards do not require function notation in grade eight, it is appropriate to expose students to it. The function notation $f(x)$ simply means "the function whose input is x."

In the Classroom

The National Council of Teachers of Mathematics' algebra standard for grades six through eight emphasizes that all students should "identify functions as linear or nonlinear and contrast their properties from tables, graphs, or equations" (NCTM 2000, 222). Few students have experience working with the notation of sets and the concept of domain and range. Since it is important that students understand that for every x-value there is one and only one y-value, it is helpful to work with contextual examples of functional relationships before moving into the mathematical representations.

One teacher begins her work with relationships using familial situations and asks her students if they believe each relationship is a function. She presents the following situations: {(father, children)}; {(Parker, his age)}; {(Jill, her height)}. The class discusses the fact that the {(father, children)} relationship is not a function because the father may have more than one child; {(Parker, his age)} is a function since Parker can have only one age at any one point in time; and {(Jill, her height)} is a function since there is only one height for the person Jill at any one time. This teacher reads the last example as "the set of Jill and her height" as a way of modeling the vocabulary. She also rephrases the way in which her students talk about functions and set notation using mathematically appropriate terminology until her students adopt its use. She challenges her students to make a list of other functional relationships. One student reports that the relationship between classmates in his group and each of their favorite colors would be represented as {(Joe, red), (Billy, blue), (Angie, green), (Grace, yellow), (Isabel, blue), (Simon, red), (Jose, blue)}. The students discuss the list and agree each student has only one favorite color, so the relationship is a function. The teacher then explains some mathematical terminology: the *domain* is the input and the *range* is the output.

This teacher arranges a gallery walk with samples of graphs and tables and asks the students to identify whether they represent functions. (See figures.) If they are functions, the students must indicate whether they are linear or nonlinear.

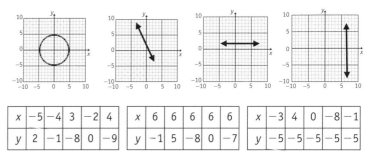

After an allotted period of time, the class discusses the students' responses. Next, the teacher directs each group of students to solve the problem found on the *Name That Function* reproducible on page A37 in the appendix. Students must use all six clues to solve this problem. The teacher passes out two clues to each of the three students in a group. Group members orally share the information provided on their two clues, decide the order in which to use the clues, and work collaboratively to identify whether they have a function and what it is.

Meeting Individual Needs

For students who struggle with the vocabulary and symbolic notation, provide a graphic organizer for recording the terminology. Encourage students to write the term; show a graphic, tabular, and symbolic representation of the term; identify what strategy they might devise to help them remember the term; and finally write a definition in their own words. Be sure to check the definitions for accuracy.

REFERENCES/FURTHER READING

Billings, Esther M. H., and Charlene E. Beckmann. 2005. "Children's Literature: A Motivating Context to Explore Functions." *Mathematics Teaching in the Middle School* 10 (9): 470–478.

National Council of Teachers of Mathematics (NCTM). 2000. *Principles and Standards for School Mathematics*. Reston, VA: Author.

You, Zhixia. 2007. "Investigating Students' Thinking About Functional Relationships." *Mathematics Teaching in the Middle School* 13 (5): 312–315.

Mathematical Focus

- Identify linear functions in tables and graphs.
- Solve linear functions for given sets of domains.

Potential Challenges and Misconceptions

"Horizontal" development of a concept of functions occurs through exposure to multiple representations and indicates breadth of understanding (DeMarois and Tall 1996). Students often confuse these representations with functions themselves and believe that *function* is another name for a graph or an equation. Others find it difficult to translate among equations, tables, and graphs.

"Vertical" development of a concept of functions occurs through building up understanding from a cognitive root or base and indicates depth of knowledge (DeMarois and Tall 1996). Students who are not afforded the experiences of building conceptual understanding of functions often struggle as the mathematics becomes more challenging.

Ideally, students gain both horizontal and vertical concepts of functions to develop a "two-dimensional" cognitive representation of what a function is.

In the Classroom

One teacher begins by posing this *range question: Given y = 5x − 3, make a list of everything you know.* He intends to assess the range of understanding that his students have about linear functions. He listens for mathematical terminology, including statements such as "The slope is 5," "The y-intercept is (−3)," "The equation is linear," "The equation is of the form y equals mx plus b," "It is a function," "For any given value of x, we substitute that number into the equation," and "Multiply by 5, then subtract 3." After debriefing the student responses, he poses the following situation.

> Marisol planted a tomato plant in her patio garden. When she planted the tomato plant, it measured 3.5 inches. The following week when she measured it, the plant was 4.0 inches tall, and it was 4.5 inches at the end of week two. If this represents the average growth rate per week for the plant, what function best represents its growth? How tall will the plant be in three weeks? Five weeks? Seven weeks? Identify the domain and make a graph to illustrate this function.

He walks around the room, listening as his students discuss how best to represent the problem. He pauses to ask one group why they are beginning their table at (0, 0) when the plant was already 3.5 inches when it was purchased. He asks a second group to explain to him how they are going to include the domain if they write an equation in the form y = mx + b. He asks yet another group to explain why their graph has a line representing the data rather than a ray. This teacher provides each group with easel-size graph paper and instructs the students to record the function and the graph. They hang the graphs around the room. He focuses the class discussion on similarities and differences among the functions and the graphs.

To ensure all his students are proficient in working with functions, this teacher sends as many students as fit at one time to the board and dictates various functions with specific domains. He may announce, for instance, $y = \frac{-2}{3}x - 5$ with a domain of {−3, −6, 3, 9}. Students must record the function and solve for the range that corresponds to the dictated domain. For a second challenge, he might give them the domain {(−1, 5), (0, 2), (1, −1), (2, −4)}. Students record the ordered pairs and write an appropriate function. Students who are not at the board record the same information on their individual whiteboards and find the range or function. As the students work on the solutions, the teacher observes and intervenes with individual students as soon as they make an error.

To give students additional practice with linear functions, assign the *Do I Represent a Constant Change?* reproducible on page A38 in the appendix.

Meeting Individual Needs

To ensure he has an understanding of what his students have learned about functions, this teacher assigns an *exit card* on which he asks the students to tell him in their own words what a function is, what the domain represents, and what the range represents. He uses the information in the exit cards to group his students in order to provide support as necessary and to reinforce their developing understanding before moving on to nonlinear functions.

REFERENCES/FURTHER READING

Clement, Lisa L. 2001. "What Do Students Really Know About Functions?" *Mathematics Teacher* 94 (9): 745–748.

DeMarois, Phil, and David Tall. 1996. "Facets and Layers of the Function Concept." In *Proceedings of the 20th Annual Conference for the Psychology of Mathematics Education*, Vol. 2 (Valencia, Spain): 297–304.

Solving Problems Using Ordered Pairs

Mathematical Focus

- Interpret the meaning of slopes and intercepts in real-world situations.
- Identify two given points within a problem situation.
- Create an equation of the line containing two given points.

Potential Challenges and Misconceptions

Given sufficient practice, many students become proficient at finding an equation for a line containing two given points when the points are identified in their coordinate form, for example, $(3, 5)$ and $(-1, -9)$. Yet many of these students struggle when the points are embedded within a word problem. Students may not be sure which data represent the x-values and which represent the y-values or which variables are independent and which are dependent.

Once students are able to identify the relevant coordinates, they can apply their known procedures to find the equation containing these two points. Often, students are not asked to relate their finding back to the context of the problem. Students rarely have opportunities to interpret the meanings of slope and intercepts or identify the relevant domain and range within a variety of contexts, to build their conceptual understanding of algebraic constructs.

In the Classroom

One teacher presents the following problem to his students.

> Massie joins the Fitness Sports Club. She pays an initiation fee and is charged a monthly fee at the end of each month. After four months her total cost of membership is $265. At the end of a year, her total cost is $545.

The teacher asks the students to work alone or with a partner to find the equation that will allow them to determine Massie's cost, given the number of months she has been a member of the Fitness Sports Club. A few students suggest that there is not enough information in the problem to do this. Several students make a table, but a few enter 1 for the x-coordinate associated with $545. Some students apply arithmetic thinking. They subtract $265 from $545 to determine that the additional 8 months added a cost of $280. They then divide by 8 to determine the monthly fee of $35. At this point, some students are surprised to find that $35 \times 4 \neq \$265$. Finally, a few students suggest that the difference between 35×4, or $140, and $265 must be the initiation fee, which is $125.

The teacher asks, "So how could we find out what Massie paid after eight months?" Many of the students are familiar enough with the context to suggest multiplying $35 and 8 and then adding $125. Then Eric asks, "Can we just double the cost at four months?" The students try both techniques and several are surprised that the outcomes are not the same.

The teacher asks, "What are you really doubling here?"

Juanita says, "Oh, I get it. Eric's way is 125 dollars too much because we doubled the initiation fee, too, and you only pay that once."

Next the teacher asks about the total cost after fourteen months. This time the students all agree, and when he asks about n months, they identify the equation as $C = \$35M + \$125$. He then asks them to identify the slope and the y-intercept and what they each represent in this problem.

Next the teacher asks, "How do we find an equation for a line?" The students identify that they need two points or a point and the slope. He directs them back to the problem and asks students to identify the two given points. He calls on a volunteer to use these points to determine the slope. Another volunteer shows how to use a point and the slope to find their equation.

Finally, he uses his overhead graphing calculator to show the line. He asks, "Can every point on this line tell us the months and associated cost of membership?" With further questions, they recognize that for this context, the domain would be limited to whole numbers and that realistically they would be less than 1,000. Bella adds, "The range would also be all positive integers because you don't pay for parts of months."

The teacher distributes copies of the *Problem Solving with Points* reproducible on page A39 of the appendix. He says, "Remember that if you can identify two points, you can determine the equation for the line that contains them."

Meeting Individual Needs

Graphic organizers can help students who continue to struggle with identifying the relevant data points within a story problem or with determining which variable is independent and which is dependent. Consider using the *Graphic Organizer for Linear Equations* reproducible on page A40 of the appendix with students who you think need such scaffolding. You may also wish to encourage students to use calculators so that they can focus on the interpretation of their findings.

REFERENCES/FURTHER READING

Koedinger, Kenneth R., Martha W. Alibali, and Mitchell J. Nathan. 2008. "Trade-Offs Between Grounded and Abstract Representations: Evidence for Algebra Story Problems." *Cognitive Science* 32 (2): 366–397.

Stephens, Ana C. 2003. "Another Look at Word Problems." *Mathematics Teacher* 96 (1): 63–66.

Mathematical Focus

- Identify a table of data as quadratic based on the finite differences in the table.
- Recognize the sum of consecutive odd integers beginning with 1 is a square number.

Potential Challenges and Misconceptions

Many students struggle to connect one concept to another and often do not realize that geometric representations can be made for both numeric and algebraic concepts. When students are introduced to quadratics, they hear the term *squared* but many do not connect the fact that a square number can actually be represented as a square. To help students make connections between previously learned concepts and quadratics, it is important to carefully select activities that prompt those connections and to represent quadratics algebraically as well as geometrically.

In the Classroom

To introduce square numbers, one teacher begins by distributing a handful of colored discs to each of his students and modeling a triangular pattern using the discs on his projection device. He instructs his students to copy the pattern on their tables. The pattern consists of consecutive odd integers. (See figure.)

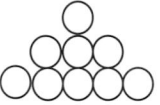

He challenges his students to tell him what the total number of discs would be, if the pattern continued, for seven rows. He reminds them that they must support or prove their conjectures. As the groups work on building the seven rows, the teacher walks around, observing and asking questions. He asks one group, "What do you notice about how the rows grow?"

He listens as another group discusses whether to break the problem down into a smaller problem. He hears one member say, "But if we do one row there is only one disc, but if we do two rows there are four discs. I bet we'll see a pattern if we make a table with the row and number of discs."

He observes yet another group rearranging the discs and poses a *clarifying question*: "What are you thinking as you rearrange the discs?"

One student in the group responds, "I think that if we move the discs around, we might make a shape other than a triangle and that might help us." When this teacher facilitates the summary of the investigation, he focuses the class's attention on the table that one group made and asks the students to identify any patterns they notice. (See figure.)

Row Number	1	2	3	4	5	6	7
Number of Discs	1	4	9	16	25	36	49

One student responds, "When I looked at the number of discs, I saw they increase by different amounts, so I know this is not a linear function."

A second student adds, "I saw that also and wrote *plus 3, plus 5, plus 7, plus 9, plus 11, . . .* and saw these are consecutive odd numbers."

A third student points out, "If you do that subtracting one more time for the output, $5 - 3 = 2$; $7 - 5 = 2$; $9 - 7 = 2$; and $11 - 9 = 2$, you get plus two, plus two, plus two, plus two."

Next the teacher asks the group that was rearranging the discs to describe what it discovered. A student shares the fact that the group was able to make squares. The teacher facilitates a discussion about squares and consecutive odd integers by asking, "Do you think that always works? How can you tell? Let's write an equation for this phenomena and graph the data from the table. What information does the graph provide?"

We can make quadratics relevant to students through problem solving and relating graphs to those problem situations. For example, one teacher poses the following problem:

> Grade-eight students are enlarging a drawing to make a mural for their school. They know the length must be $1\frac{1}{3}$ times the height. If the mural will cover 192 square feet, what will the dimensions be?

Students work in small groups to solve the problem. Jesse's group comes up with the following equation for solving the problem: $l \times w = A$ so $(1\frac{1}{3}w)w = 192$. This group solves the equation by first applying the distributive property to get $\frac{4}{3}w^2 = 192$. Their second step is to use the multiplicative inverse, which yields $w^2 = 144$. Their solution is $w = \pm 12$. They discuss whether they need both the positive and negative 12. They agree that it is not possible to have a negative length or width so they need only the solution $w = 12$ feet. From there, the students substitute 12 into the equation for the width and get a length of 16 feet. The class discusses the problem before moving on to the problems on the *Am I Square?* reproducible on page A41 in the appendix.

Meeting Individual Needs

Many students find using algorithms without organized data from which they can see relationships too abstract. It is helpful to direct these students to record their data in a table and to graph the data in the table. Once the students see the shape the data make, they may be more likely to determine whether the graph is linear or nonlinear. Encourage all students to sketch the graphs using paper and pencil before checking their work with their graphing calculators.

REFERENCE/FURTHER READING

Roy, Jessica A., and Charlene E. Beckmann. 2007. "Mathematical Explorations: Batty Functions: Exploring Quadratic Functions Through Children's Literature." *Mathematics Teaching in the Middle School* 13 (11): 52–56.

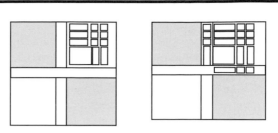

Mathematical Focus

- Use algebra tiles to model quadratic expressions.

Potential Challenges and Misconceptions

Many teachers tell students to use FOIL as they work on representing the factored form of a quadratic expression in expanded form. However, the widespread use of this acronym prevents many students from being able to expand their thinking when it is time to multiply a trinomial by a binomial. Using the appropriate mathematical property and calling it *the distributive property* empowers students as they work with more complex multiplication involving variables.

In the Classroom

Providing concrete and pictorial representations and contextual situations involving quadratics helps most students gain a deeper understanding of the differences between the factored form of a quadratic and its expanded form. It is extremely beneficial to begin the exploration of quadratics using algebra tiles. You can use the *Algebra Tiles Template* reproducible on page A3 in the appendix along with the *Algebra Mat for Modeling Quadratics* reproducible on page A42 in the appendix for this activity. One teacher displays a copy of the mat on her projection device and directs the class to model with her the expression "the quantity of b plus three times the quantity of b plus three," as shown in the figure on the left below.

No one did, so she directs the students to record the expression and sketch the algebra mat and product in their notebooks. If someone had mentioned a different answer, she would have reviewed how to model the factors and product.

Next, she presents an example that includes negatives: $(b + 2)(b - 3)$. She invites a volunteer to the overhead to model the factors, as in the first figure below, and a second volunteer to demonstrate the product $b^2 - 1b - 6$. After students identify the product, as shown in the second figure below, she directs her students to record a pictorial and a symbolic representation in their notebooks.

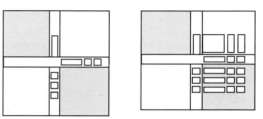

Then the teacher challenges her class to model a story problem: *The dimensions of a square patio are changed so that the width, b, is shortened by 2 feet while the length is increased by 2 feet. What is the change in the area?* Lauren shares her work. (See figures below.)

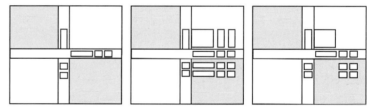

She explains that the final product left two squares—one in the first quadrant, which is positive, and one in the fourth quadrant, which is negative, for a result of $b^2 - 4$. She explains the original area has decreased by 4 square units.

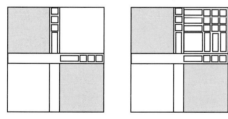

The class discusses how the algebra tile representation (shown in the figure on the right above) relates to the partial product multiplication of $(b + 3)(b + 3)$, represented as $b^2 + 3b + 3b + 9$. The class then agrees the final product is $b^2 + 6b + 9$. The class practices a few more examples until students demonstrate confidence with the model and its relation to the distributive property. Before moving on, the teacher directs her students to analyze the shape the product makes. It is important to this teacher that her students recognize that a binomial times a binomial will always make a rectangle or, in this case, the special rectangle, a square before the expression is simplified.

Next, the class moves on to factoring a given trinomial. This teacher challenges her students to model the product and to write the symbolic representation for the factors of $b^2 + 5b + 6$. After an allotted period of time, she invites a volunteer to the projection device to model the product. When the volunteer completes the product as shown in the following figure, the teacher asks if anyone got a different answer.

Meeting Individual Needs

Many students need assistance to see the differences between perfect square trinomials and the difference of two squares. They should have ample experiences to build each type until they can recognize the difference easily. You might also direct students who have moved to symbolic notation to occasionally check their solutions with the algebra tiles. Including the tiles for all students removes any stigma that students who need the tiles might feel.

REFERENCE/FURTHER READING

Leitze, Annette Ricks, and Nancy A. Kitt. 2000. "Algebra for All: Using Homemade Algebra Tiles to Develop Algebra and Prealgebra Concepts." *The Mathematics Teacher* 93 (6): 462–468.

Mathematical Focus

- Model and factor trinomials.
- Solve quadratic equations.

Potential Challenges and Misconceptions

Students who work with quadratics written in standard form and who have a lot of practice factoring are usually adept at solving equations such as $x^2 - x - 6 = 0$ and correctly compute $(x - 3) = 0$ or $(x + 2) = 0$, identifying the x-intercepts or roots of the equation as 3 and -2. The challenge for many students begins when the equation is not set equal to 0. For instance, when solving the equation $x^2 - x - 6 = 12$, many incorrectly believe that $(x - 3) = 12$ or $(x + 2) = 12$. Many students also mistakenly think that the vertex is a minimum point when the parabola opens downward and a maximum point when the parabola opens upward. Teachers can often correct this misconception if they relate graphs to a contextual situation.

In the Classroom

Because not all students relate well to modeling with algebra tiles, one teacher introduces an area model for multiplying binomials and factoring trinomials. The area model is familiar to many students from their work with partial products in the earlier grades, and the teachers finds the transition to using it with quadratics is seamless. She begins by modeling the expression $a^2 + 5a + 6$, as shown in the following figure.

a^2	$3a$
$2a$	6

Then she directs her students to determine the factors. After a short period of time, she asks a volunteer to share his work. He displays the area model with the binomial factors. (See figure below.)

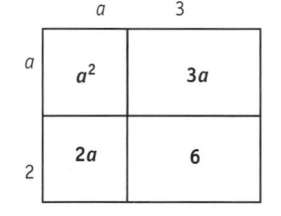

The student explains that he found the factors by working first with the terms a^2 and 6. He explains the only way to get a product of a^2 is to multiply a by a, and he is going to work with the positive a's so he places those factors first. He then notes that to find the product of 6, he has two choices: either 3×2 or 6×1. Because the terms $1a$ and $6a$ cannot combine to make $5a$ if both are positive, he recognizes he must use $+3a$ and $+2a$ to produce the middle term, $5a$. The original factors have to be the quantity of $(a + 3)$ and the quantity of $(a + 2)$. This teacher asks if anyone found anything different. When no one responds, she directs the students to model the trinomial $a^2 + 7a + 12$. She instructs her students to use either the area model or their algebra tiles to represent the trinomial and to identify the factors. She is not surprised when many students state their preference for a

algebra tiles. She assures them they may use whichever method makes the most sense to them. After ensuring that all students correctly identify the binomial as $(a + 3)(a + 4)$, she challenges them to represent and solve a contextual problem:

> Conor is designing a skateboard park. Its length is 3 yards less than its width. Its area is 180 square yards. What are the dimensions of the skateboard park?

Students work in small groups. While the students work, this teacher walks around, observing, listening, and asking probing questions. She notices that most students set up the correct equation: $w(w - 3) = 180$. She asks one group to explain to her what information it has. Renee responds, "We have the length, width, and area. We know that length times width equals area. We have two factors and the product." The teacher further asks Renee to explain what she thinks her first step will be. Renee answers, "If we use the distributive property we will have the product w^2 minus $3w$ equals 180."

The teacher listens in to a member of another group, who is saying, "We need to find two factors that are pretty close together to get a difference of 3 but when they are multiplied equal 180. Let's list the factors of 180." The group makes an organized list of factors, which includes 20×9 (difference: 11); 18×10 (difference: 8); and 15×12 (difference: 3).

As she moves among the other groups, she overhears Angel explaining, "We have w^2 minus $3w$ equals 180. When we did the factors with the algebra tiles, the product had three terms; remember it was called a trinomial? I think what we need to do is subtract the 180 from both sides of the equation to get the three terms. Then we'll have w^2 minus $3w$ minus 180 equals 0." This teacher praises Angel for his clear explanation and asks other members of his group if they can explain to her what Angel just said. Because both Ramon and April are able to tell her in their own words, she is convinced they can follow Angel's reasoning. The group members model their trinomial using algebra tiles. They factor the trinomial and find that $(w - 15)(w + 12) = 0$. They solve for w and announce the width is 15 yards and that it is not possible to have a negative length. They go back to the statement in the problem that says the length is 3 yards less than the width and subtract 3 yards from 15 yards, for a length of 12 yards. Their teacher asks them to check their results using their graphing calculator. She asks April to enter the binomials and Ramon to enter the trinomial and compare and discuss the results.

After discussing the problem and its solution, the class works on the *Solving Quadratics* reproducible on page A43 in the appendix.

Meeting Individual Needs

It is very beneficial to introduce all students to several ways of representing the multiplication of binomials and factoring of trinomials. Students should experience each representation and be allowed to choose the one they understand best. Often when subtraction is included in the trinomial, students choose to use algebra tiles; otherwise, most students use the area model as they transition to working symbolically.

REFERENCE/FURTHER READING

Cramer, Kathleen. 2001. "Using Models to Build an Understanding of

Mathematical Focus

- Examine patterns that grow exponentially.
- Model situations with exponential growth and decay.

Potential Challenges and Misconceptions

One of the most prominent challenges students face when graphing exponential data from a table is labeling the axes. Many students commonly use the exact data from the tables to label the y-axis without accounting for the proportional relationship from one data point to the next. That is, if they were graphing $y = x^2$, they would place a 9 one unit from a 4 and a 16 one unit from the 9. The result would be a linear graph. This misconception is often due to lack of experience and can be resolved by solving more problems with exponential growth and decay.

In the Classroom

Most students have little experience with exponential patterns and do not comprehend how quickly a value will grow or decay when exponents are involved. One teacher assigns the *How Many Rectangles?* problem to introduce exponential growth. Students take one piece of $8\frac{1}{2}$-by-11-inch paper and fold it in half repeatedly to determine the total number of rectangles they can make if they fold the paper 1, 2, 3, 4, 5, or n times. The students record their data in a table and in a graph. The teacher also challenges them to write an equation to represent what is happening in the table and graph. As the students work on the problem, this teacher walks around the room, listening for accountable talk and observing how they are recording their data. She overhears a member of Tamara's group say, "It is impossible to fold a piece of paper ten times. Why don't we take the number of rectangles after five folds and double it?"

The teacher asks the group a *refocusing question*: "Did you get double the number of rectangles from two folds to four folds?"

Tamara responds, "No, we got four rectangles when we folded the paper twice and sixteen when we folded it four times. The paper gets thicker and thicker and harder and harder to fold. We struggled to fold it five times. There's no way we can fold it ten times."

The teacher moves on and listens to Grace's group discuss how to label the y-axis on their graph. She hears Grace say, "The numbers are getting really big really fast, so we need to figure out what to count by."

Another member of the group says, "Just use the number of total rectangles after each fold."

The teacher asks a *clarifying question*: "When you are making a graph or number line, do you just use the data points in your tables or do you need to ensure the intervals are the same?"

Then she listens to Julian's group struggle to write an equation. Julian says, "We have a starting value of 1 piece of paper, and each fold doubles the amount of rectangles from the one before, so we have to use the 1 and the 2. I don't know what else to do." The teacher suggests they make a third column in their table and write the prime factorization of the total number of rectangles they found. The adjusted table helps this group complete the equation. (See figure.) Their notation is $r = 1(2)^f$.

Number of Folds	Number of Rectangles	Prime Factorization	Exponential Notation
0	1		2^0
1	2	2	2^1
2	4	2 × 2	2^2
3	8	2 × 2 × 2	2^3
4	16	2 × 2 × 2 × 2	2^4
5	32	2 × 2 × 2 × 2 × 2	2^5
n			2^n

After an allotted period of time, the groups report their findings. During the debriefing, the teacher refers to the 2 in the previous equation as the *growth factor*. She leads a discussion on the difference between a growth factor and a growth rate, reinforcing students' understanding that the growth rate is a percent of growth while the growth factor is a constant factor that multiplies itself over time.

Following is another problem this teacher uses:

- *The Switcheroo Problem*: See the *Switcheroo* reproducible on page A44 in the appendix for the instructions for playing this game. In this problem students use two different-colored counters or discs, which are represented here by four lined and solid circles on a sample game board. Four counters of one color (the lined circles) are located on one side of an empty square, and four counters of a different color (the solid circles) are located on the opposite side of the empty square (see figure below).

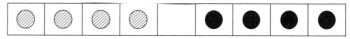

The goal of the problem is to switch the location of all lined discs with all solid discs by moving one disc at a time into a blank space or by jumping one disc at a time onto a blank space. At no time are the students allowed to move a disc backward (that is, they can move the lined discs only to the right and the solid discs only to the left). Students are challenged to write a mathematical rule for the most efficient number of moves it takes to complete the switch.

Meeting Individual Needs

These problems are often easiest to understand if students break them down into simpler problems and record the data in an organized list. The changing sides game is best solved starting with one counter on a side, then two counters, etc. It is very helpful to encourage students who struggle with recognizing the base and the corresponding exponents to make a three-column table labeled Number, Amount, and Prime Factorization, similar to the table shown in the "In the Classroom" section. The inclusion of the prime factorization enables students to determine the base for the exponential function and examine the exponent to calculate the relationship of the output to the input.

REFERENCE/FURTHER READING

Lappan, Glenda, James T. Fey, William M. Fitzgerald, Susan N. Friel, and Elizabeth Difanis Phillips. 2005. *Growing, Growing, Growing: Exponential Relationships*. Saddle River, NJ: Prentice Hall.

Exponential Decay

Mathematical Focus

- Recognize exponential decay in graphs, tables, and equations.
- Write equations for exponential decay functions.
- Solve exponential decay problems.

Potential Challenges and Misconceptions

Often students who demonstrate misconceptions with negative slopes also have difficulty discerning between exponential growth and exponential decay. Graphing exponential functions challenges some students who struggle to understand the concept that a graph may approach zero but never quite reach it. Although students at this level do not formally work with asymptotes, the work on exponential decay introduces the concept of limits.

In the Classroom

A half-life is the amount of time it takes half of a sample of material to decay. One teacher gives each pair of students 100 pennies as the starting sample of "centarium." To determine the half-life of centarium, each pair of students places the 100 pennies into a plastic drinking cup. They shake the cup and pour the pennies onto their table. They count and remove any pennies that have tails facing up. They record the number of pennies, the number of tails removed, and the number of heads in a chart, as shown in the following figure.

# of Coins	Toss #	# of Tails	# of Heads
100	1	43	57
57	2	26	31
31	3	15	16
16	4	9	7
7	5	3	4
4	6	3	1
1			

The experiment continues until there is one or no pennies left. Because the probability of getting heads or tails is one-half, the half-life for centarium is one-half.

Since the students are working with experimental data, the results will probably come close to the theoretical decay but will not be exact. The decay can be represented either as a fraction $\left(\frac{1}{2}, \frac{1}{4}, \frac{1}{8}, \frac{1}{16}\right)$ or with negative exponents $(2^{-1}, 2^{-2}, 2^{-3}, 2^{-4})$.

After discussing the results of the experiment, the teacher tells the pairs to write an equation to best represent the half-life of centarium and sketch a graph of the half-life on easel-size paper. She asks Taylor to explain her thinking. Taylor says, "I know that there is a fifty-fifty chance of getting a head or a tail, but I don't understand how that probability relates to this problem. When we tossed the hundred pennies the first time, only ten were heads. Why do we write that as half when it is a tenth?"

The teacher asks Taylor's partner what she thinks. Madelyn responds, "I think our results were abnormal. If we combined the data for the whole class, the results would be closer to one-half than to our one-tenth. I think it is like doing a probability experiment when the more the trials, the closer you get."

Taylor nods her head and interjects, "I think I get it. Our equation should be 100 times the quantity of 1 minus 0.5, raised to the power of x. Does this mean if we used a number cube and removed cubes that had a 1 facing up, we would write the equation to show

that there is a one-sixth chance of decaying, so it would be 100 times the quantity of 1 minus $\frac{1}{6}$, raised to the power of x?" The class agrees that Taylor's thinking is correct.

The class determines that the greatest differences are in the scales used on the y-axis. One graph (see the figure below) stands out as totally different from the exponential graphs of the rest of the class. The teacher challenges the class to determine why this graph looks so different.

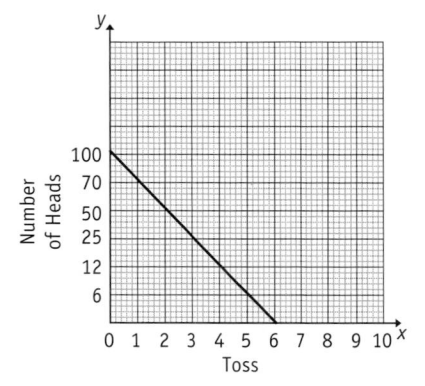

This teacher has discovered that when her students engage in error analysis, they become more highly aware of potential mistakes and it helps her uncover some of their misconceptions. She also finds her students are more likely to double-check their work to ensure their solutions are reasonable. The teacher also asks Taylor to explain her thinking about why she needed to use the equation $100(1 - 0.5)^x$ even though her experimental data did not match it.

Next, this teacher challenges her students to determine how much money they would have left if they invested $1,000 and it lost 5 percent compounded annually for ten years. Upon completion of their work, she encourages her students to use their graphing calculators to check the accuracy of their tables and graphs. She suggests they set the window settings to align with the scales they used on their hand-drawn graphs. She directs them to write a reflection on how the simulation of the half-life experiment relates to the loss of money in the investment problem. Students then work on the *Growing Smaller* reproducible on page A45 in the appendix.

Meeting Individual Needs

To understand what it means to come close to but never reach zero, it helps students to see what happens if you promise them a five-dollar bill if they can reach you while following a certain set of rules. Have students start at one end of the room while you stand at the opposite end. Instruct them to move half the distance to you.

For students who prefer a visual representation of the decay rate, suggest they line up the pennies they remove in columns. If forty pennies showed tails on the first toss, the students should line them up in a column. Next to that column, they should line up the number of pennies showing tails on the second toss. Have them continue aligning the discarded pennies in order to visualize how the sample is breaking down. This visualization together with the recording sheet enables students to deepen their understanding of the breakdown of a sample.

REFERENCE/FURTHER READING

Lappan, Glenda, James T. Fey, William M. Fitzgerald, Susan N. Friel, and Elizabeth Difanis Phillips. 2005. *Growing, Growing, Growing: Exponential Relationships.* Saddle River, NJ: Prentice Hall.

APPENDIX

Copy this reproducible on heavy stock, cut out the cards, and laminate them if possible. Give one complete set of cards to each pair of students.

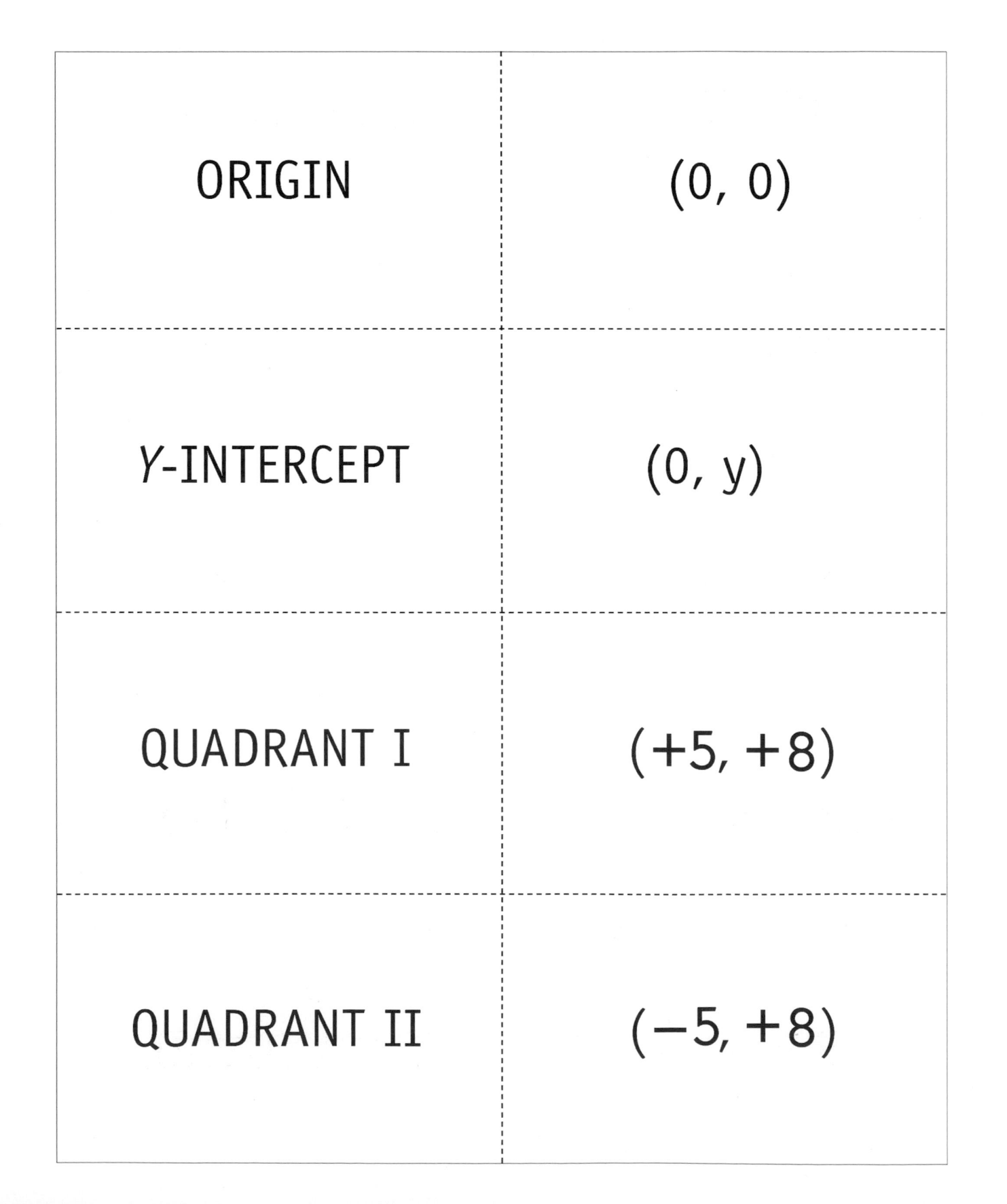

ORIGIN	(0, 0)
Y-INTERCEPT	(0, y)
QUADRANT I	(+5, +8)
QUADRANT II	(−5, +8)

QUADRANT III	$(-5, -8)$
QUADRANT IV	$(+5, -8)$
ABSCISSA	X-AXIS
ORDINATE	Y-AXIS
X-INTERCEPT	$(X, 0)$

ALGEBRA TILES TEMPLATE

Copy this reproducible on heavy stock and cut out the tiles. Each student should receive all of the tiles shown below. Notice that the square unit tiles do not fit evenly along the rectangular variable tiles. This is by design so the students may not say that the rectangular tile equals 3.

Before students work with the tiles, allow them to take a few minutes to examine the relationship among the three tile sizes. Notice the rectangular variable tile is the same width as the side length of the unit tile. Also notice that the large square has the same length and width as the length of the rectangular variable tile.

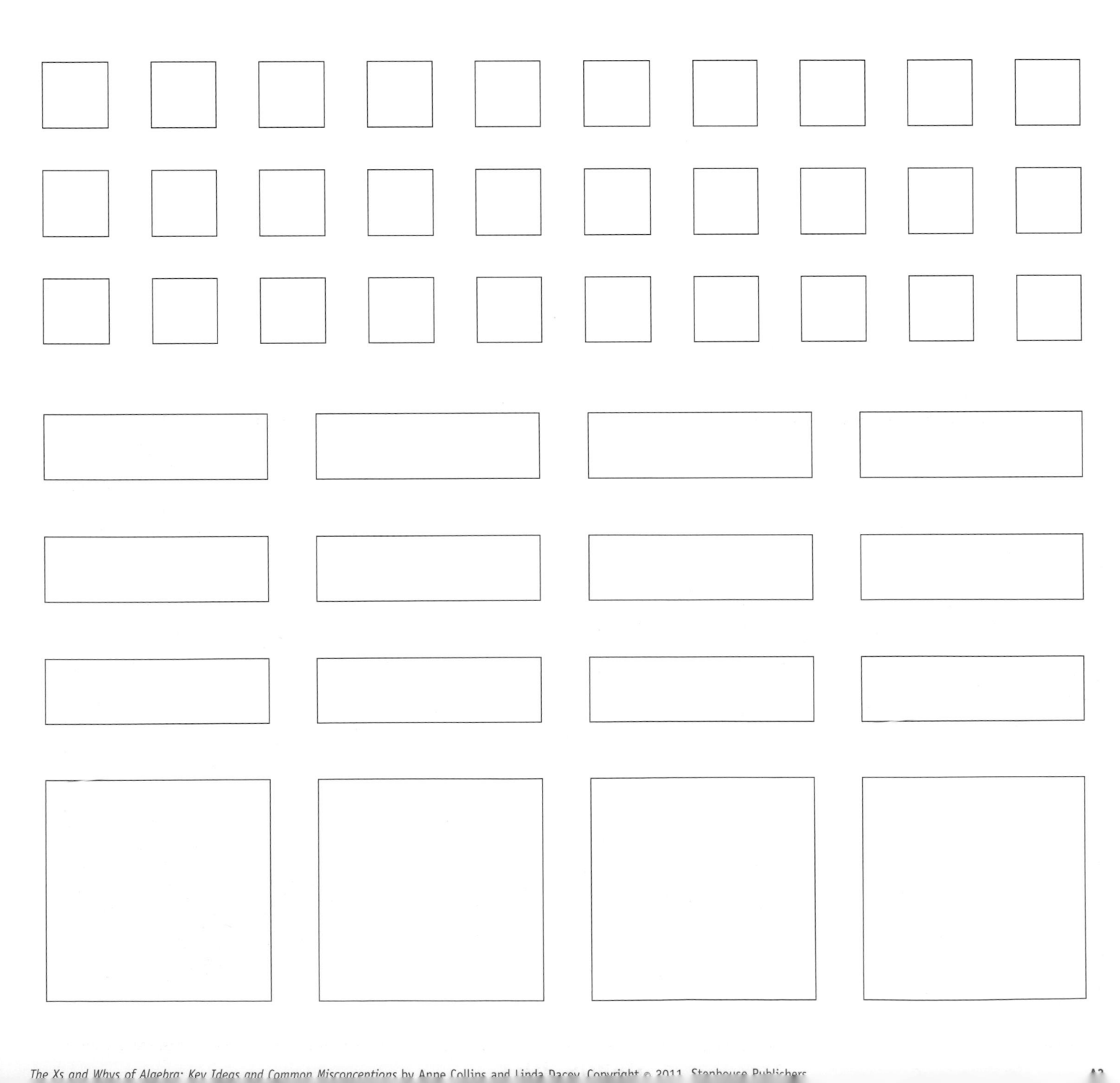

Name: Date:

Directions:

1. Group your students into trios.

2. Assign all students the number 1, 2, or 3.

3. Instruct the students with the number 1 to go to the board.

4. Dictate an expression, which these students should record on the board. For example:

$$3(2) - 4 + 8(-5) + 8$$

5. The students with the number 1 do one step to simplify the expression and sit down.

$$6 - 4 + 8(-5) + 8$$

6. The students with the number 2 go to the board and do one more step and sit down.

$$6 - 4 - 40 + 8$$

7. The students with the number 3 go to the board and do one more step and sit down.

$$2 - 40 + 8$$

8. The students with the number 1 go back to the board and do one more step and sit down.

$$-38 + 8$$

9. The students with the number 2 go back to the board and do one more step and sit down.

$$-30$$

10. Dictate another expression and instruct the students with the number 3 to go to the board and record the new expression and do the first step.

The Xs and Whys of Algebra: Key Ideas and Common Misconceptions by Anne Collins and Linda Dacey. Copyright © 2011. Stenhouse Publishers.

Name: Date:

Part I: Find the area of the following figures. Write an expression for your area in factored form and in expanded form.

1.

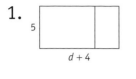

2.

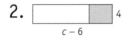

3.

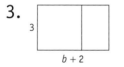

Part II: Draw a pictorial representation of each expression below and write the product in expanded form.

4. $3(-2 + b)$

5. $-2(d - 7)$

Name: Date:

For each set of figures, complete the following and attach your work to this sheet.

1. Talk with a partner about how Figure 5 will look.
2. Draw Figure 8.
3. Find the number of triangles in Figure 25.
4. Find the number of squares in Figure 15.
5. Write two expressions: one that tells the total number of triangles and one that tells the total number of squares in any given figure number.
6. Write how to see your expression in the figures.

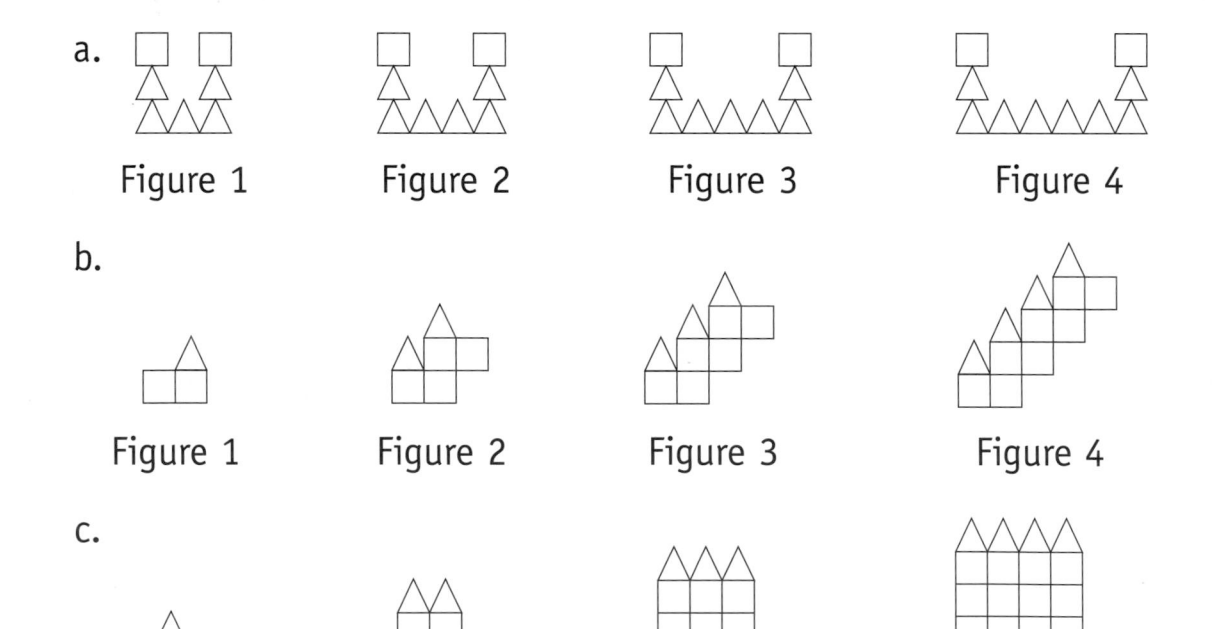

a. Figure 1   Figure 2   Figure 3   Figure 4

b. Figure 1   Figure 2   Figure 3   Figure 4

c. Figure 1   Figure 2   Figure 3   Figure 4

The Xs and Whys of Algebra: Key Ideas and Common Misconceptions by Anne Collins and Linda Dacey. Copyright © 2011. Stenhouse Publishers.

Copy this reproducible on heavy stock, cut out the cards, and laminate them. Give each student group a complete set of cards, and instruct them to shuffle the cards before they begin playing the game.

$4a + 8 - 2a - 14$	$4(a + 2) - 2(a + 7)$
$3(a - 4) - 2(a + 7)$	$3a - 12 - 2a - 14$
$3(a - 4) - 2(a - 7)$	$3a - 12 - 2a + 14$
$-5 - (a - 4) - 2 + (a - 7)$	-10

$-3a - 9 - 2a - 14$	$-3(a + 3) - 2(a + 7)$
$6 + 2(a - 4) - 2(a + 7)$	-16
three more than four times the quantity of some number and eight	$4a + 35$
$7a + 9 - 2a - 3$	$5a + 6$

The Xs and Whys of Algebra: Key Ideas and Common Misconceptions by Anne Collins and Linda Dacey. Copyright © 2011. Stenhouse Publishers.

Seth sold forty-five less than three times as many tickets (a) as Ben	$3a - 45$
thirty-five dollars less than twice Zac's salary (a)	$2a - 35$
six more than three times a number a minus four	$6 + 3a - 4$
eight increased by five times a number a	$8 + 5a$

Copy this reproducible on heavy stock, cut out the cards, and laminate them. Give each student one or two cards and play the game as a class.

I have $n + (n + 1) + (n + 2)$ Who has **the difference of a number and eight, divided by ten**?	I have $\frac{(n - 8)}{10}$ Who has n^2?
I have $4 + 3(n + 4)$ Who has **the sum of three consecutive integers**?	I have $\frac{1}{2}n(n + 1)$ Who has **four more than three times the sum of a number and four**?
I have $1 + 3 + 5 + 7 + 9 + (2n - 1)$ Who has **Isaiah has two more stickers than three times as many as Sam**?	I have $2 + 3n$ Who has **six less than the product of five and y plus three**?
I have $(n - 2)180$ Who has **four times a number cubed decreased by seven**?	I have $4n^3 - 7$ Who has **the perimeter of a square**?

I have $5 + (n - 9)$

Who has **the perimeter of a parallelogram**?

I have $4n$

Who has **the sum of the interior angles of a polygon**?

I have $-28, -26, -24, -22$

Who has **the area of a circle**?

I have $\pi r^2 - n^2$

Who has **five more than the quantity of nine less than some number**?

I have $\frac{1}{2}n(n + 1) - n^2$

Who has **six less than seven times the quantity of some number n minus three**?

I have $7(n - 3) - 6$

Who has $n, n + 2, n + 4, n + 6$?

I have πr^2

Who has **the difference between the area of a circle and the area of a square**?

I have $2(n + m)$

Who has **a triangular number minus a square number**?

I have $1 + 4 + 9 + 16 + 25$

Who has **the area of a triangle**?

I have $\frac{1}{2}nm$

Who has **three times the quantity of a number n minus three**?

I have $2^n - 1$

Who has **triple the sum of some number less one**?

I have $3(n - 3)$

Who has **the sum of squares**?

I have $6n - 3$

Who has **an expression for 1, 3, 6, 10, and 15**?

I have $2(7 - 3n)$

Who has **an expression for 3, 7, 15, and 31**?

I have $3(n - 1)$

Who has **three less than six times a number**?

I have $(5y + 3) - 6$

Who has **double the quantity of seven minus three times some number**?

Name: Date:

1. The Home Station Store is having a sale on carpet for stairs. The sale price is $8.95 per yard plus $145.00 for installing the carpet. Make a table that shows five inputs and outputs for getting carpet for your stairs. Pick one of the pairs and tell what it means in this situation.

2. Mark's son is two years less than one-third of the age of his father. Make a table that shows five reasonable values for the ages (in years) of Mark and his son. Write an expression that allows you to find the age of Mark's son, given the age of his father. Make a sketch of a graph of this equation. Why don't all of the points in the line make sense in this situation?

3. The area of a square is found by squaring the length of that square. Make a table listing the areas for squares with side lengths of 1–6 feet and then sketch a graph of these points. Why do you think the points are not in a straight line?

A14

Name: Date:

Solve the following problems. Be sure to identify the problem-solving strategy you are using.

1. Stephanie and Ramon are playing a *Guess My Number* game. Stephanie says her number is the sum of three consecutive even numbers. What expression might Ramon write to represent the middle number?

2. Dee built a rectangular grid that is 30 toothpicks long and 10 toothpicks wide. She filled it with squares made of 1 toothpick by 1 toothpick.

   a. What is the total number of toothpicks Dee used?

   b. If *l* represents the number of toothpicks in the length and *w* represents the number of toothpicks in the width, write an expression representing the total number of toothpicks in the figure. Justify your answer.

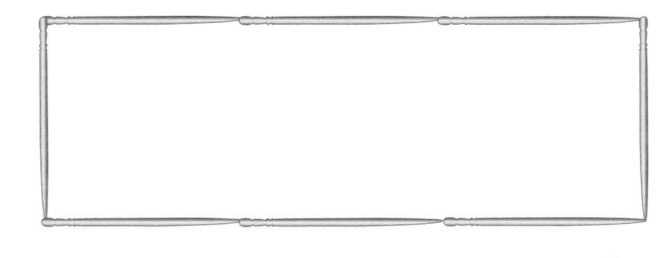

3. Jason works at a gym. He decided to glue a triangular stack of tennis balls together to advertise a special tennis workshop. If he continued stacking the balls in this fashion, how many tennis balls would he need to make seven rows? Ten rows? *N* rows?

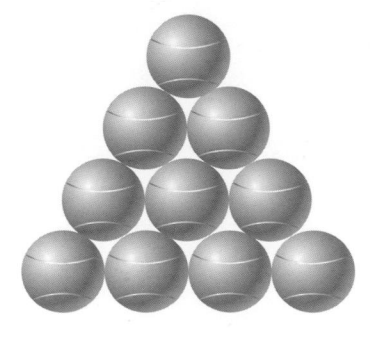

4. Students in Mrs. Sullivan's math class have to present their investigations on Thursday. If there are 5 groups presenting, in how many different orders might they make their presentations? How many orders for *n* groups? Justify your response.

Name: Date:

1. Consider the following pattern and create an appropriate problem to go along with it.

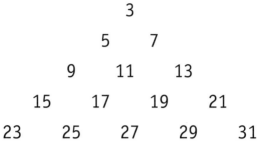

```
                    3
               5        7
          9        11        13
     15        17        19        21
23        25        27        29        31
```

2. Consider the following charts and create an appropriate problem to go along with them.

Input	Output
1	5
2	10
3	15
4	20
5	25
6	
7	
8	
n	

Input	Output
1	1
2	2
3	4
4	8
5	16
6	
7	
8	
n	

Input	Output
1	25
2	50
3	75
4	100
5	125
6	
7	
8	
n	

3. Consider the following graph and pose an appropriate problem for it.

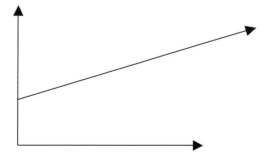

Name: Date:

Solve each problem for *x*. Record your thinking in drawings, words, and symbols.

1.

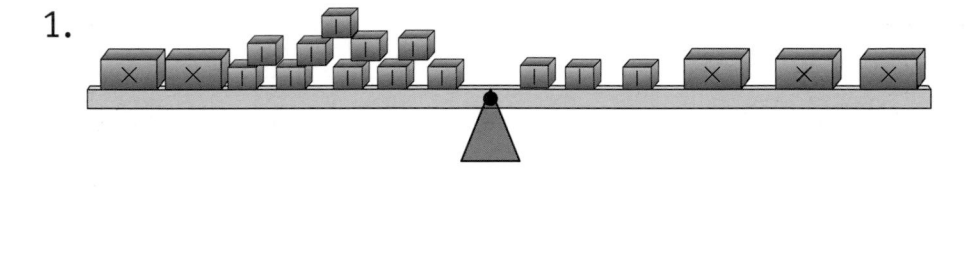

2.

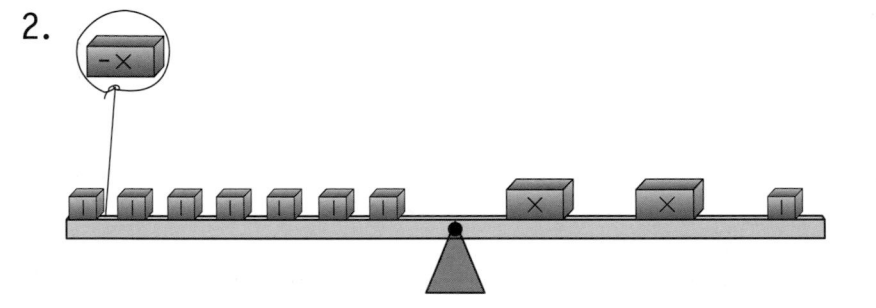

3.

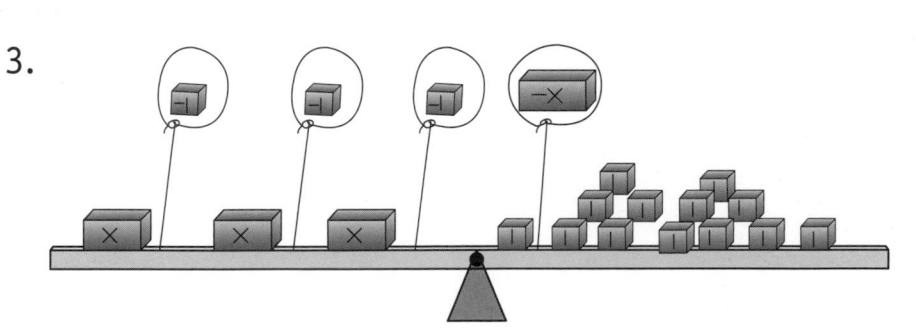

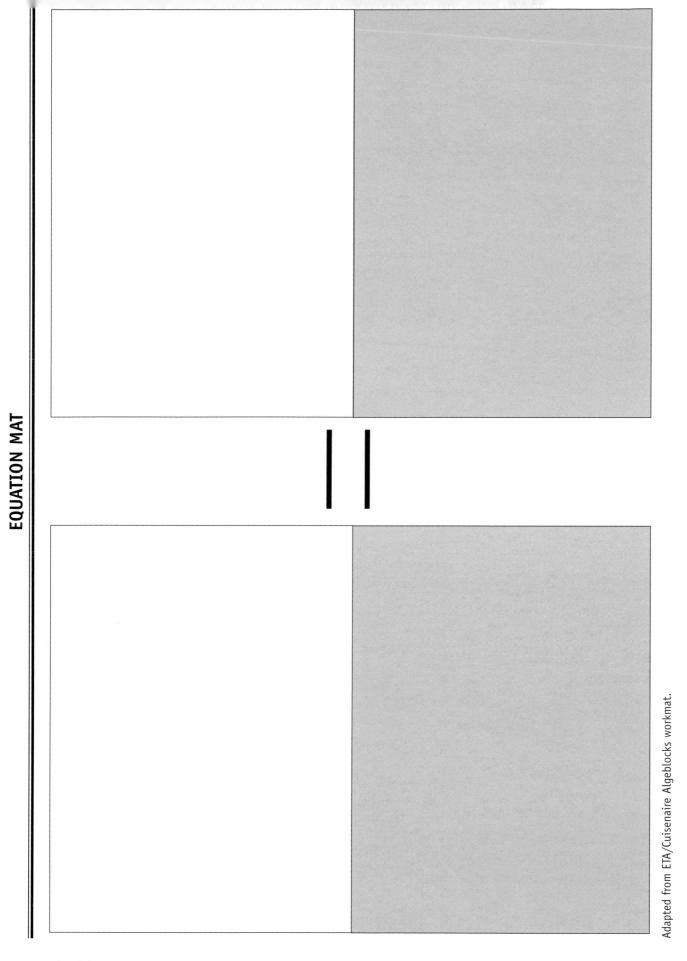

EQUATION MAT

$$=$$

Adapted from ETA/Cuisenaire Algeblocks workmat.

		Free Space		

EQUATION BINGO

For teachers only. Use in random order.

1. $3c + 5 = -4$ (answer: $c = -3$)

2. $5d - 6 = 4$ (answer: $d = 2$)

3. $-7b + 4 = -3$ (answer: $b = 1$)

4. $8 + 2c = 16$ (answer: $c = 4$)

5. $13 = -13 - 2b + 4$ (answer: $b = -11$)

6. $\frac{c + 1}{4} = -2$ (answer: $c = -9$)

7. $\frac{a - 7}{5} = -3$ (answer: $a = -8$)

8. $2\left(d + \frac{1}{2}\right) = 15$ (answer: $d = 7$)

9. $-3(c + 5) = 2c + 15$ (answer: $c = -6$)

10. $-4(c - 8) = -8$ (answer: $c = 10$)

11. $2b + 10 = -3b - 15$ (answer: $b = -5$)

12. $-6c - 4 = -5c - 3$ (answer: $c = -1$)

13. $8a + 5 = 7a + 3$ (answer: $a = -2$)

14. $2b - 4 + 3b = -4$ (answer: $b = 0$)

15. $8 - 2b - 10 = 22$ (answer: $b = -12$)

16. $-4c + 7 + c = -5$ (answer: $c = 4$)

17. $-3 - 5b = -6b + 8$ (answer: $b = 11$)

18. $3 + 4b + 4 = -3 + 6b$ (answer: $b = 5$)

19. $-5 - 3a = 5 - 2a$ (answer: $a = -10$)

20. $2 - 4b + 24 = 8 + 2b$ (answer: $b = 3$)

21. $\frac{a}{4} - 2 = 3a + 9$ (answer: $a = -4$)

22. $3a + 7 = -14$ (answer: $a = -7$)

23. $3b - 6 + 2b = 24$ (answer: $b = 6$)

24. $-5(a - 4) = -25$ (answer: $a = 9$)

Name:

Date:

Table	Graph

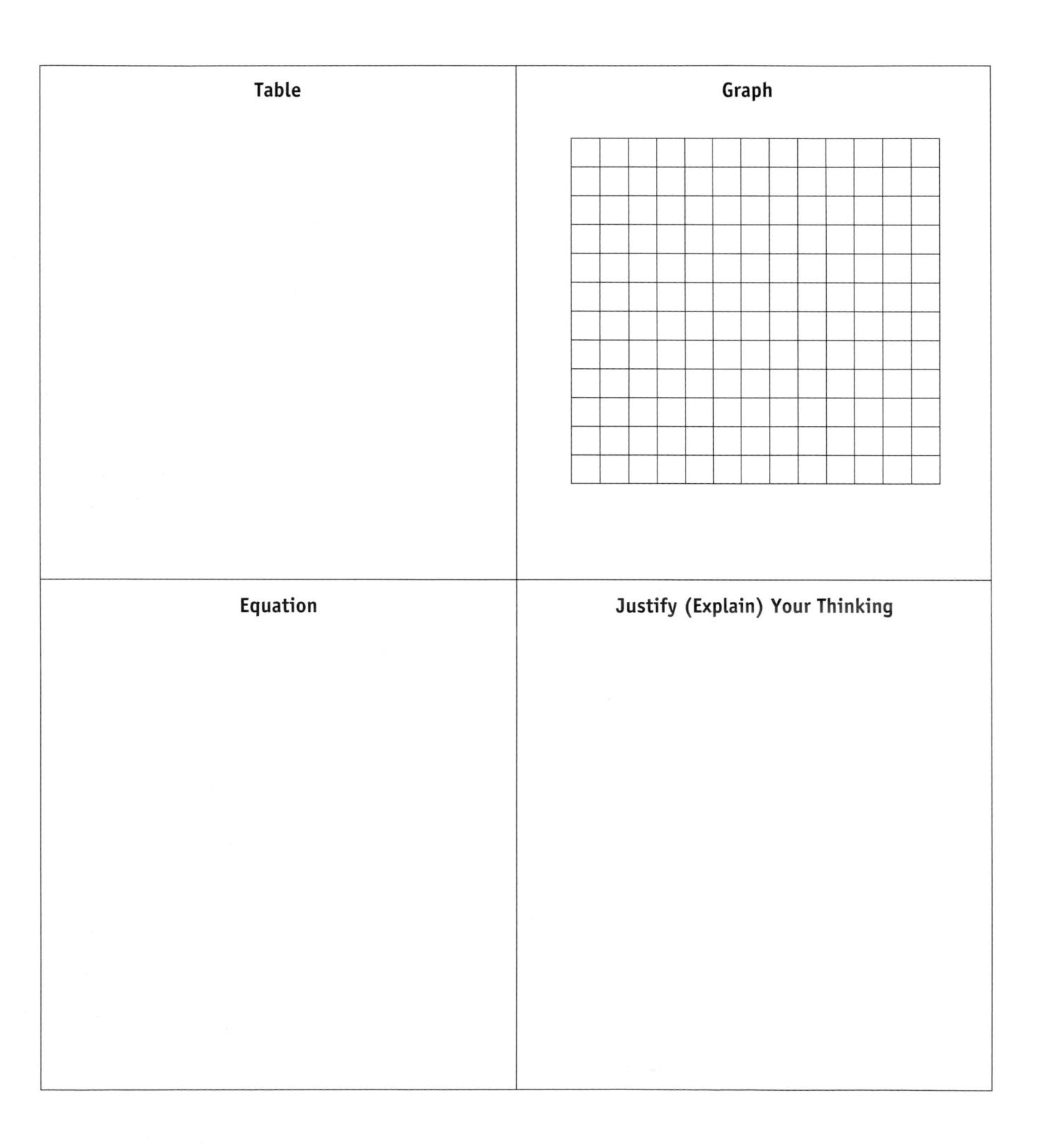

Equation	Justify (Explain) Your Thinking

Name: Date:

Use graph paper for all graphs.

1. Write an equation and draw a graph to represent the data in the table.

Input	Output
−8	−6
−4	−3
0	0
4	3
8	6

2. Make a table and a graph to represent the equation $y = -4x + 3$.

3. Write an equation and make a table for the following graph.

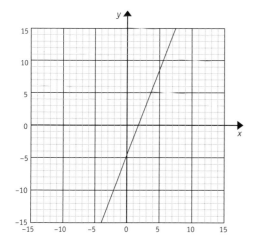

Name: Date:

Number of Cups	Height of Cups

Describe the relationship between the number of cups and the height of the cups.

_____

_____

_____

_____

_____

Name: Date:

Miles	Money

Describe the relationship between the number of hours walked and the money raised.

_____

_____

_____

_____

_____

_____

Copy this reproducible on heavy stock, cut out the cards, and laminate them. Randomly pass out the cards to your students. Instruct them to each find a student with an equivalent value to the one displayed on their card.

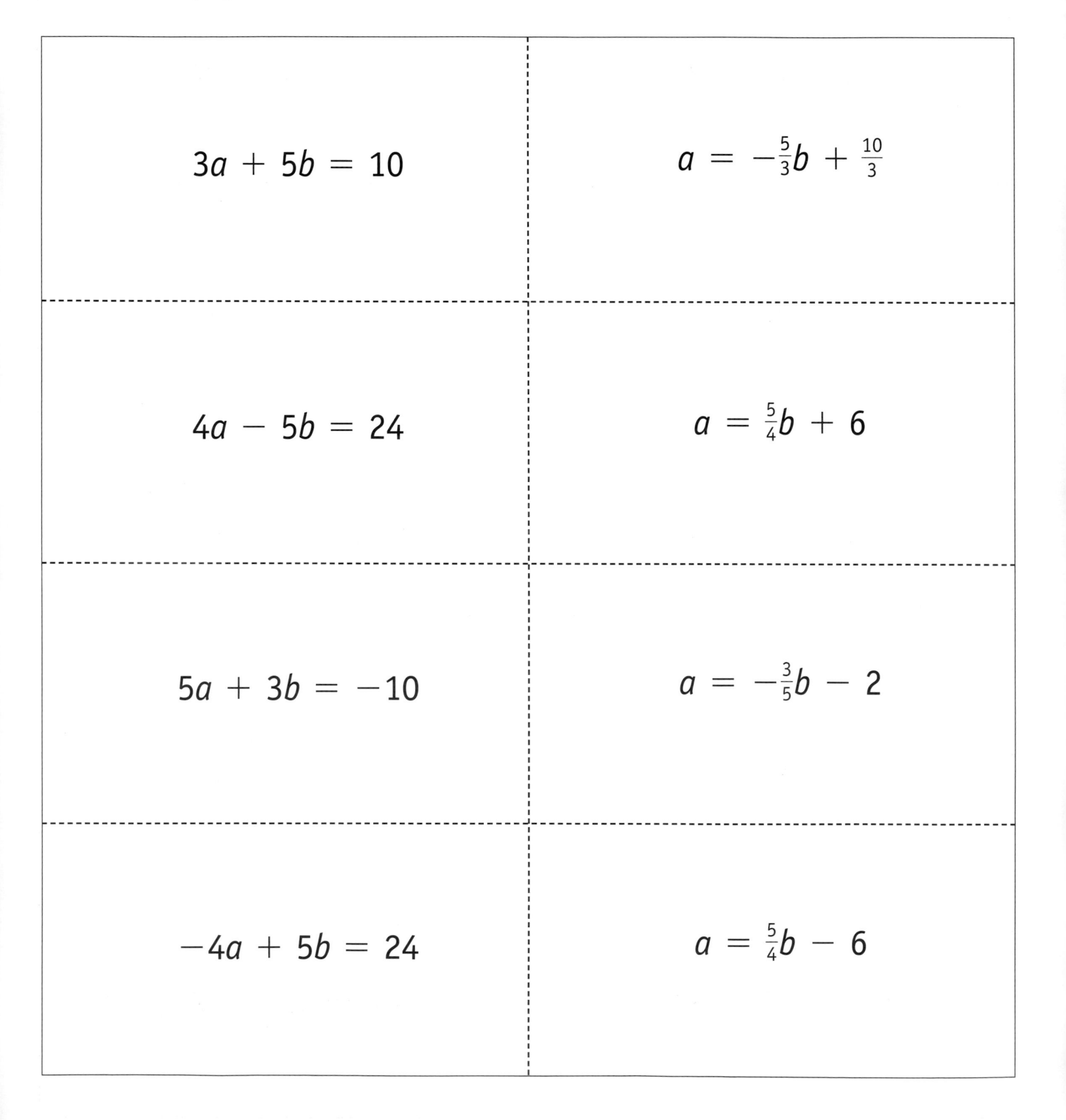

$$3a + 5b = 10$$

$$a = -\frac{5}{3}b + \frac{10}{3}$$

$$4a - 5b = 24$$

$$a = \frac{5}{4}b + 6$$

$$5a + 3b = -10$$

$$a = -\frac{3}{5}b - 2$$

$$-4a + 5b = 24$$

$$a = \frac{5}{4}b - 6$$

$3a - 7b = 12$	$a = \frac{7}{3}b + 4$
$-3a - 7b = 12$	$a = -\frac{7}{3}b - 4$
$-3a + 7b = 12$	$a = \frac{7}{3}b - 4$
$-7a + 3b = 12$	$a = \frac{3}{7}b - \frac{12}{7}$
$7a - 3b = 12$	$a = \frac{3}{7}b + \frac{12}{7}$

Name: Date:

Use graph paper for all graphs.

1. A bicycle rider pedals at a constant rate of speed. After every eight minutes, she completes an additional half mile. Make a table, draw a graph, and identify the slope.

2. Examine the following graph, which depicts mixtures for camp bug juice.

   a. Identify the slope of each of the lines.

   b. Write an equation for each line.

   c. Which line represents the juicier mixture?

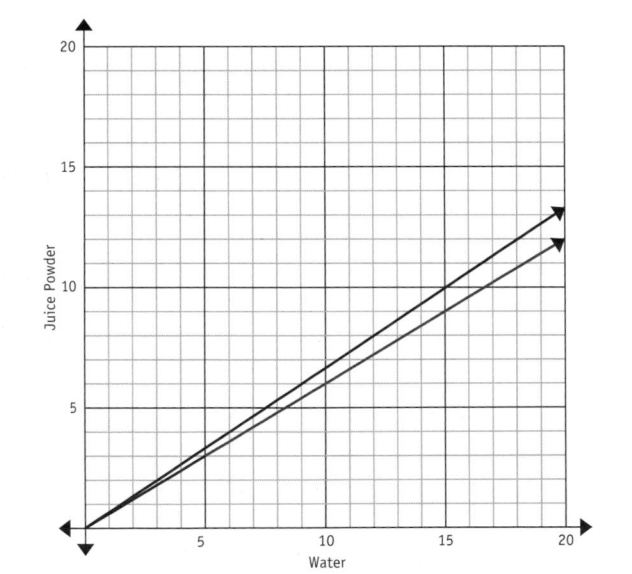

Name: Date:

Directions:

1. Fold up the long sides of your 4-by-11-inch strip of cardstock by a half inch on each side to create curbs, then lean the strip against a textbook or block of wood to serve as a ramp.

2. Measure the height in centimeters from the table to the top of the textbook. Record it in the chart below.

3. Place a small toy car at the top of the ramp and let it go.

4. Measure how far from the bottom of the ramp the car travels. Record it in the chart below.

5. Continue to add one textbook or block at a time to the support and repeat the experiment.

Trial 1

Books or blocks	0	1	2	3						
Height (cm)										
Distance (cm)										

Trial 2

Books or blocks	0	1	2	3						
Height (cm)										
Distance (cm)										

What do you notice about the distance the car travels as the height of the ramp increases?

_____

_____

_____

_____

Name: Date:

1. The following graph illustrates the time it takes to drain a 40-gallon aquarium.

   a. What is the rate at which the water is draining?

   b. Write an equation that best describes the change in the water volume over time.

   c. At what rate might the aquarium finish draining in 7 hours?

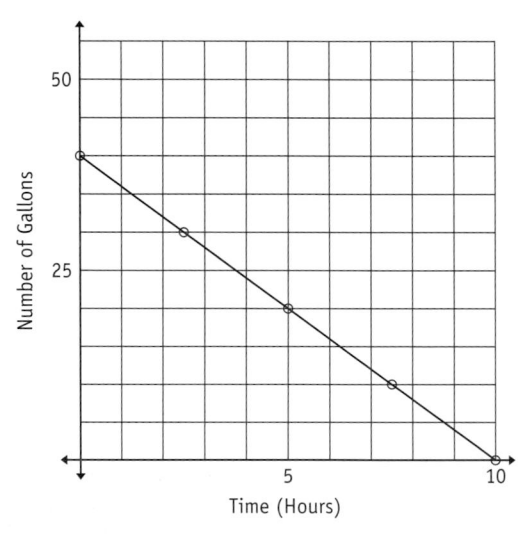

2. A 50-gallon aquarium is draining at a rate of 2 gallons every 4 hours. Write an equation and draw a graph to illustrate this situation. Justify your response.

3. Based on the graph below, which aquarium is draining at a faster rate? Justify your answer.

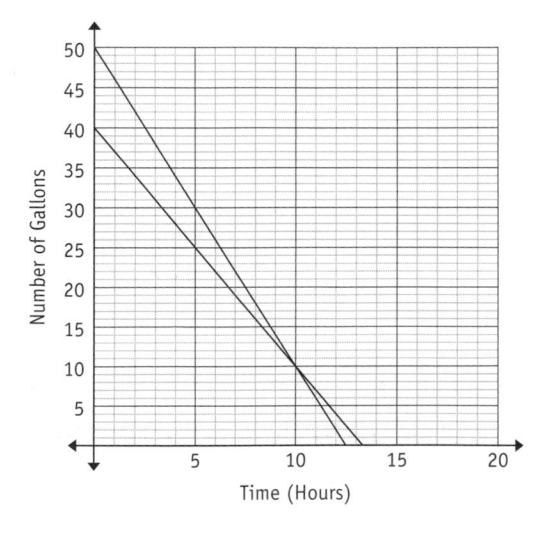

Name: Date:

Talk about each graph in your group and create a few stories that could match it. Be sure to refer to each change in the graph, to identify the unit of time, and to label the *y*-axis.

1. Choose one of your ideas to share with the class. Practice telling the story so that it will be told well, no matter which group member is called on to report.

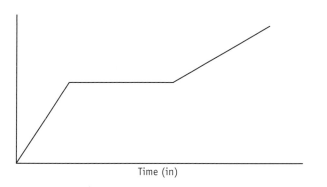

Time (in)

2. This time each group member should choose one of the group's stories to write. You may each choose a different scenario or some of you may choose to write about the same one. Feel free to add details to the story as you write your individual interpretation.

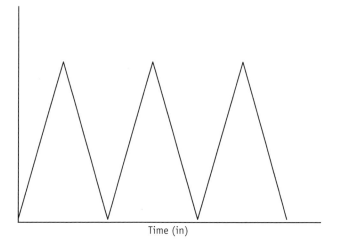

Time (in)

The Xs and Whys of Algebra: Key Ideas and Common Misconceptions by Anne Collins and Linda Dacey. Copyright © 2011. Stenhouse Publishers.

Name: Date:

Solve these problems using any method that is reasonable. Use a graph to check your answers.

1. The admission fee at the Harvest Fair is $3.50 for children and $8.00 for adults. On a certain day, 2,200 people enter the fair and $15,575 is collected. How many children and how many adults attended?

2. The owners of Greenscape Landscaping bought 23 bushes and 9 trees for a total of $864. They then purchased 9 bushes and 3 trees for a total of $312. The bills do not list the per-item prices. What were the costs of one bush and one tree?

3. The middle school students decided to join the Walk for Hunger in April. Grade eight students decided to charge their sponsors $5.00 plus $1.25 per mile for every mile they walked. Grade nine students agreed to ask their sponsors for $3.00 plus $2.50 per mile walked. Which grade will make the most money if they walk the same distance? Justify your response. What makes the greater difference, the amount per mile or the up-front charge? Support your answer with data.

Name: _____   Date: _____

1.

2.

3.

4.

Cut out each square, mix the squares up, and match each inequality situation to a symbolic representation and to a graphical representation. Then glue the matching squares into your notebook.

Liam scored more than 10 points but fewer than 45 points during a basketball tournament.		$10 < x < 45$
Jose owes at least $10 and less than $45, depending upon whom you ask.		$10 \leq x < 45$
Jessa works less than 10 hours or she works more than 45 hours if it snows.		$x < 10 \text{ or } x > 45$
Maria earns at most $10 when she baby-sits her sister but earns at least $45 on other jobs.		$x \leq 10 \text{ or } x \geq 45$

Name: _____   Date: _____

Pose a problem situation that could be answered by each of the following representations.

1. Be sure to add numerical values to this number line.

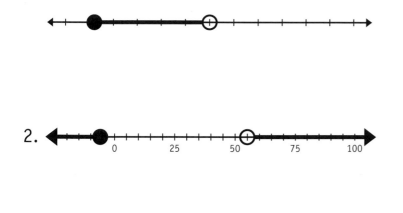

2.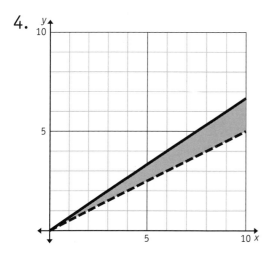

3. $5 < m \leq 70$

4.

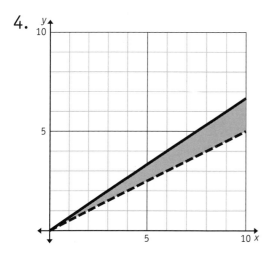

Name: Date:

For each situation below, label the number line appropriately, write an absolute value equation, solve it, and represent each solution on the number line.

1. Mrs. Collins challenged her class to determine her starting location on the number line if she moved a distance of 3 units from -7 on the number line.

<----+----->

2. Jeremy has an after-school job at his uncle's store. He tries to earn $50 each week. Last week he earned $12 more or less than his target salary. What are the most and least amounts of money that Jeremy might have earned?

<----+----->

3. The normal temperature in Billings during the month of February is 29.8°F. Last night a meteorologist announced that the temperature varied 14.9°F from the normal temperature. What might the temperature have been?

<----+----->

Name: Date:

1. If I traveled fewer than 18 units from 5 less than some starting point on the number line, where might I have started? Show your answer on the number line below, and write and solve an equation to represent the situation.

<————+——+——+——+——+——+——+——+——+——+——+——+——+——+——+——+——+——+——+————>

2. Write an absolute value inequality to describe each graph.

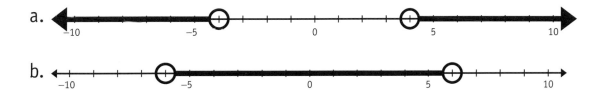

3. Solve this inequality and graph the solutions on a number line.
$$|a - 5| \geq 9$$

NAME THAT FUNCTION

Cut out each of the six puzzle pieces. Pass two pieces to each of the three students in a group. Students read their clues and then orally share their information with their group. They may not pass around the clues. Each clue is necessary to solve this one problem.

A

Line *l* has an *x*-intercept of −5.

Help your group write the equation for line *l* and draw its graph.

B

Line *l* never passes through the first quadrant. Based on this clue alone, what can you say about the slope of the line?

Your group's job is to write the equation for line *l* and draw its graph.

C

Point E is at (−6, −6) and does not rest on line *l*.

Write the equation for line *l* and draw its graph.

D

Point A is at (−9, 5) and rests on line *l*.

Help your group write the equation for line *l* and draw its graph.

E

The slope of a line perpendicular to line *l* is 25/20.

Write the equation for line *l* and draw its graph.

F

The line passing through point E goes through the origin.

Your group's job is to write the equation for line *l* and draw its graph.

Name: Date:

1. The Crunchy Snackfood Company published a table to represent the efficiency with which it produces corn chips.

Corn Chip Production	
Time in Minutes	Number of Corn Chips
3	30
4	40
15	150
25	250

   a. Does this table represent a linear or nonlinear relationship? Justify your answer by representing the data in a graph.

   b. If this is linear, write a function to represent the relationship between the time and the number of corn chips.

2. The Tansey family received an estimate for their family cell phone plan. They will pay $25 a month plus $0.15 per minute. Write a function for the cost (C) in terms of the minutes (m) used. Graph your function. Is it linear or nonlinear? Justify your answer.

3. A large middle school had 2,546 students in 2004 and 2,702 students in 2006. Assume that the enrollment follows a linear growth pattern. Let $t = 0$ correspond to 2,000 and let $f(t)$ represent the enrollment in year t.

   a. Assume that $f(t)$ is linear. Using the data given, find the slope of $f(t)$.

   b. What does the slope of $f(t)$ signify in terms of enrollment growth?

   c. Find an equation for $f(t)$ and use it to predict the enrollment of the school in 2009.

Name: Date:

1. The eighth-grade students decided to hold a car wash to raise relief money to send over-seas. They bought their supplies, and their school said they could use water at no cost. After washing 12 cars, they had made a profit of $40.35. After washing 45 cars, their profit was $221.85.

   a. At the end of the day they had washed 89 cars. How much profit did they make?

   b. What was the cost of their supplies?

   c. What is the domain of this linear function?

2. The length of a person's femurs, or thighbones, is directly related to that person's height. In fact, anthropologists and forensic scientists who measure the length of a femur can fairly accurately estimate the original height of the person. One anthropologist, Dr. Jessie Finder, discovered two femur bones in a new site. One bone was 19.00 in. long and the doctor estimated that it was from a woman who had been about 67.73 in. tall. The other bone was 17.50 in. long and the doctor estimated that this bone was from a woman who had been 64.91 in. tall. What equation did Dr. Finder use to estimate these heights?

3. Jason was doing some experiments. He lit a new candle. After the candle burned for 30 minutes, it was 26.25 cm tall. After it burned for a total of 2 hours, it was 21.00 cm tall. Jason found that there was an inverse linear relationship between the height of the candle and the time it had burned.

   a. How did the candle's height change per hour?

   b. How tall was the candle before Jason lit it?

   c. What is the x-intercept of the equation that predicts the length of this candle based on the amount of time it has burned? What does this intercept tell us about this problem situation?

Name: _____   Date: _____

Take
a
look...

at what changes in the problem

The two things that change are _____ and _____.

Take
a
look...

at the question

You are to find the number of _____, given the number of _____.
                          (dependent)   (independent)

Take
a
look...

at the specific data in the problem

	Dependent x	Independent y
Point 1		
Point 2		

Name: Date:

1. Given an 8-by-8-square checkerboard, count all the different-size squares there are.

   a. How many total squares are there?

   b. What strategy did you use to ensure you counted all squares?

   c. How do you know you have not missed any or double counted any squares?

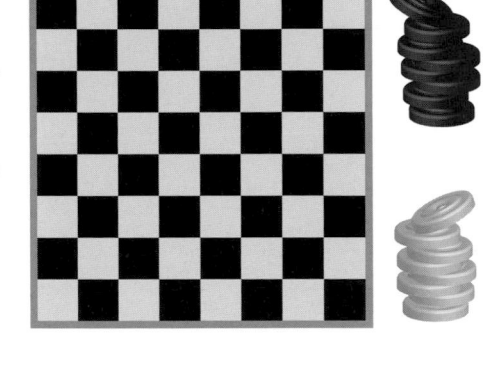

2. The following domain values were put through a special function machine.

$$\{-4, 8, -5, 0, -9, 6, 12\}$$

   The following range values were outputted after going through the function machine.

$$\{26, 74, 35, 10, 91, 46, 154\}$$

   a. Identify the function for this special function machine.

   b. Graph the ordered pairs that represent each domain with its resulting range.

3. The length of a vegetable garden is three times its width. If the area of the garden is 75 square meters, what are the length and the width?

Name: _____   Date: _____

1. Complete the tables.

a	b
0	0
1	−3
2	−4
3	−3
4	0
10	
20	
n	

x	y
0	4
1	−1
2	−6
3	−11
4	−16
10	
20	
n	

a	b
0	0
1	3
2	8
3	15
4	24
10	
20	
n	

2. For her birthday, Gracie received a new puppy. She wants to build a rectangular dog pen for him. If she has 150 feet of fencing and wants only whole number values for the length and width, what dimensions will give the puppy the largest area in which to run around? Justify your solution.

3. Find the number of dots in each figure. These are called pentagonal numbers. If the following pattern continues, how many dots will be in the 7th, 10th, and nth terms?

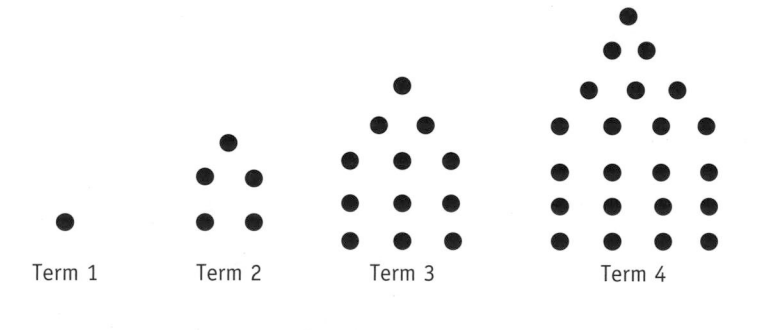

Term 1   Term 2   Term 3   Term 4

Name: Date:

In this game for two, you must exchange the discs that are on the right side with the discs on the left side (an example of the board appears below). You must follow these rules:

• You may move only one disc at a time, alternating turns.

• You may move only forward, toward the opposite side.

• You may jump only one disc in a move, as long as you land on an empty space.

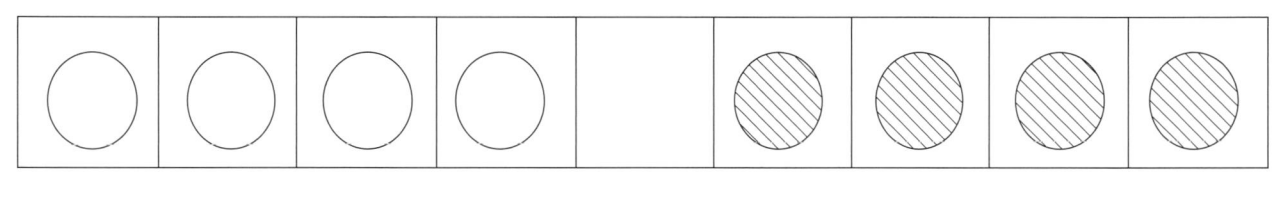

Your goal is to completely exchange the discs in the *fewest* moves possible.

Use the game board below to play the game. Consider how you know you have identified the most efficient way to exchange the discs.

   Based on your discovery of how to most efficiently exchange the discs, how many moves will it take to exchange seven discs on each side? Ten discs? *N* discs?

Name: Date:

1. Which of the following graphs represent an exponential function? Tell whether the function is a growth or decay function.

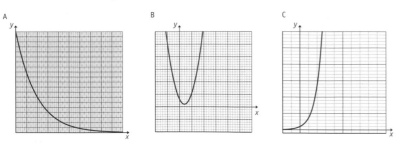

2. Find the missing values:

   a. Decay rate: 15%   Decay factor:

   b. Decay rate: Decay factor: 0.35

   c. Decay rate: $7\frac{1}{2}$%   Decay factor:

3. Suppose the half-life of a radioactive substance is 2 hours. If there are 1,600 unstable atoms (atoms that have not yet decayed) at the starting point, how many unstable atoms will there be after 8 hours? Make a table and a graph to illustrate the half-life.

4. The depreciation rate of most automobiles averages about 20% per year. If you buy a luxury car for $45,000, what might the car's value be after five years? Make a table and a graph to illustrate the depreciation.

Match It Cards

origin: $(0, 0)$
y-intercept: $(0, -4)$
quadrant I: $(+x, +y)$
quadrant II: $(-x, +y)$
quadrant III: $(-x, -y)$
quadrant IV: $(+x, -y)$
abscissa: x-axis
ordinate: y-axis
x-intercept: $(6, 0)$

Algebra Tiles Template

No answer.

Chip Board

No answer.

Equivalent Expressions Round-Robin

No answer.

Working with Expressions

1. $5d + 20$; $5(d + 4)$
2. $4c - 24$; $4(c - 6)$
3. $3b + 6$; $3(b + 2)$
4. $-6 + 3b$;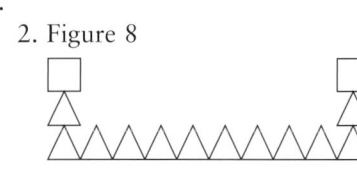
5. $2d + 14$;

See the Pattern

a.
2. Figure 8

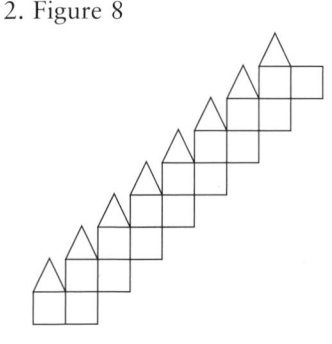

3. 29 triangles
4. 2 squares
5. $t = n + 4$; t represents triangles, n represents term
   $s = 2$; s represents squares
6. Multiple answers are possible.

b.
2. Figure 8

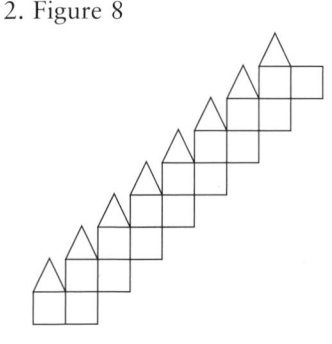

3. 25 triangles
4. 30 squares

5. $t = n$; t represents triangles, n represents term
   $s = 2n$; s represents squares, n represents term
6. Multiple answers are possible.

c.
2. Figure 8

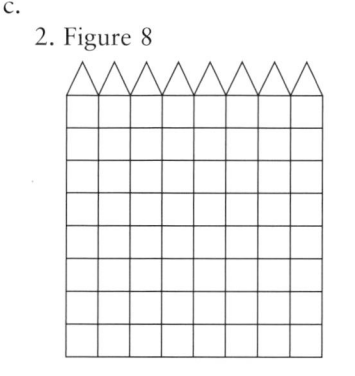

3. 25 triangles
4. 15^2, or 225, squares
5. $t = n$; t represents triangles, n represents term
   $s = n^2$; s represents squares, n represents term
6. Multiple answers are possible.

Do You Have a _____?

$4a + 8 - 2a - 14 = 4(a + 2) - 2(a + 7)$
$3(a - 4) - 2(a + 7) = 3a - 12 - 2a - 14$
$3(a - 4) - 2(a - 7) = 3a - 12 - 2a + 14$
$-5 - (a - 4) - 2 + (a - 7) = -10$
$-3a - 9 - 2a - 14 = -3(a + 3) - 2(a + 7)$
$6 + 2(a - 4) - 2(a + 7) = -16$
three more than four times the quantity of some number and eight $= 4a + 35$
$7a + 9 - 2a - 3 = 5a + 6$
Seth sold forty-five less than three times as many tickets (a) as Ben $= 3a - 45$
thirty-five dollars less than twice Zac's salary $(a) = 2a - 35$
six more than three times a number a minus four $= 6 + 3a - 4$
eight increased by five times a number $a = 8 + 5a$

I Have _____; Who Has _____?

Who has the difference of a number and eight, divided by ten?
$\frac{(n - 8)}{10}$
Who has the sum of three consecutive integers? $n + (n + 1) + (n + 2)$
Who has Isaiah has two more stickers than three times as many as Sam? $2 + 3n$
Who has four times a number cubed decreased by seven? $4n^3 - 7$
Who has n^2? $1 + 3 + 5 + 7 + 9 + (2n - 1)$
Who has four more than three times the sum of a number and four? $4 + 3(n + 4)$
Who has six less than the product of five and y plus three? $(5y + 3) - 6$
Who has the perimeter of a square? $4n$
Who has the perimeter of a parallelogram? $2(n + m)$
Who has the area of a circle? πr^2
Who has six less than seven times the quantity of some number n minus three? $7(n - 3) - 6$
Who has the difference between the area of a circle and the area of a square? $\pi r^2 - n^2$
Who has the sum of the interior angles of a polygon? $(n - 2)180$
Who has five more than the quantity of nine less than some number? $5 + (n - 9)$

Who has n, $n + 2$, $n + 4$, $n + 6$? -28, -26, -24, -22
Who has a triangular number minus a square number? $\frac{1}{2}n(n + 1) - n^2$
Who has the area of a triangle? $\frac{1}{2}nm$
Who has triple the sum of some number less one? $3(n - 1)$
Who has an expression for 1, 3, 6, 10, and 15? $\frac{1}{2}n(n + 1)$
Who has three less than six times a number? $6n - 3$
Who has three times the quantity of a number n minus three?
$3(n - 3)$
Who has the sum of squares? $1 + 4 + 9 + 16 + 25$
Who has an expression for 3, 7, 15, and 31? $2^n - 1$
Who has double the quantity of seven minus three times some number? $2(7 - 3n)$

It's a Relationship

1. Multiple answers are possible. Following is one example:

Yards	Cost	Total Cost
5	$44.75	$189.75
10	$89.50	$234.50
15	$134.25	$279.25
20	$179.00	$324.00
25	$223.75	$368.75

(10, 234.50) means that for 10 yards of carpet, the total cost of the carpet and the installation is $234.50.

2.

Mark (f)	Mark's Son (s)
33	9
36	10
39	11
42	12
45	13

$s = \frac{1}{3}f - 2$, where s represents the age of the son and f represents the age of the father

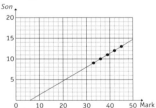

3.

Length	Area
1	1
2	4
3	9
4	16
5	25
6	36

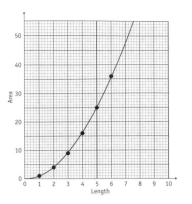

There is not a constant rate of change.

Express It

1. $n + 2$; n is even
2.
   a. 640 toothpicks
   b. $n = l(w + 1) + w(l + 1) = 2lw + l + w$
3. 28 balls, 55 balls, and $\frac{1}{2}n(n + 1)$ balls
4. There are 5!, or 120, different ways for five groups. There are $n!$ orders for n groups.

So What's the Problem?

1. Multiple answers are possible. Appropriate questions include the following:
   How do the values change from row to row?
   What is the sum of each row?
   What patterns do you notice?
2. Multiple answers are possible. Appropriate questions include the following:
   Which of the tables shows a linear relationship?
   What are the missing values?
   What is the expression that best represents the relationship in each table?
3. Multiple answers are possible. Appropriate problems include the following:
   What situation might the graph represent?
   What might account for the fact that the line begins above the origin?
   Is this a linear or nonlinear relationship?

In Balance

1. $x = 7$. Multiple representations are possible.
2. $x = 2$. Multiple representations are possible.
3. $x = 4$. Multiple representations are possible.

Equation Mat

No answer.

Equation Bingo

No answer.

Sample Bingo Equations

No answer.

Multiple Representations

No answer.

1. $y = \frac{3}{4}x$

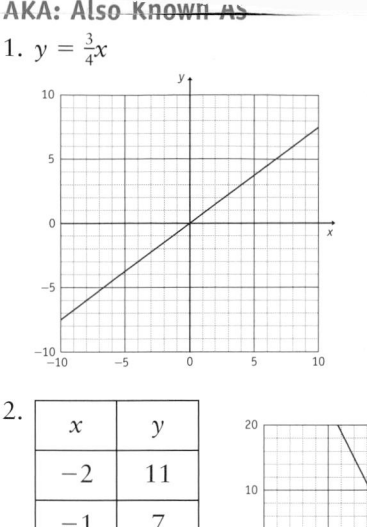

2.

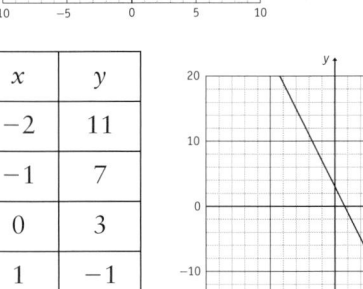

x	y
-2	11
-1	7
0	3
1	-1
2	-5

3. $y = \frac{8}{3}x - 5$

x	y
-3	-13
0	-5
3	3
6	11

Stacking Cups

Multiple answers are possible. The lip height of the cup is the slope, and the base height is the y-intercept.

Pet Health Awareness Walk

Multiple answers are possible, but be sure the slope is positive.

Equivalence Cards

$3a + 5b = 10$ is equivalent to $a = -\frac{5}{3}b + \frac{10}{3}$

$4a - 5b = 24$ is equivalent to $a = \frac{5}{4}b + 6$

$5a + 3b = -10$ is equivalent to $a = -\frac{3}{5}b - 2$

$-4a + 5b = 24$ is equivalent to $a = \frac{5}{4}b - 6$

$3a - 7b = 12$ is equivalent to $a = \frac{7}{3}b + 4$

$-3a - 7b = 12$ is equivalent to $a = -\frac{7}{3}b - 4$

$-3a + 7b = 12$ is equivalent to $a = \frac{7}{3}b - 4$

$-7a + 3b = 12$ is equivalent to $a = \frac{3}{7}b - \frac{12}{7}$

$7a - 3b = 12$ is equivalent to $a = \frac{3}{7}b + \frac{12}{7}$

Slippery Slopes

1.

Time in Minutes	Miles
0	0
8	$\frac{1}{2}$
16	1
24	$1\frac{1}{2}$
32	2

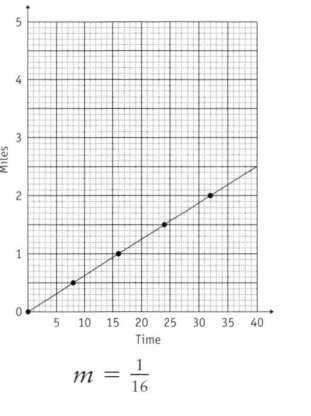

$$m = \frac{1}{16}$$

2.

   a. top line: $m = \frac{10}{15}$ or $\frac{2}{3}$; bottom line: $m = \frac{3}{5}$

   b. top line: $y = \frac{10}{15}x$ or $y = \frac{2}{3}x$; bottom line: $y = \frac{3}{5}x$

   c. $y = \frac{10}{15}x$ is the juiciest because it is the steeper line.

Investigating Ramps and Travel Distance

Multiple answers are possible. The steeper the line up to a point, the greater the distance. As the ramp approaches a vertical line, the cars crash. The vertical line has an undefined slope.

Aquarium Problems

1.

   a. rate of 4 gallons per hour

   b. $w = -x + 40$

   c. rate of 5.71 gallons per hour

2. $w = -2x + 50$

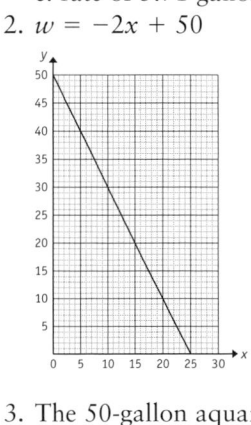

3. The 50-gallon aquarium is draining at a faster rate because the line is steeper.

Tell a Story

1. Settings and stories will vary, but they should each identify the x-axis and three distinct periods within the graph: a shorter period of increase at a constant rate, a longer period of no change, and a similar longer time of increase at a constant rate, but one that is less than the rate of the first increase.

2. Again, settings and stories will vary, but all should indicate three cycles of an increase and decrease (or six alternating changes). Each change is at the same rate. Possible ideas include the height someone is off the ground when jumping three times or the distance from home of someone who changes his mind three times about whether to walk to the library.

Systems, Strategies, and Solutions
1. 450 children and 1,750 adults
2. $18 per bush and $50 per tree
3. Up to 1.6 miles, grade eight ($1.25m + 5$) will make more, but after 1.6 miles, grade nine ($2.50m + 3$) will make more.

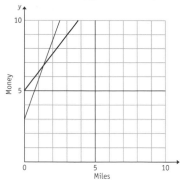

The greater difference is the amount per mile.

Number Lines
No answer.

Matching Inequalities
Liam scored more than 10 points but fewer than 45 points during a basketball tournament.

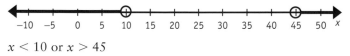

$10 < x < 45$

Jose owes at least $10 but less than $45, depending upon whom you ask.

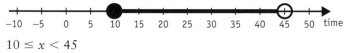

$10 \leq x < 45$

Jessa works less than 10 hours or she works more than 45 hours if it snows.

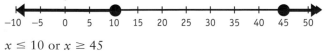

$x < 10$ or $x > 45$

Maria earns at most $10 when she baby-sits her sister and at least $45 on other jobs.

$x \leq 10$ or $x \geq 45$

Problem-Posing Representations
Multiple answers are possible for all of these problems but should include the following data.
1. Something is greater than or equal to ____ but less than ____.
2. Something is less than or equal to −5 or greater than 55.
3. Something is greater than 5 and less than or equal to 70.
4. Somet...

Distance Is Always Positive
1. $|x - (-7)| = 3$ $x = -4$ or $x = -10$

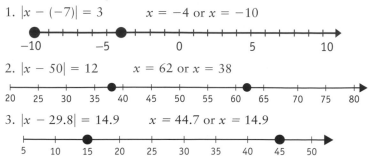

2. $|x - 50| = 12$ $x = 62$ or $x = 38$

3. $|x - 29.8| = 14.9$ $x = 44.7$ or $x = 14.9$

What Is My Range?
1. $|x - 5| < 18$, so $x < 23$ or $x > -13$

2.
   a. $|x| > 4$, so $x > 4$ or $x < -4$
   b. $|x| < 6$, so $x < 6$ and $x > -6$
3. $a \leq -4$ or $a \geq 14$

Name That Function
$y = -1.25x - 6.25$

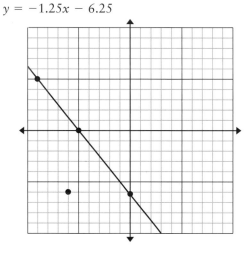

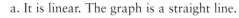

Do I Represent a Constant Change?
1.
   a. It is linear. The graph is a straight line.

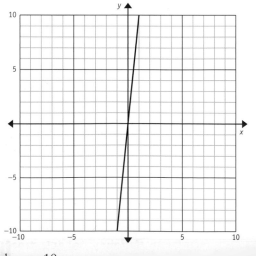

Algebra Mat for Modeling Quadratics

No answer.

Solving Quadratics

1. (10, 60); (20, 320); $(n, n^2 - 4n)$
   (10, -46); (20, -96); $(n, -5n + 4)$
   (10, 120); (20, 440); $(n, n^2 + 2n)$

2. The greatest area is the area formed as a square. 150 = Perimeter; $2l + 2w = 150$. $2l = 150 - 2w$, $l = 75 - w$. If $l = 38$ then $w = 37$; these two dimensions are closest to a square. 37 feet × 38 feet = 1,406 square feet.

3. 70 dots; 145 dots; $n^2 + \frac{1}{2}n(n - 1)$

Switcheroo

One disc per side requires a minimum of 3 moves.
Two discs per side require a minimum of 8 moves.
Three discs per side require a minimum of moves.
Four discs per side require a minimum of twenty-four moves.
Seven discs per side require a minimum of sixty-three moves.
Ten discs per side require a minimum of 120 moves.
N discs per side require a minimum of $n(n + 2)$ moves, or $(n + 1)^2 - 1$ moves.

Suggestions for solving this problem:

1. Solve a similar but simpler problem, using one disc on each side, which requires three moves.
2. Solve a similar but simpler problem, using two discs on each side, which require eight moves.
3. Solve a similar but simpler problem, using three discs on each side, which require fifteen moves.

Growing Smaller

1. Graph A is an exponential decay function; graph C is an exponential growth function.

2.
   a. Decay factor: 0.85
   b. Decay rate: 65%
   c. Decay factor: 0.925

3. There will be 100 atoms left after 8 hours.

Hours	Atoms
0	1,600
2	800
4	400
6	200
8	100

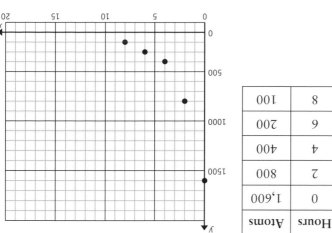
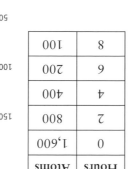

---

2. $C = 0.15m + 25$. The function is linear. The graph is a straight line.

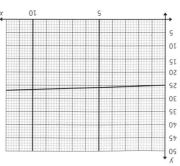

3.
   a. $m = \frac{156}{2}$, or $m = 78$.
   b. The slope indicates that for every year after 2000, there will be an additional 78 students.
   c. $f(t) = 78t + 2,234$; the population in 2009 would have been 2,936 students

Problem Solving with Points

1.
   a. $463.85
   b. $25.65
   c. whole numbers 0–89

2. H (height in inches) = 1.88 × F (length of femur in inches) + 32.01
   Note that the formula for the estimation of female heights in inches is $height = 1.880 \times femur\ length + 32.010$. The annexed zeros indicate accuracy to the thousandths place. Students will not be able to identify these zeros from their calculations but may be interested in learning of the level of accuracy possible.

3.
   a. decreased by 3.50 cm per hour
   b. 28.00 cm
   c. The x-intercept is 8, which is the total number of hours the candle could burn before being completely melted.

Graphic Organizer for Linear Equations

No answer.

Am I Square?

1.
   a. 204 squares
   b. Counted each 1-by-1, 2-by-2, 3-by-3, 4-by-4, 5-by-5, 6-by-6, 7-by-7, and 8-by-8 square.
   c. The sum of the squares from 1^2 to 8^2 gives the total number of squares.

2.
   a. $y = n^2 + 10$
   b.

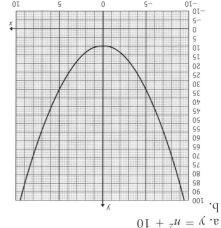
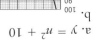

3. $l = 15$ meters, $w = 5$ meters

4. The car's value would be $14,745.60.

Years	Value
0	45,000
1	36,000
2	28,800
3	23,040
4	18,432
5	14,745.60

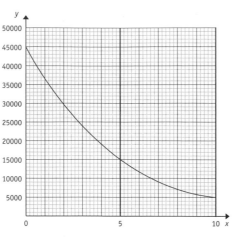